OXFORD MEDICAL PUBLICATIONS

Infection

OXFORD GENERAL PRACTICE SERIES

Editorial Board

Godfrey Fowler, Jacky Hayden, Iona Heath, and Clare Wilkinson

Infection

Oxford General Practice Series • 40

Lesley Southgate
Professor of General Practice, Centre for Health Informatics and Multiprofessional Education (CHIME), UCL Medical School, London

Cameron Lockie
General Practitioner, Rother House Medical Centre, Stratford upon Avon; Honorary Senior Lecturer, Department of Public Health, University of Glasgow

Shelley Heard
Dean for Postgraduate Medicine, North Thames; Consultant Medical Microbiologist, Homerton Hospital NHS Trust

Martin Wood
Consultant Physician, Birmingham Heartlands Hospital, Birmingham

Oxford : New York : Tokyo

OXFORD UNIVERSITY PRESS

1997

Oxford University Press, Great Clarendon Street, Oxford OX2 6DP

Oxford   New York

Athens   Auckland   Bangkok   Bogota   Bombay
Calcutta   Cape Town   Dar es Salaam   Delhi
Florence   Hong Kong   Istanbul   Karachi
Kuala Lumpur   Madras   Madrid   Melbourne
Mexico City   Nairobi   Paris   Singapore
Taipei   Tokyo   Toronto   Warsaw

and associated companies in
Berlin   Ibadan

Published in the United States
by Oxford University Press Inc., New York

A catalogue record for this book is available from the British Library

Library of Congress Cataloging in Publication Data
(Data applied for)

ISBN 0 19 262092 4

Typeset by Palimpsest Book Production Limited,
Polmont, Stirlingshire
Printed in Great Britain by Biddles Ltd, Guildford, Surrey

CONTENTS

Contents

FOREWORD

Hardly a week goes by without some media headline about infection, killer bugs, or deadly viruses. The public are presented with plagues and epidemics, doomsday scenarios, and miracle cures. But I suspect that it has always been the case. In the early part of this century, the emphasis was on the diagnosis of new organisms to explain signs and symptoms and the pathogenesis of disease. The treatment was limited but included immunological techniques and serum therapy and by the middle of the century antibiotics were being rapidly discovered and developed. By the 1970s there was a sense of complacency, the problems were being solved. Apart from a few tropical infections we didn't need to worry. HIV infection changed all that, and with the identification of transmissible spongiform encephalopathies, antibiotic resistant organisms, the emergence of new infections, and a resurgence of old ones, the stage is set for a new look at communicable disease. The rise in world travel means that no person, no country is immune. Communicable disease is a problem for all of us.

The general practitioner (GP) has a central role in the control of infection. The GP is in the frontline, from the diagnosis, through treatment, to dealing with the consequences for the patient and the carers. Health promotion and the protection against infectious disease by immunization forms an important part of this work. The early diagnosis may be critical, but difficult, as in meningitis, and handling the implications of serious infections such as HIV and hepatitis can be very taxing and require specific skills. The GP is seen as a source of advice and help on all forms of communicable disease, and keeping up-to-date with travel-related infections, new antibiotics, and diagnostic tests, or even new diseases, is not easy.

This book combines the science background with clinical practice. The first few chapters set the scene, and the remainder deal with specific infections. As would be expected from a group of authors with significant educational experience, the background is illustrated by relevant case histories and the judicious use of summaries. It covers a wide area of clinical practice.

In an age of bigger and bigger science and complicated equipment and tests, it is useful to be reminded sometimes of the importance of clinical skills. This is nowhere more so than in dealing with infection. Taking a history, careful observation, and meticulous examination are all relevant.

There is a need to understand the natural history of the disease and know when there is something 'not quite right'. This is where the experience of the GP is crucial. A high index of suspicion is essential, as is the curiosity to find out more and explain the symptoms and signs. Communication of all of this to the patient and carers is an integral part of the process and for both acute and chronic infections a major part of the GP's function. The problems are all different and whether the illness affects a child, an adult, or an elderly person, individual care is required. The GP with the family and social background available, and with continuity of care over a period of time, is in a unique position to help.

We expect a great deal from our GPs and the primary care team. We expect them to be kind, compassionate, and caring; to be up-to-date and practise the best medicine; to link effectively with colleagues in specialist practice and to communicate and explain to the patient the diagnosis, prognosis, and treatments available. This is a tall order, but it is done regularly and effectively in all surgeries across the country every day of the year. That infection and its control form part of this has already been emphasized. This book, as a practical reference source, will help in the process.

K. C. Calman
London
June 1997

CHAPTER ONE

x2

A history of infection

Since time immemorial infection and infectious diseases have played an established and important role in the history of mankind. The biblical ten plagues included both a scourge of boils and the slaying of the first-born, which was likely to have been an acute, devastating infection. The New Testament is replete with references to individuals afflicted with infection who are saved, by the intervention of Christ from an inevitably fatal outcome. In antiquity, Plato wrote of maintaining both a pure mind and body and recognized only a limited role for doctors in treating acute illness or injuries incurred in battle.

The ancient Greeks were clearly well aware of the devastation of infection, having experienced a cyclical recurring and remitting outbreak of plague in Athens during the Peloponnesian War between 430 and 426 BC. Thucydides' graphic and detailed account of its effect indicates that the infectious nature of the illness was quickly appreciated by the physicians of the time.

> . . . for a while physicians, in ignorance of the nature of the disease, sought to apply remedies; but it was in vain, and they themselves were among the first victims, because they oftenest came into contact with it. No human art was of any avail, and as to supplications in temples, enquiries of oracles, and the like, they were utterly useless . . . Too appalling too was the rapidity with which men caught the infection: dying like sheep if they attended on one another: and this was the principal cause of mortality which physicians have ever given names . . .

Concern with infection and infectious diseases has long been part of man's historical perspective. In literature and art it is a theme which has rivalled and has often been blended with both love and war as a subject worthy of repetition, variation and exploration. In the Bible, the Book of Leviticus is the first ancient text which specifically describes a contagious disease, arguably leprosy or some form of infectious skin disease, and recognizes that the means of controlling its spread was by isolation of the victim from the rest of the community.

Philip Rhodes has argued that 'the success story of the twentieth century has been the near conquest of infections of many kinds'. Prior to this time most infections could only be controlled by attempting to avoid the spread of the infection by isolating the patient. The infection then ran its course and the outcome was dictated by the natural history of the infective process. The

1

integrity of the host was all that was available to deal with the infection and, as Plato had recognized centuries before, 'the art of medicine [was] for the benefit of people of sound constitution who normally led a healthy life, but had contracted some definite ailment'.

The increasing understanding of the necessity for safe, hygienic food and water supplies following John Snow's important observations on the spread of cholera (1854) and subsequently, Lister's fundamental observations concerning antiseptics (1867) followed by the discovery of antibacterials beginning early this century (1906), made it possible to envisage a time when infections could no longer decimate a population and threaten whole families with extinction. Since the concept of immunity or protection against disease had already became formalized with Jenner's vaccine work (1796), the triumvirate of infection control, antibiotics, and immunization were established as the fundamental principles in the management of infectious diseases.

The effectiveness of this three-pronged attack can be counted by its successes and, paradoxically perhaps, by its impact on modern medicine. The large fever hospitals of the Industrial Revolution set the style of medicine for the first three-quarters of this century. They were built in order to isolate and treat epidemic diseases such as tuberculosis, smallpox, and diphtheria. They dictated a style of medicine that relied heavily on the provision of acute care which was both doctor and hospital orientated. With the control and, indeed, abolition of these great killers and the increasing emphasis on more chronic diseases such as heart disease, renal failure, and cancer, it is becoming increasingly possible to ask whether this style of medicine, dictated almost entirely by the nature and ravages of acute infectious disease is any longer appropriate to the requirements of modern health care.

The changes in the management of infectious disease as a result of better control accounts in part for the declining requirement for acute hospital care in the UK. Along with the demographic and technological changes that have characterized the approaching end of the twentieth century, the control of epidemic infectious diseases has resulted in an increasingly elderly population characterized by chronic illness. Care strategies of a different type are required to cater for these new problems and it is the recognition of this change that underlies the recommendations for changes in health care in the UK.

But what then of infectious disease? As a world-wide generic medical problem it is clearly not a thing of the past, but because its management is now governed in developed countries by vaccination programmes, antibiotic treatment, and public health control, its impact on acute medical care has apparently diminished. Nonetheless, many diseases which have been recognized as new in the last 20 years are infectious diseases. These include Lassa fever, legionnaires' disease, toxic shock syndrome, and acquired immune deficiency syndrome (AIDS). None of these, however, have had the impact of the great epidemics of the nineteenth and early-twentieth centuries. Even the advent of AIDS has not necessitated the massive use of acute hospital resources that epidemics of tuberculosis, smallpox, or polio required for large acute wards which served both as treatment and as control areas. The reasons for this are clear; the study of the epidemiology of human immunodeficiency virus (HIV)/AIDS has defined the relatively limited conditions by which this illness is spread. Moreover, its chronic clinical course allows for the development of innovative approaches to its management in both hospital and community settings.

It might, of course, be argued that this latter-day plague has only been controlled by good fortune. Had HIV been spread say, by the respiratory route, its containment might have been much more difficult. Its scale of spread is already very considerable, particularly in North America and in Africa, with some estimates placing the size of the epidemic by the turn of the century at some 30 million infected patients world-wide. This pandemic—caused by an organism which almost seems to be a reflection of the sophistication of the late twentieth century in its ability to illustrate many of the 'new' immunological principles which elucidate host/organism interactions—serves as a warning of the continuing capability of the microbiological world to impose its variety and its force on the human world. It reminds us that the study of infectious agents and the diseases they cause—a study as old as the ancient world—is not an academic issue but reflects the vitality and adaptability of microorganisms as they compete for a place within the biological world.

History, modern medicine, and the philosophy of this book

One of the fundamental aims of this book is to explore this tension between old and new—old and new organisms, old and new understandings of the basis of infection, and old and new approaches to decision-making and the delivery of health care. The authors have tried to achieve a balance between the art of medicine and clinical care and the evidence base for making treatment and resource decisions. The tension between using scientific knowledge for decision-making and delivering health care in the primary care setting is explored in a recent report on the 'Nature of general medical practice' from the Royal College of General Practitioners.[1]

Patient: Why should I take this blood pressure treatment when I feel quite well?
Doctor: It will reduce your risk of having a stroke
Patient: Hmm . . . by how much?
Doctor: (after referring to the latest clinical effectiveness report): After treating 100 people like you for 10 years at least 3 strokes will be prevented.
Patient: I'll take my chance without treatment because I know I'm one of those 97.

As the scientific basis of infection becomes better understood, interruption of the process by the use of antibiotics, by public health interventions, and by modulation of the immune system will continually be subject to evidence-based evaluation. This is, of course, right and proper and should determine the direction of the investigation and management of disease wherever possible. This approach must, however, be tempered by the recognition that medicine also involves experience,[2] pattern recognition, and intuition particularly in primary care, where the interaction between the disease, the individual and the environment make the results of randomized clinical trials difficult to apply.[3,4] The National Health Service Executive has also recognized the importance of expert opinion and past experience, especially in the absence of randomized trials.[5] In an editorial about the purpose and place of evidence based-medicine, Sackett et al.[6] state

The practice of evidence based medicine means integrating individual clinical expertise with the best available external clinical evidence from systematic research.

It is for this reason that the authors of this book have come together as general practitioners, hospital doctors, and scientists to recognize that a blend of evidence, case histories, and experience in dealing with patients offers the best approach to discussing these important issues. All of the chapters are the product of discussion and writing between all the authors. Sometimes, this has led us to question the conventional wisdom of general practice; sometimes, we could not resolve differences between ourselves despite examining available evidence and we have allowed the text to reflect this debate.

References

1. The nature of general medical practice: report of a working party. *Reports from general practice 27*. RCGP London (January 1996)

2. McCormick J. The place of judgement in medicine. *Brit J Gen Pract* (1994) **44**: 50–1

3. Pringle M, Churchill R. Randomised controlled trials in general practice. Gold standard or fool's gold. *BMJ* (1995) **311**: 1381–2

4. Charlton B. Practice guidelines and practical judgement: the role of mega-trials, meta-analysis and consensus. *Brit J Gen Pract* **44**: 290–1

5. *Promoting clinical effectiveness: A framework for action in and through the NHS.* NHS Executive (1996)

6. Sackett D, Rosenberg W, Muir Gray J *et al.* Evidence based medicine: what it is and what it isn't. *BMJ* (1996) **312**: 71–2

CHAPTER TWO

The prevention of infections

[handwritten: look at page 181]

Infectious diseases are still a major cause of mortality and morbidity in the modern developed world. The changing picture is complicated by frequent international travel for business and pleasure and population movements as people seek better conditions for themselves and their families. The advent of antibiotics and good public health practice (Appendix 1) have had a major impact but their use is only a part of the approach which should be adopted in general practice where most infections present and are managed. In this chapter the strategies of health education, immunization, and prophylaxis are examined with practical suggestions to enable the primary health care team to maximize their impact on the incidence of infection.

Health education

The contract for general practitioners, which came into force in April 1990, emphasized the attainment of immunization targets compatible with the World Health Organization's targets for the European Region and encouraged health education and health promotion. Also, the modern emphasis on cost containment and drug budgets has led to mounting pressure on general practitioners and other health professionals as they attempt to care for an increasingly informed public with cash-limited resources. These factors indicate that an optimum use of scarce resources in managing infection in general practice will be achieved by a high coverage of immunization and effective advice on prevention. *[handwritten: educating needed]*

The traditional model of the doctor–patient relationship in which the patient is a relatively passive participant has been described as a barrier to involvement in changing lifestyles. Since the 1980s, changes in the nature of the relationship have taken place which emphasize the personal responsibility and participation of the patient and enable informed choices about lifestyles and habits. The patient requires information, sensibly presented, and the opportunity to discuss and modify health beliefs.[1]

Case history

A middle-aged woman consulted with an offensive vaginal discharge. The general practitioner asked her what she thought it might be due to. The patient replied that it smelled fishy and that she wondered if it was related to the salmon

5

> sandwiches she had eaten two days ago. While this was a reasonable attempt to make sense of her symptoms she readily accepted the explanation for the smell associated with bacterial vaginosis.

The enhancement of patient autonomy in the pursuit of health must, however, exist side by side with opportunities for patients to temporarily surrender autonomy should they wish. The timing, pacing, and reinforcement of health promotion must be sensitive to these other needs or the effect will be the opposite of that which was intended. The potential to discuss sexually transmitted disease with a 17-year-old youth consulting for acne certainly exists, the practice may have decided this as a priority for health education, but the insensitive implementation of the policy may result in poor compliance with treatment for acne and a resolve to avoid doctors in the future.

General practitioners may chose to offer opportunistic health promotion within a patient-initiated consultation in two broadly different ways. The discussion may be related to the presenting problem or it may be tailored to the patient's age, sex, and lifestyle and may cover a range of problems which the patient had not expected to discuss on that occasion. The latter approach, in particular, requires well-developed consultation skills and a clear under-standing of the purpose and impact of the conversation on the patient.

Prevention and health promotion are more easily carried out within special sessions arranged for the purpose, as the patient's expectations will be different. Unfortunately, those individuals who are the least informed and the least able to exercise choice in lifestyle and health behaviours, due to such factors as poverty or language barriers, are also those least likely to attend such sessions. Health promotion by GPs for these individuals remains, initially, within the consultation although receptivity of patients may principally be determined by factors outwith the influence of the practice team.[2]

The development of the primary health care team and a more coherent approach to prevention enables the work of the general practitioner within the consultation to be co-ordinated with that of the practice nurse, district nurse, midwife, and health visitor, in the surgery and in the patient's home. The relationship between patients and nurses is often described as more equal and hence more conducive to mutual exchange and patient participation. As teamwork develops within a practice a common approach to prevention must be fostered, with individuals concentrating on those areas in which they have particular expertise. Health professionals will base their activities on a sound knowledge base and an appreciation of the ethical aspects of prevention so that choice is improved, anxiety appropriately constrained, and the consequences of professional activities, such as how to deal with the results of screening tests, anticipated before they cause harm.

Prevention of infection

The prevention of infection through health education follows logically from an understanding of sources of infection and the potential portals of entry of *gives a few examples in essay*

Table 2.1 *Sources of infection, and portals and vehicles of entry*

Sources of infection:

People: with an active infection, convalescent but excreting the organism, or a symptomless carrier

Animals: either with an active infection, convalescent but excreting the organism, a symptomless carrier or via an arthropod vector

Environment: airborne, soil, contaminated food or water

Portals and vehicles of entry:

Alimentary: contaminated food, water, contaminated hands, eating utensils

Respiratory: droplet nuclei, secondary aerosols

Contact: skin or mucosa (including the eyes) of an individual to their own skin or mucosa or that of another person. Sexual contact of all kinds is included in this category. Indirect contact with infectious agents may occur via water and surfaces (fomites)

Tissue penetration: bites, minor injuries, non-sterile injections, blood transfusions, and surgical procedures

Congenital: transplacental or from the birth canal

---

pathogens into the human body. For an alternative authoritative discussion the reader is referred to the Bible, Leviticus, chapters 11–15. Some infections seen in UK general practice are shown together with their source and portal of entry in Tables 2.1 and 2.2. In the sections that follow examples are given which demonstrate how primary health care professionals, with a knowledge of the method of spread of an infectious disease, can provide health education tailored to the needs of individuals and groups. Pregnant women, travellers abroad, people with children who keep domestic pets are obvious examples.

Sources of infection

The alimentary tract

Infections spread by the faecal–oral route are common, particularly in conditions of poor hygiene, overcrowding, and poor sanitation. Many of the agents that are spread by this route cause diarrhoea, hence enhancing their potential for transmission. The spread may be via contaminated fingers, eating utensils, or food and water. Although most adults in the UK will have received some education about avoiding these infections, members of the primary health care team should be ready to reinforce the advice and have fact sheets available in the practice to hand to patients.

Changes in eating habits in the UK with new catering methods and the increased use of convenience foods have also been accompanied by a rise

Table 2.2 *Sources of infection and portals of entry of some infections*

Portal of entry	Source		
	Human	Animal	Environmental
Alimentary tract	*Shigella* dysentery Polio	Salmonellosis *Campylobacter*	Hepatitis A
Respiratory tract	Influenza Tuberculosis *H. influenzae*	Psittacosis	Legionellosis
Contact	Impetigo Herpes simplex	Tinea Orf	Plantar warts
Tissue penetration	Hepatitis B HIV	Rabies Malaria	Tetanus Erysipelas Leptospirosis
Congenital	Rubella Cytomegalovirus (CMV)	Toxoplasmosis	Listeriosis

in the incidence of food-borne disease,[3] including the emergence of *Listeria*, *Campylobacter*, *Cryptosporidium*, *Escherichia coli* and *Salmonella* as public health hazards. While legislation addresses standards for food safety, the primary health care team can contribute by informing the public about proper standards for the preparation, cooking and storing of food. If the guidelines shown in Table 2.3 are observed then infections are unlikely: they will need adapting to the individual circumstances of some patients, such as elderly people living alone or families in temporary accommodation, but can be used as a basis for patient information handouts.

The respiratory tract

The old rhyme 'coughs and sneezes spread diseases, use your handkerchief!' is good advice. Microorganisms in the mouth, throat, and respiratory tract can be released during coughing, sneezing, and speaking, to form droplet nuclei which may remain airborne for long periods. Other particles may settle on surfaces and then be dispersed as secondary aerosols which may subsequently be inhaled. Overcrowding, active and passive smoking, coughing, spitting, and sneezing all enable the spread of these infections which include most of the viral exanthems, respiratory syncytial virus (RSV), *Haemophilus influenzae*, *Streptococcus pneumoniae*, influenza, and the common cold. Patients seen in practice with acute symptoms of upper respiratory infections should be told to stay away from other people if at all possible: 'working through' a streaming cold is, for the most part, an antisocial rather than noble action![4]

Table 2.3 *Guidelines for domestic food safety*

Shopping
- Avoid shops that appear dirty, where the staff have dirty hands or nails, or are eating or smoking while selling goods
- Avoid food which is past the sell-by date or is in damaged containers
- Do not buy cracked eggs
- Ensure that fresh meat is wrapped and cannot contaminate other foods
- Take food home and store it appropriately immediately. Do not leave it in the boot of a car for several hours

Storage
- Make sure the fridge is cold enough: below 4 °C
- Store different types of food separately
- Do not allow meat, fish, and poultry to drip on to other foods
- Freezers should be at or below 0 °C

The kitchen
- Keep the kitchen clean
- Separate cooked and uncooked meats
- Do not allow pets on the work surfaces or near to food.
- Wash hands with soap and warm water before touching food and after touching pets, the waste bin, dirty nappies, or going to the lavatory
- Do not prepare food if you have diarrhoea or vomiting
- Cover cuts and abrasions
- Wash worktops with hot soapy water and dry with paper towels
- Use a different board for raw meat, cooked foods, and vegetables; and wash knives and utensils between different stages of food preparation
- Wash fruit and vegetables thoroughly, peel raw foods before eating
- Keep kitchen linen and cloths clean

Preparation and cooking
- Follow manufacturer's instructions on pre-cooked food
- Defrost frozen food fully in the fridge or microwave prior to cooking
- Defrost poultry completely before cooking
- Cook meat thoroughly, use a meat thermometer to ensure the centre has reached 70 °C
- Raw or lightly cooked eggs may harbour *Salmonella* and should be avoided
- Pregnant women and the very young or old should avoid soft cheeses and meat pâté
- Do not reheat food more than once and ensure that it is hot right through
- Observe microwave standing times
- Discard cooked food that has been in the fridge for more than 2 days

---

Direct contact

This route is particularly important for the spread of skin, mucocutaneous, and sexually transmitted infections and infestations. Mothers of young children with impetigo or conjunctivitis, for example, will need explanations of the route of spread so that they can cover the lesions if appropriate, prevent close contact with other children, and supervise the family bathroom to prevent shared use of flannels and towels. Sleeping arrangements and shared clothes are another source of transmission (e.g. threadworms, scabies) and the recent fashion for whirlpool baths and hot tubs provides further opportunities for the spread of infections.

Sexual contact

Infections transmitted primarily by sexual contact are among the commonest of health problems world-wide and cause immeasurable misery to individuals and families and consequences for society. Although most of these infections can be cured, with the present exception of AIDS, many patients remain undiagnosed with the development of chronic ill health and infertility. Primary prevention of sexually transmitted disease (STDS) requires individuals to modify their behaviour in circumstances where the power of sexual feelings often make it difficult to behave rationally. Unless the individual is well informed it is easy to deny the risk or let it weigh lightly against the immediate pleasure of ignoring it (See Table 2.4).

General practitioners and other members of the practice team frequently have difficulty in talking to patients about sex, and in particular, talking in detail about sexual practices. Individual prejudices and personal beliefs can impair the effectiveness of health education in this situation and it is important to ensure that the practice team receives training. Recent studies have shown that particular difficulty occurs in discussing the sexual practices of homosexual men and women, and that younger and female doctors show the greatest anxiety. Many approaches have been used as sex health education interventions for young people but few have been rigorously evaluated.[5,6] Effective interventions have included a school programme aimed at increasing knowledge and student–parent communication, and work with young homeless adolescents directed at individual barriers to safe sex. However, harmful intervention was reported: a programme aimed at younger adolescents, which promoted premarital abstinence through information about reproduction and the implications and risks of sexual behaviour, resulted in none of the desired changes in attitudes and behaviour. Boys in the intervention group were more likely to become sexually active than the control group.

The ability of any infection to establish itself depends on the virulence of the organism and the size of the inoculum in relation to the host's defences. Advice given in primary care to prevent STD is directed to reducing exposure and reducing the inoculum. The transmission to a woman of a specific STD, such as *Chlamydia*, occurs, for example, as the result of virulent organisms

Table 2.4 *Strategies for protection from sexually transmitted diseases (STDs)*

• Review sexual activity	*No risk*: abstinence; one lifetime partner who has had only one partner *Low risk*: serial monogamy with uninfected partners *High risk*: multiple partners, especially unfamiliar partners
• Use barrier contraceptives; male and female condom, diaphragms	Reduce risk if used with a spermicide Not effective if infectious lesions are not covered. May be used in addition to other contraception to prevent infection
• Practice safe sex	Avoid sexual practices which cause trauma to skin or mucous membranes and which increase the direct inoculation of pathogens. Avoid receptive anal intercourse, oral–anal contact, and practices that cause bleeding Avoid sex during menstruation
• Ensure sexual partners comply with diagnosis and treatment of STD	50% of partners of patients with gonorrhoea and *Chlamydia* are infected, many asymptomatically
• Periodic screening	Go for screening tests if at higher risk

being deposited on or near the cervix where they invade the endocervical cells to cause infection. The chances of infection, therefore, are related to the nature and frequency of contact with an infected partner as well as the condition of the cervix and the patient's immune state. Consideration of these factors enables sensible advice about prevention (i.e. avoid intercourse with infected partners and use barrier contraception). Because the combined oral contraceptive pill causes cervical changes which increase susceptibility to *Chlamydia* infection, further advice should include the use of a condom as well as the pill if there is a risk of catching a sexually transmitted disease.

An understanding of how the common and important sexually transmitted diseases cause infection will enable the GP to develop the skills to discuss the relevant sexual behaviour with patients of both sexes, all ages, and differing sexualities.[7] The discussion must be in sufficient detail to allow an informed choice to be made the next time the patient is tempted to take a risk. The necessary skills include the development of self-awareness, sensitivity about the timing and circumstances of the discussion, and the use of language that the patient can understand.

Tissue penetration

Intact mucous membranes and skin can be penetrated by some infectious agents such as *Leptospira* from rats' urine. Blood transfusions, surgical procedures, organ transplantation, and non-sterile needles carry the risk of infection from blood-borne diseases, such as hepatitis-B, cytomegalovirus, and human immunodeficiency viruses (HIV), especially in countries with poor facilities. Intravenous drug-users who share needles may develop hepatitis-B or HIV infection. Animal bites and those of arthropod vectors transmit many infections such as rabies, malaria, Lyme disease, and dengue.

Avoidance of infection from blood products in the practice setting

Between 1980 and 1984, 361 cases of acute hepatitis-B occurred in health service staff out of a total of 6696 reported. In a study of 598 GPs, Kinnersley[8] found that only half had been vaccinated against hepatitis-B. The majority gave the reason for non-compliance as 'I just haven't got round to it'. Doctors and nurses working in general practice and carrying out practical procedures are at risk of infection from blood products which enter the body through minor cuts and abrasions or from needlestick injuries. Hepatitis-B and HIV infection may both be transmitted in this way. Training for all team members who carry out any practical procedure or who clear up afterwards must ensure that the following advice is followed:

- Keep cuts and abrasions covered with a waterproof dressing
- Wear gloves
- Do not re-sheath needles
- Dispose of sharps directly into a sharps' bin
- Wash off splashes; irrigate splashes in the eyes or mouth with plenty of water
- *Spills*: blood spills should be covered in 1:9 thick household bleach for 2 minutes and then thoroughly mopped up and washed down using the bleach preparation. Gloves should be worn throughout and ventilation of the area should be adequate. Bleach should be stored safely and away from areas of patient access
- Use a steam autoclave which reaches a temperature of 134 °C to sterilize instruments

A protocol for the management of needlestick injury is shown in Appendix 2. Each practice should display a copy of such a protocol in all the relevant areas.

Congenital infections

These infections occur either as a result of transplacental spread or from the birth canal either during pregnancy or labour. Infections that cross the placenta may be acquired by the mother via any of the portals of entry already discussed, making advice to susceptible pregnant women about food preparation (e.g. *Listeria*), [9]domestic pets (e.g. toxoplasmosis), and contact with infected individuals (e.g. chickenpox) particularly important.

Sexually transmitted infections can be passed from the mother to the fetus during pregnancy and labour. Primary prevention involves the avoidance of intercourse with infected partners during pregnancy. Some studies have suggested that the continuance of intercourse to the end of pregnancy also increases the risk of perinatal infection. Family doctors are sometimes aware of situations where there is a risk to an unborn child through the sexual activity of either parent. It is important that the individual be informed of the potential danger for the baby. Such consultations require skill in communication, in which concern for the child is properly balanced by an understanding of the factors leading to the behaviour of the adult. Once trust is established and information given it is often possible to modify risky behaviour and enable screening of the other partner without fatal damage to the relationship.

Perinatal bacterial infection is acquired during pregnancy or during delivery in up to 5 in 1000 births. In the UK, bacterial infections are about three times more common than viral or protozoan infections.

Apart from the modification of sexual activity the other strategy employed to protect the fetus is screening of the mother and early treatment if appropriate. In the UK, all women are screened for syphilis, and selective screening for *Chlamydia* and gonorrhoea is carried out. Other potentially dangerous maternal infections which are sexually transmitted include hepatitis-B, human papilloma virus, HIV, herpes simplex virus (HSV), and cytomegalovirus. Management of these infections in pregnancy, including screening, is included in the relevant sections on each individual infection (See below).

Case study: The prevention of congenital toxoplasmosis

The final part of this section on health education comprises a detailed consideration of the prevention of congenital toxoplasmosis. The material is included here to enable the reader to synthesize the preceding sections; some practices might like to base a clinical meeting for team members on its contents. It is a particularly good example for enabling discussion of ethical issues in prevention, the use of health care resources and to demonstrate how knowledge of portals of entry can lead to sensible advice to patients. Approaches to the prevention of toxoplasmosis illustrate many of issues that must be resolved before embarking on a prevention programme in general practice.[10]

The organism has a complicated life cycle in the cat, other animals, and man. It can cause infection of the unborn child which is potentially devastating, difficult to treat, but is also uncommon. There are opposing views on the implementation of screening in the UK.[11] The subject has received increasing media attention and women now frequently ask their general practitioners for screening. These issues were highlighted by a written reply to a Parliamentary Question in November 1990 on the introduction of screening which stated that the procedure would not be introduced in the UK because of uncertainty about the natural history of the disease, the accuracy of tests, and the efficacy of possible treatment (*The Independent*, 14 November 1990).

Congenital infection with *Toxoplasmosis gondii* only occurs if a pregnant

---

woman acquires an acute infection and the infective organisms enter the fetal blood circulation. This situation can only occur once in the woman's lifetime and subsequent pregnancies will not be affected. Infection early in pregnancy may lead to abortion, although most congenitally infected infants are asymptomatic at birth and may either remain so or develop ocular impairment later in life. Retinochoroiditis, hydrocephalus, and intracranial calcification, the 'classic triad' of congenital infection with *T. gondii* is extremely rare in the UK. Although the prevalence of antibodies to *Toxoplasma* is about 33% world-wide with wide variations, the incidence of congenital toxoplasmosis is not known with any certainty despite a number of surveys. The rates vary between countries and may in part be due to different dietary practices, such as eating undercooked meat and attitudes to household pets. The reported UK incidence of toxoplasmic uveitis, which is considered to be a congenital infection, is ten times greater than that of congenital toxoplasmosis, demonstrating that congenital infection is certainly under-reported in the UK. Recent estimates of the incidence of maternal infection are 2/1000 pregnancies, the maternal–fetal transmission rate is about 40%, and the middle estimate of congenital infection is about 1/1000 live births.

The prevention of congenital toxoplasmosis is controversial. In France and in the US state of Oregon, tests for toxoplasmosis in pregnancy are compulsory and in Austria refusal leads to the withholding of full maternity benefit. In the UK facilities for the detection of toxoplasmosis are not widely available and there is no general agreement on the need to screen pregnant women. Public awareness of the problem is increasing and general practitioners and midwives are now being consulted by women who may request a test for immunity to the infection. While this may be justified in particular instances (e.g. women employed in veterinary work, or packing raw meat), the implications of a negative antibody test must be fully understood by the professional and patient before screening is embarked on. These might include, in appropriate circumstances, a plan to supplement general advice with regular retesting to detect acute infection. If an infection occurs in the first trimester, when treatment cannot be used, the woman may seek an abortion. Although infection later in pregnancy may be modified by treatment this assertion is not supported by controlled trials. It is essential, therefore, that the patient understands these facts before screening is carried out and that care is taken not to provoke undue anxiety. The discussion of such a complex matter must be underpinned by excellent communication skills and an appreciation of the ethical issues involved. If the antibody status of a pregnant woman is unknown, as is the case for the vast majority of UK women, then she should receive specific advice about prevention which is derived from an understanding of the life cycle of the organism.

There are two distinct life-cycles of *T. gondii*: (1) an entero-epithelial cycle which occurs in the small intestine of the cat and which leads to oocyst production; and (2) an extra-intestinal cycle involving proliferative forms and tissue cysts, which can take place in any warm-blooded animal including man.

Cats shed oocysts 3–21 days after ingesting any of the forms of *T. gondii* and during feline infection over one thousand million oocysts may be shed. Oocytes must sporolate after shedding to become infective and although they are excreted only once in the lifetime of the cat they may retain infectivity in moist soil for over a year. Anywhere that cats may defecate, such as garden soil or children's sandpits, may contain oocysts which can then result in an acute infection in individuals who ingest them.

The extraintestinal cycle of *T. gondii* infection takes place in any warm-blooded animal after the ingestion of oocysts and tissue cysts. The infective organism liberated from the cysts by digestion may enter the lymphatic system and are disseminated inside white blood cells. The chronic stage which follows acute infection is characterized by the formation of tissue cysts which occur in skeletal and cardiac muscle, the eye, and visceral organs, as well as in the central nervous system. Intact tissue cysts may persist throughout the lifetime of the host and are probably harmless although they represent a large reservoir of infection should the host become immunocompromised and are the source of acute infection should the host's flesh be consumed by another animal including man.

All pregnant women should be advised of the need for care in handling and cooking meat and in handling cats, particularly cat litter. Specific advice, based on the life cycle of *T. gondii*, is shown in Table 2.5.

Table 2.5 *Advice to pregnant women for the prevention of congenital Toxoplasmosis*

- Wash hands and kitchen surfaces after handling raw meat and poultry
- Do not touch eyes or mouth while preparing raw meat and poultry
- Cook meat completely; heat to at least 65°C
- Do not clean cat litter boxes or, if unavoidable, wear gloves
- Wear gloves when gardening
- Cover children's sandpits when not in use
- Do not feed raw meat to cats
- Wash or peel fruit and vegetables

Immunization

Immunization against disease has transformed the health of populations in the developed world. The scandal of mortality in lesser developed countries due to vaccine-preventable disease is one of the great moral issues of the 1990s: it reminds those of us working in UK general practice of our duty to ensure the immunization of individuals who should receive it given that we are fortunate to live in a society where it is freely available. The purpose of immunization programmes is to protect individuals and to produce a high level of herd immunity which benefits vulnerable unprotected groups such as the immunosuppressed and the new-born.

The scientific basis of immunity

Many GPs who regularly immunize patients against infection would be hard put to explain the scientific basis for the procedure except in very general terms. However, an understanding of the mechanisms whereby immunity develops leads to careful clinical practice and safe administration of live and killed vaccines. Some important concepts are included in the section on the body's response to infection (Chapter 3).

Immunization can be *passive,* by providing temporary protection from administration of preformed antibody to the infectious agent, or *active,* with stimulation of the body's immune mechanisms through administration of a vaccine. The antibodies used to provide passive immunization may be obtained from humans, from animals actively immunized with the infectious agent, or through the use of molecular genetic techniques. Antisera produced in animals are less successful because the foreign globulins are cleared rapidly (within about 10 days) from the recipient and there is a danger of the foreign protein producing hypersensitivity reactions such as serum sickness or even anaphylaxis. Human antibodies do not produce hypersensitivity and persist in the circulation, providing protection, for several weeks. Human antibodies are available in two preparations: (1) normal immunoglobulin; and (2) hyperimmune globulins.

Normal immunoglobulin is an intramuscular preparation of the gamma-globulin fraction of blood pooled from a large group of blood donors and contains antibody to many common, naturally occurring diseases. Intravenous immune globulin is a special preparation which is used for replacement therapy in immunodeficiency states rather than for immunization. Specific hyperimmune globulins are obtained from the blood of individuals who have either recently recovered from natural infection or who have been hyperimmunized to produce very high antibody titres to one specific agent. The immunoglobulin preparations currently available are shown in Table 2.6.

Active immunization can be provided by means of vaccines containing living attenuated (avirulent) organisms, killed or inactivated organisms or fractions thereof, or with toxoids (bacterial toxins that have been modified to render them safe but still immunogenic).

Live vaccines produce an immune response that is very similar to that following natural infection with a rapid development of both local and humoral immunity. The initial antibody production is IgM, shortly followed by IgG. One dose of live vaccine generally confers durable, often lifelong,

Table 2.6 *Immunuglobulin preparations*

- Human normal immunoglobulin (antibodies to varicella, measles, hepatitis A)
- Anti-varicella-zoster virus
- Anti-hepatitis B
- Anti-tetanus
- Anti-rabies

protection. Live vaccines are, in general, contraindicated in pregnancy or in immunocompromised individuals because even an attenuated organism may be sufficiently virulent to cause infection dangerous to the fetus or the immunosuppressed individual.

Inactivated vaccines, on the other hand, provide immunogenicity without infectivity but the immune response is less marked and they must be given parenterally and in repeated doses (and boosters) to induce permanent immunity. Adjuvants are used in some vaccines containing inactivated microorganisms or toxoids. This improves the immune response, probably by mobilizing phagocytes and delaying antigen release, but an adjuvant-containing vaccine must be given intramuscularly since local irritation and necrosis can result from subcutaneous administration.

The immune response to most protein vaccines depends upon an interaction between B and T lymphocytes but some vaccines composed of polysaccharide antigens from microorganisms (e.g. *Haemophilus influenzae* type b vaccine, can induce antibody responses without involvement of T cells). Unfortunately, such responses are poor in infants and children under the age of 18 months and the lack of a T-cell response means that memory is poor and booster responses are not seen after repeat administration. Such vaccines are often linked to a protein molecule in order to convert them to T-cell-dependent antigens. The currently available vaccines are shown in Table 2.7.

Practical approaches to immunization

Immunization against infection is a safe and well-tried procedure, and is a routine part of general practice. All the members of the practice team should be familiar with the roles and responsibilities of each person involved whether it be clinical or administrative. There are certain basic principles which should underlie any immunization programme, namely, excellent clinical practice supported by multidisciplinary education and training, and proper regard for patient autonomy achieved by explanation and informed consent.

Drugs and equipment necessary for an immunization session

The first requirement for excellent clinical practice is that the premises are adequate for safe immunization to be carried out. Equivalent equipment for domiciliary immunization should be available if the procedure is carried out by the practice. The equipment required is:

- Refrigerator (with maximum–minimum thermometer)
- Examination couch
- The latest edition of *Immunisation against infectious disease*. HMSO, (London)
- Small portable oxygen cylinder
- Airways: adult and paediatric sizes

Table 2.7 *Vaccines available in the UK*

Live vaccines	Non-living vaccines
Measles	Pertussis
Mumps	Cholera
Rubella	*H. influenzae* polysaccharide
Polio (oral)	Hepatitis B
Typhoid (oral)	Hepatitis A
Yellow fever	Polio (intramuscular)
Japanese B encephalitis	Influenza
Tuberculosis (bacillus	Meningococcal polysaccharide
Calmette–Guérin, BCG)	Pneumococcal polysaccharide
	Rabies
Toxoid vaccines	Typhoid (parenteral)
Whooping cough	Tick-borne encephalitis
Plague	
Diphtheria	
Tetanus	

- Emergency drugs to include:
  1:1000 adrenaline (1 mg/ml), hydrocortisone sodium succinate, chlor-pheniramine maleate

Storage of vaccines. The manufacturer's recommendations on storage must be followed or the potency of the vaccine cannot be guaranteed. In general, vaccines must be stored in the centre of a reliable refrigerator. They must not be placed in the freezing compartment nor must they be left out of the refrigerator. Vaccines must be replaced immediately at the end of a session. Should transport between buildings or clinics be necessary they must be placed in a reliable cold bag containing freezer packs. They should be warmed before use. On completion of a vaccination session all prepared or open vaccines together with syringes, needles, and used ampoules are disposed of for future incineration. In general practice they are conveniently placed in a sharps container which is then sealed and removed for incineration.

Hunter (1989)[12] conducted a survey of storage of vaccines in general practice. The majority of the practice nurses who responded did not know at what temperature their refrigerator was operating; in addition, many practices gave patients vaccines to store at home where the care would likely be even worse. Hunter makes the following recommendations which are in line with guidelines from the UK department of health:

1. Every fridge should contain a maximum–minimum thermometer Ideally, use a special fridge with a preset thermostat and external temperature gauge.

2. The temperature should be read twice per day and always at the beginning of each vaccination session. Normally, it should be within the range 2–8°C

and should not fall below freezing. Human normal immunoglobulin (HNIG) must be stored at 0–4°C.

3. The storage of other items in fridge should be kept to a minimum.

4. Regular defrosting (store vaccines in another fridge).

5. Phials containing single doses should be used if possible. If these are not available, then opened multiple dose phials should be discarded at the end of a session.

6. The manufacturer's instructions for shelf-life and correct storage temperatures must be strictly observed at all times.

A study of 45 general practices and 5 child health clinics[13] reported that only 16 respondents were aware of the recommended storage conditions for the vaccines that they administered. The authors monitored the temperatures of fridges in 8 practices using maximum and minimum thermometers: in 6 centres the vaccines were exposed to temperatures which would reduce their potency. Another study of 29 practices reported that the potency of some vaccines in 10 of 26 deliveries of live vaccines became suspect due to breaks in the cold chain.[14] Readers might like to reflect on these findings since there is no point in meeting immunization targets if the vaccine that is administered has lost its effectiveness. (A fact sheet on refrigeration equipment can be obtained from: Supplies Technology Division, Product Group 1B, 14 Russell Square, London WC1B 5EP.)

Administration of vaccines

The role of nurses

Both doctors and Registered General Nurses administer vaccines in general practice although the responsibilities taken by nurses in organizing and administering the service varies considerably. Within general practice the development of the primary care team and the employment of practice nurses has led to many nurses working in an extended role and gaining considerable job satisfaction from doing so. Despite these changes there is still a reluctance for some doctors and nurses within practice to encourage nurses to take full responsibility for immunization either of children or adults. The reluctance of nurses to immunize in the absence of a doctor appears to be based on anxiety about their ability to manage anaphylaxis and about taking responsibility for ensuring that the patient is fit for the procedure. Anaphylaxis is an extremely rare event and there is no evidence that a well-trained nurse will be less competent at initial management than a doctor.[15]

Some practices have advocated the use of checklists for nurses running immunization sessions for children as a way of increasing confidence.[16] Nicholl et al.,[17] in an authoritative review of the reasons for poor uptake of childhood immunization in the UK in the 1980s, state that immunization is a nursing activity. The current consensus is, they feel, that an immunization course can be prescribed by a doctor after which there is no legal or medical bar to the immunization being given by a nurse with or without a doctor present in the building. This approach holds equally well for the immunization of children and adults.

Each general practice team should debate the issues raised by the changing role of the nurse in vaccination practice. The aim should be to ensure that individuals are well trained and competent to carry out their clinical responsibilities with frequent opportunities to discuss any situation that causes anxiety should it be necessary.

The following advice is given by the Department of Health.[18]

A doctor may delegate responsibility for immunization to a nurse providing the following conditions are fulfilled:

1. The nurse is willing to be professionally accountable for this work.

2. The nurse has received training and is competent in all aspects of immunization including the contraindications to specific vaccines.

3. Adequate training has been given in the recognition and treatment of anaphylaxis.

If these conditions are fulfilled and nurses carry out the immunization in accordance with accepted district health authority, NHS trust, or health board policy, the authority trust/board will accept responsibility for immunization by nurses. Similarly, nurses employed by GPs should work to agreed protocols including all above conditions.

Injection technique and site of injection

Intradermal injections

BCG (bacillus Calmette–Guérin) vaccine is always given intradermally; rabies, cholera, and typhoid vaccines may also be given this way.

Technique. Nurses and doctors must be trained in the correct technique and should practice with intradermal saline if necessary. The skin of the subject should be stretched between thumb and forefinger of one hand while the other hand is used to insert the needle (size 25G), bevel upwards, for about 2 mm into the superficial layer of the skin, almost parallel with the surface. A successful technique results in a raised, blanched bleb showing the tips of the hair follicles. There is resistance to the injection which is absent if the injection is too deep. In this situation, the needle should be removed and reinserted before any further vaccine is administered. A bleb of 7 mm in diameter is approximately equal to 0.1 ml.

Sites:

BCG. Over insertion of left deltoid muscle. The tip of the shoulder must be avoided as keloid formation is more likely in that area.

Mantoux or Heaf. Middle of flexor surface of forearm but this site should not be used for injecting vaccines.

Intradermal rabies. Behind posterior border of distal portion of deltoid muscle.

Subcutaneous and intramuscular injection in infants

Infant immunizations are best given in the antero-lateral aspect of the thigh or upper arm. Some practitioners prefer to use the buttock; if this site is chosen the risk of sciatic nerve damage is avoided by using the upper outer quadrant. Injection into fatty tissue of the buttock has been shown to reduce efficacy of hepatitis B vaccine.

Immunization emergencies

Anaphylactic reactions following immunization are extremely rare. No deaths from this cause were notified to the Office of Population, Censuses, and Surveys (OPCS) during the period 1978–89. During the same period the Committee on Safety of Medicines were notified of only 18 anaphylactic and anaphylactoid reactions, while at the same time 25 million childhood immunizations were given.

The possibility of these reactions engenders anxiety among those responsible for immunization and may on occasion predispose a professional to advise that immunization be postponed or avoided on the basis of a false contraindication such as atopy or a dislike of eggs. Specific training in the recognition and management of anaphylaxis improves the confidence of those administering vaccines.[19] In the general practice setting, doctors and nurses who immunize should train together and regularly review the procedures to be followed should an emergency arise. All the staff should be proficient in cardio-pulmonary resuscitation and the general management of the unconscious patient. An easily accessible alarm should be installed in all rooms where injections are given in order to summon assistance without leaving the patient. The location of paediatric and adult airways, oxygen, and the emergency drugs' tray should be known to all, and the availability and expiry dates of all necessary drugs checked regularly. The treatment of choice for clinical anaphylaxis is adrenaline and the range of doses for adults and children should be prominently displayed near to the emergency drugs' tray. Nebulized salbutamol and intravenous steroids are indicated for bronchospasm.

The majority of reactions following immunization are simple fainting attacks which are particularly common in adolescents and young adults. Infants and small children rarely faint: if they lose consciousness after an immunization they should be presumed to be suffering from an anaphylactic reaction. A strong carotid pulse persists during a faint and during a convulsion which may occur if a vaso-vagal attack is prolonged. The carotid pulse is weak and difficult to palpate during an anaphylactic reaction.

Guidelines for safe administration of vaccines

Before an immunization is given a careful history must be taken to assess suitability for the procedure. Contraindications are discussed fully later in this chapter, but in planning any programme the following guidelines will be useful.

1. Two or more live vaccines may be given simultaneously (but oral polio and oral typhoid vaccines should *not* be given together and should be separated by 2 weeks).

2. If live vaccines are *not* given simultaneously, 3 weeks should elapse before the second vaccine is administered to prevent the immune response to the first impairing the response to the second.

3. Live vaccines must not be given in pregnancy.

4. Gamma-globulin may be given at the same time as a live vaccine if given together. If not given simultaneously, they must be separated by 21 days and the live vaccine should be given first.

5. If yellow fever is given first, then there is no need to wait for 21 days before giving gamma-globulin purchased in the UK.

6. Gamma-globulin must not be given together with a BCG vaccination.

7. Vaccination should be avoided if the recipient has an acute febrile illness.

8. Most live vaccines contain small traces of antibiotics such as neomycin and polymyxin. If there is a history of sensitivity to such antibiotics, then particular caution is advised.

Informed consent

No child or adult should be vaccinated without informed consent being obtained at the time of each immunization. Written consent at the time that primary vaccination for children or other immunization programmes (e.g. for travellers abroad) are first discussed and planned is always to be supplemented by express consent when the immunization is given (see Department of Health (1996). *Immunisation against infectious disease.* HMSO, London). The nature of informed consent is such that the patient (or patient's parent/guardian) has a right to know the risks and benefits of the procedure including a discussion of common and serious side-effects. Individuals, including older children,[20] must be given an opportunity to ask questions and health professionals have a duty to provide accurate, unbiased answers. The giving of this information in a way that does not provoke unfounded anxiety is a core skill required from health professionals who immunize and its absence is a major reason for the inadequate coverage of primary vaccination in many districts in the UK.[21,22] The basis for a confident approach to obtaining informed consent springs from the training of health professionals in all aspects of immunization practice. The use of role play and videotape to examine consultations with real or simulated patients in which consent for immunization is obtained can be a powerful learning tool. This approach is frequently used in many general practices to study a range of consultations and the approach might form the basis of practice team-training to improve immunization uptake.

Record-keeping

As in any aspect of clinical practice good record-keeping is fundamental to good vaccination programmes. For each individual who is immunized the exact nature and dose of the vaccine, the batch number and date of injection must be recorded. The record should demonstrate that informed consent for the procedure has been obtained. Any reactions must be carefully documented; accuracy avoids false contraindications to future immunizations arising from exaggerated accounts of reactions. It is important that the medical records contain this information as well as the clinic and health visiting notes; sometimes, logistic difficulties must be overcome if a child is immunized in a health authority clinic and then presents the next day to the GP. Problems may be overcome by asking the mother to hold an immunization record for her child.

All children will be offered a complete immunization programme via the community child health service. Unfortunately, co-ordination with general practice is not always optimal, particularly in areas with highly mobile populations. Computerized call and recall systems running within practices, co-ordinated with the Regional or District Health Authority database, are particularly efficient for childhood immunization, but are not yet available to all practices.

Immunization of children

In the developed world the introduction and widespread use of vaccines in childhood has had a profound effect on the mortality and morbidity due to infection. In 1988, reports from the 32 European countries stated that 26 were free from poliomyelitis, 25 were free from neonatal tetanus, and 20 reported no cases of diphtheria. In addition pertussis and measles have both declined sharply. The success of these programmes have led some countries to work for the elimination of certain infections: both former Czechoslovakia and the former German Democratic Republic set the target of measles elimination in 1976, and by 1985, 98% of Czech children had been immunized against measles.

The World Health Organization Expanded Programme on Immunization set a target of 90% primary vaccination cover for Europe by 1990 as part of the policy of achieving health for all by the year 2000. The aim of the initiative is the elimination of diphtheria, poliomyelitis, neonatal tetanus, measles, and congenital rubella by the year 2000. Although many European countries have already reached the target, the performance of the United Kingdom, by the beginning of the 1990s, was among the worst in the region and was bettered by some developing nations. For example, in 1990 completed DPT (diphtheria, pertussis, tetanus) vaccination rates were higher in Kuwait, Singapore, Costa Rica, Chile, and Argentina than they were in the UK.[23]

The average uptake in England for children born in 1984 and immunized by the end of 1986 was 85% for third diphtheria, 67% for third pertussis, and 71% for measles. A description of the COVER scheme (Cover of Vaccination Evaluated Rapidly) in England and Wales reported a modest improvement by May 1988.[24] In the 126 participating districts the average coverage was 84% for third diphtheria, 73% for third pertussis, and 77% for measles. There were, however, disturbing differences between districts within regions where the range of uptake varied between 42% and 93% for measles, 46% and 87% for third pertussis, and 51% and 96% for third diphtheria.

In proposals for a national health strategy, the UK government (*Health of the Nation* 1991) included a target for 95% coverage for the childhood immunization schedule by 1995. The COVER data for 118 districts for February 1991 showed further improvements for the three sentinel antigens: diphtheria 92.1%, 88.4%, pertussis 86.0%, 82.4%, measles 90.3%, 86.3%.[25] The figures are percentages, the first being districts with low deprivation scores and the second being high deprivation districts. While coverage has continued to improve throughout the 1990s it remains lowest within deprived areas.

Reasons for poor performance within general practice

Several studies published in the late 1980s have shown that a low uptake of immunization is associated with the over-crowding and higher population density, which is particularly a feature of the UK's inner cities.[26] These factors were independent of the organization of primary care services in influencing immunization rates and make an important contribution to the difficulties experienced by primary health care teams in reaching targets in deprived areas. Recent studies have shown that despite the organizational changes consequent on the British health reforms of the 1990s the inverse care law still applies.[27] In Glasgow, in 1992, a disproportionate number of practices achieving higher coverage were in affluent areas whereas a higher than expected proportion of practices in the most deprived areas did not meet targets or achieved only the lower level.[28]

Poor organization

Many other factors do, however, contribute to low immunization rates. The organization of primary care in the UK leads to vaccination programmes being carried out by the community health services at child health clinics or schools and also by GPs in their own surgeries. This may lead to confusion if meticulous records and communication are not maintained. Ideally, each GP should achieve more satisfactory rates by efficient administration and immunization of the practice population. There is some evidence that the immunization uptake rate is better in general practices than child health clinics in inner city, suburban, and rural areas.[29]

Jarman *et al.* found that low uptake of immunization from the years 1983 to 1985 was associated with the practices of GPs who were elderly, single-handed, or with large list sizes. These doctors have often given a devoted service to ill patients but have not placed a priority on prevention and health promotion. In the absence of computerization and team work some have expressed hopelessness at their ability to meet the targets for vaccination for which payment will be made. These practices may then decide not to offer immunization at all and to ask their patients to be seen at the local district health authority (DHA) clinic. Lack of resources and unfilled health visitor posts in some districts compound the problem leading to inadequate provision for immunization within some DHA clinics which may themselves be situated in the same neighbourhood as ineffective general practices.

Inaccurate registers

Many practices who are committed to achieving an excellent coverage experience difficulties because of the inaccuracies of the DHA and former family health service authority (FHSA) and health board registers. Age–sex registers based on a computer download from the FHSA are usually 10% or more inaccurate and this figure can rise to 30% in inner city areas with a mobile population.[30] Although the situation is improving since the introduction of targets for immunization in the GP contract there is still room for improvement.[31]

A study of one Birmingham practice found the DHA register recorded that 40% of the children aged 2–3 years were completely immunized, the practice computer recorded 51%, and the practice notes 56%. When the information was combined the coverage was in fact 73%.[32] There is often poor exchange of information between the various groups immunizing in a locality who may even feel competitive towards each other. On the whole, computerized records held in general practice now give the most satisfactory results and the need to meet contract targets has improved the situation even more. Developments within the NHS child health system, which became fully interactive in the early 1990s should lead to a closer integration of district and practice registers which will in turn result in better coverage and the promotion of team work within a district.

False contraindications

Action Research for the Crippled Child (1989), commissioned a national study on factors influencing immunization uptake. Information was obtained from some 2000 health professionals and more than 3000 parents in 16 DHAs in England and Wales. There was an excellent response rate of almost 90%. An important finding was that the GPs knowledge of contraindications to vaccinations had a profound affect on vaccine uptake.[33]

When parents were questioned about why their children (a total of 400), had not been given immunization against measles, the most important reason stated was that the advice given by the doctor or health visitor had implied that the vaccination was contraindicated. Further inquiry revealed that in almost all instances the decision was based on inaccurate advice. The survey also highlighted the parents' misconception, described in other studies, that a potentially dangerous vaccine was being used to prevent a trivial illness.[34,35]

In common with many developed countries, improvements in vaccination coverage in the UK are hindered by fear of rare complications and a long list of contraindications, many of which are spurious. Despite statements issued by the Expanded Programme on Immunization and supported by statements within individual countries that minor upper respiratory illness are not a contraindication to immunization, the procedure is often postponed by apprehensive health care providers on these grounds. As the incidence of an infection decreases so the relative importance and attention given to possible serious consequences increases. Sensational reporting of adverse effects and the lack of a rapid unified response by the profession and the Department of Health, further undermine the confidence of parents and health workers alike. Worries about responsibility for damaging a healthy child by vaccination may be conveniently dealt with by adding to the few recognized contraindications and avoiding or postponing vaccination.[22]

Several studies in the 1980s demonstrated that there was a low commitment to vaccination on the part of health professionals. This stemmed from a poor understanding of the target diseases (in particular a view that measles and pertussis are not serious infections), fear of adverse effects, and a belief in mythical contraindications.[32] Such anxiety and low commitment easily communicates itself to the parents who are then glad to avoid immunization which they regard as a high-risk activity which health professionals would rather avoid. (Table 2.8 shows a good practice checklist for achieving immunization targets.)

Klein et al.,[36] in a study of 184 children admitted to hospital, reported that 106 were not completely immunized. In 91 of these children there was no recommended contraindication: two false contraindications (mild intercurrent infection and atopy) accounted for a third of the failures to immunize, and a further third were due to the failure of professionals to refute false beliefs held by parents.

Targets for childhood immunization: The general practitioner contract

Since 1990, the payment of GPs for carrying out childhood vaccinations has depended on meeting target levels of coverage rather than on an item for service basis. This approach recognizes the public health benefits of a coverage of more than 90% which is the level necessary to meet the WHO Regional target for the elimination of vaccine preventable diseases. Fewer than 1% of parents refuse consent for their child to be immunized and only 1% of children

Table 2.8 *Checklist for achieving immunization targets*

- Check practice records, identify all under-5-year-olds and remove any 'ghost records'
- Create and maintain manual or computerized age–sex register
- Close co-operation with health visitor (vaccination records, parent education, surgery displays, information packages)
- Full understanding of system of payment
- For 2-year-olds, target levels represent average cover levels across:
  - diphtheria, tetanus, and polio (3 doses)
  - pertussis (3 doses)
  - MMR (mumps/measles/rubella) (1 dose)
  - Hib (*H. influenzae* type b)
- From birth date prepare quarterly cohorts, which will constantly change and require continuous updating
- Discuss and devise call-up system
- Encounter vaccinations, memory triggers:
  (1) Encourage practice nurse to ask parents about children's status even if not attending with offspring
  (2) Make use of home postnatal visit to ensure child is registered and parents know date of first vaccination
  (3) At postnatal examination and/or 6-week developmental assessment give date for first and subsequent vaccinations
  (4) Contraception examinations provide an opportunity to enquire into child's vaccination status
  (5) 6–8-month child health surveillance identify defaulters
- Encourage patient participation groups
- 'User-friendly' staff and premises
- Prepare and constantly update practice children's immunization status
- Home visits to defaulters
- Do not place full reliance on Authority figures without checking

---

have valid contraindications to MMR (mumps/measles/rubella) vaccination. Approximately 3.5% have valid contraindications to pertussis vaccine. In the light of these figures it would appear that all general practitioners should be able to achieve an uptake of 90% or more for all childhood immunizations.

The target population is all the children on the general practitioner's list who become 2 or 5 years of age in the year preceding the claim. The proportion of payment made is based on the work carried out under general medical services. The GP is paid for immunizations carried out either in his/her own practice or a previous practice: the GP who completes the course of immunization will receive the financial benefit. Payment is not given for courses given by community clinics. Immunizations given by attached staff or employed staff under the direction of the GP as part of general medical services, will be treated as having been performed by the GP.

The following factors make it more difficult for a general practice to reach immunization targets:

(1) mobile populations;

(2) complicated methods of claims;

(3) poor team work within general practice;

(4) lack of incentive if particular circumstances dictate a 'no hope situation!';

(5) poor record-keeping (computer almost essential);

(6) socioeconomic distribution within the practice population;

(7) widely scattered population: branch surgeries;

(8) no practice nurse;

(10) negative attitude of parents;

(11) parents given poor and inadequate information.

Practices that do not meet immunization targets must consider which, if any, of the above factors are responsible for the situation. A positive attitude to team-working and maintaining good records can work wonders! (See Table 2.9 for *false* contraindications to immunization.)

Performance indicators

The advent of payment for childhood immunization, only if targets are reached and the requirement of practices to submit an annual report in which the performance is recorded, leads to the conclusion that comparative performance review in the health service will inevitably be applied to general practice. It will be important that the indicators of success be determined by the social context and the rate of improvement as well as by absolute coverage, lest excellent practices who fail to reach targets and hence receive income, lose enthusiasm or remove 'difficult' families from their lists.[37]

Needs of special groups

Ethnic minorities

Several studies have shown that the uptake of immunization among minority ethnic children born in the UK is higher than that for the local indigenous population.[38] This is not true, however, for the first-generation immigrants many of whom are severely disadvantaged in using the health service because of language and cultural barriers. These children are at particular risk of polio, diphtheria, and tuberculosis if they visit relatives abroad. Most minority ethnic communities have workers who can act as interpreters and health advocates and district health authorities take the ethnicity of the local

Table 2.9 *False contraindications to immunization*

- The child (or family member) has a past or present history of asthma, eczema, or hay fever
- Baby with nappy or heat rash
- Premature baby: immunization should not be postponed[69]
- Low birth weight baby
- History of neonatal jaundice
- Receiving antibiotics (if acute phase of illness is over)
- The baby is said to have had the illness (e.g. whooping cough or measles—the disease may have been wrongly diagnosed. It is safe to immunize
- Receiving low dose topical or inhaled steroids
- Chesty or snuffly baby who is apyrexial and not acutely ill
- Down's syndrome
- Mother is breast-feeding
- The child is over two years of age. (All missed immunizations, including pertussis and a single dose of Hib should be given)
- Interrupted course. It is not necessary to recommence the course. Continue as if no break has occurred. If the child is over 13 months start with MMR
- Mother is pregnant. Any immunization may be given to the child
- Child with stable neurological condition. If any doubt exists paediatrician or neurologist should be consulted

---

population into account when they appoint health professionals. Any GP working in such an area should if possible employ members of staff who are from local minority ethnic groups. All the health professionals engaged in vaccination should be aware of the attitudes of the local community to the procedure and the culturally determined differences that need to be recognized in order to ensure a good uptake. Members of the community might be asked to participate in staff training to foster good working relationships.

Parental refusal to have their children immunized

Any practice which looks after groups of people with religious beliefs which affect their uptake of immunization will need to make an effort to understand the basis of the parental or community view. Some parents use homeopathy for family health care and refuse immunization on the grounds that it compromises the immune system. There are no data to substantiate this view and the Faculty of Homeopathy recommends immunization of all children according to the present guidelines.[39] If it is not possible to modify attitudes then other methods of prevention of disease discussed in the previous section become particularly important.

Mobile patients, poverty, single parents

A vulnerable group of children are those who live in single parent families with a young unsupported mother who may be housed in bed and breakfast accommodation by the local authority. These children have a higher morbidity and mortality in the early years and are often not brought for immunization. It is important to form a good relationship with the mother during the antenatal period and for rigorous attention to be paid to follow-up in the first few weeks after the baby is born. Close co-operation with the health visitor, friendly reception staff, and a willingness to immunize at home, if necessary, will gain the mother's confidence. Opportunistic immunization of all the children in such a family will also improve coverage as these families often consult frequently in general practice.

Traveller gypsies

There are about 10 000 traveller gypsy caravans in the UK with an estimated minimum of three children in each family. This is a young population: 50% of travellers are under the age of 16. Although they are mainly located in Kent, East Anglia, Wales, the large Midland conurbation, Scotland, and London, they may present for care as temporary residents in any general practice.

Traveller gypsies place a high priority on child care, but poor living conditions, high mobility, and prejudice make access to high quality primary care a problem for many. Despite the fact that it contravenes the race relations act to discriminate against gypsies, a recent survey of GPs in East London[40] found that 10% of practices would not accept traveller gypsies as patients under any circumstances. In addition, immunization target levels pose a dilemma for the GP who may fail to reach target levels and hence lose considerable income if traveller families are registered with the practice and do not bring their children for immunization. Many travellers are opposed to any childhood vaccination programme and some GPs therefore will not accept them as registered patients and treat them as temporary residents in order that immunization target levels are attained or maintained. As a result of these factors there is a higher child morbidity and lower immunization rate amongst gypsy children. The few studies that have been reported show an uptake of about 20% for diphtheria and polio, and 10% for pertussis and measles. The community has shown itself receptive to sensitive initiatives to improve immunization rates, especially in the wake of illness such as polio in unimmunized children.[38] Any doctor or nurse seeing traveller women or children for any reason should enquire about the immunization status of the children of the family and offer immunization during that consultation if it is indicated. Those practices within areas with a large traveller community should make themselves aware of any local initiatives for offering primary care and participate in it. Difficulties in reaching targets while caring for travellers should be discussed informally with the local DHA who will usually show understanding

Table 2.10 *Schedule of immunization for children in the UK[a]*

Vaccine	Age	Comments
DPT, polio, and Hib[b]	2 months (1st dose) 3 months (2nd dose) 4 months (3rd dose)	Primary course
MMR	12–15 months	Can be given at any age over 12 months
Booster DPT and polio, MMR	3–5 years	If not given earlier
BCG	10–14 years, or infancy	Interval of 3 weeks between BCG and rubella
Booster tetanus and polio Diphtheria toxoid[c]	15–18 years	

[a] UK Department of Health immunization schedules.
[b] Since 1 October 1992 Hib vaccine has been offered at the same time as diphtheria, pertussis and tetanus vaccine at 2, 3, and 4 months. Children over 2 months and under 13 months should be given three doses, each 1 month apart. Children 13 months to 4 years should be given a single dose. No booster is recommended. Hib vaccine should be given in a different limb from other concurrently administered vaccine. Parents should be informed that Hib vaccine does *not* protect against any other forms of meningitis.
[c] The low dose diphtheria and tetanus boosters for school-leavers are available as a single injection (Td) and is to be preferred (*CMO's Update*. May 1994).

towards practices who are committed to offering excellent care to this marginalized group.

Schedule of immunization for children in the UK

The schedule of immunization recommended for British children is shown in Table 2.10. Ramsay *et al.* (1992)[41] have reported a decreased incidence of symptoms from this accelerated schedule than from the prolonged programme it replaced. In the section which follows the individual vaccines are discussed both in relation to their use in children but also, where relevant, in relation to their use in adult programmes. (*Information which will rapidly become outdated is not included, and the reader is referred to the latest government recommendations before administering any of the vaccines described below.*)

Professional advice against immunization

It is important to emphasize that no child should be refused immunization without discussion with the local immunization co-ordinator.[42] If a child is not immunized on the basis of poor professional advice and the child subsequently becomes ill then the parents might well have grounds for a complaint.

Notes on individual vaccines

Diphtheria

Although diphtheria is a very rare condition in the UK, cases still occur.[43] In 1940, before the introduction of diphtheria vaccine, there were over 46 000 cases with almost 2500 notified deaths. In order to sustain individual and herd immunity, immunization levels must be kept above 95%. Waning immunity in the population appears to be a major factor in the epidemic of diphtheria in Russia in which, by 1993, nearly 16 000 cases had been reported.[44]

Diphtheria vaccine is prepared from inactivated toxin adsorbed into a mineral carrier. This is usually combined with tetanus and pertussis vaccine (triple) but is also available either on its own or with tetanus only. In some high-risk individuals, it may be necessary to give a special low dose monovalent preparation that should be used for children beyond 10 years or for adults. The actual duration of immunity following a full course of diphtheria immunization is unknown. An accelerated immunization schedule for the DPT and oral polio vaccines aims for completion of protection by 4 months of age and is now recommended by the Joint Committee on Vaccination and Immunisation (JCVI).

Contraindications. If a child has an acute febrile illness then vaccination is best postponed until recovery.

Reactions. These are unusual and mild, generally involving localized reddening only.

Tetanus

Tetanus vaccine is an inactivated vaccine. It is administered by intramuscular (IM) or deep subcutaneous (SC) injection. The primary course is given at 2, 3, and 4 months. A booster is given at 4–5 years and at 15–18 years followed by booster doses every 10 years.

Contraindications. Vaccination should be delayed in acute febrile illness but not if necessitated by a deep, dirty, or penetrating wound. Thorough and careful surgical toilet of any wound is vital regardless of the tetanus immunization history of the patient.

The following are tetanus-prone wounds:

1. Six-hour interval between wound or burn and treatment.

2. Any wound or burn regardless of time since the injury that shows:

   • substantial devitalized tissue

- puncture wound
- contaminated with soil or manure
- presence of infection

If the wound is clean and the patient has had a full course or last reinforcing dose within the last 10 years no further immunization is indicated. Patients who have never been immunized should commence the full three-dose course, and those who have had their last reinforcing dose more than 10 years ago should receive a reinforcing dose of adsorbed vaccine.

Patients with tetanus-prone wounds are protected if they have had a full course with appropriate reinforcing doses. Individuals who are not immunized or who are out of date should receive a dose of human tetanus immunoglobulin in addition to active immunization.

Adverse reactions. Mild local reactions are common, especially in older children or adults. General reactions are extremely rare. Occasionally, a nodule will develop at the site of injection and may persist for some time.

Pertussis

Before 1975, when the acceptance of pertussis vaccination was greater than 75%, the national notification rate during the peak of any epidemic was very low, at less than 500 reported cases per week. By 1978, following the publicity concerning possible neurological effects of vaccination, the vaccination rate fell to about 30%. During the epidemic of 1978 between 2000 and 3000 cases were reported per week. Only 3 out of every 10 children born in 1976 had been immunized against pertussis two years later. Two major epidemics of whooping cough occurred in UK in during 1977–9 and in 1982. In the first, 100 000 cases were reported with 36 deaths and in the second, 66 000 cases with 14 deaths. Throughout the 1980s there has been an increase in the incidence of pertussis in the USA, particularly among adolescents and adults. This has been attributed to waning immunity and while the adult illness is less severe, these individuals can represent a source of infection for infants in the first weeks of life who may have a life-threatening infection.[45]

The vaccine is a suspension of killed *Bordetella* organisms, either combined with diphtheria and tetanus (triple vaccine) or as a monovalent vaccine. The primary course comprises three doses by IM or deep SC injection and is given at two, three, and four months; contraindications are shown in Table 2.11.[46]

Adverse reactions. Swelling and redness at the injection site may be accompanied by the persistence of a small firm nodule. There may be a constitutional upset involving pyrexia, and crying. Also, pallor, cyanosis, limpness, and convulsions have been reported after both adsorbed DPT and DT vaccinations. More severe reactions involving encephalopathy and prolonged convulsions resulting in brain damage or death have been reported.

Table 2.11 *Pertussis immunization: contraindications*

- Presently suffering from any acute illness
- History of severe reaction to a preceding dose
- An extensive indurated area of redness and swelling after preceding dose
- Problem histories. Where any doubt exists advice should be sought from a consultant paediatrician, district immunization co-ordinator or specialist in public health medicine. *No child should be refused immunisation without a specialist opinion*

Doubt may exist in situation such as:
- Children with a definite history of neonatal cerebral damage
- Personal history of convulsions with a convulsion occurring after the first dose
- Parents or siblings have a history of idiopathic epilepsy. The advice is that these children should be immunized

A connection between pertussis vaccination and possible brain damage has been suggested, although with a very low frequency (i.e. in the order of 1 case per 310 000 injections). This is equivalent to once in every 1500 GP or health visitor working years. The National Childhood Encephalopathy Study (NCES) in Great Britain reviewed 1182 children with serious acute neurological illnesses. Only 39 of these children had recently had pertussis vaccination and the association could have occurred by chance. The result of the study of cases in the NCES even after three years of very intensive study and research was too small to confirm conclusively whether or not the vaccine can cause cause permanent brain damage. These results and the methodology adopted have been intensively reviewed; a 10-year follow-up study, which sought to address some of the methodological problems, concluded that the balance of possible risk against known benefits supports continued use of the vaccine.[47]

Haemophilus influenzae type b (Hib)

Haemophilus influenzae is commonly present in the nasopharynx and is a cause of exacerbations of chronic bronchitis in adults and of otitis media. However, some strains have a polysaccharide capsule which renders them much more virulent. Strains with the Pittman type b capsule cause almost all of the invasive disease seen in the UK, which is primarily an infection of early childhood. *Haemophilus influenzae* type b (Hib) is responsible for a variety of serious invasive infections in children including meningitis, epiglottitis, septic arthritis, and pneumonia. In a study of patients treated in hospital in Wales, Howard *et al.* (1991)[48] reported the incidence of invasive Hib disease to be 34.6/100 000 with most patients aged under 5 years and with the highest incidence in children aged under 1 year. The principal diagnosis in over half the episodes of invasive disease was meningitis (58%). Epiglottitis (16%), pneumonia (8%), and bone and joint infections (5%) were less common manifestations. The cumulative risk for Welsh children to acquire the disease before their fifth birthday was 1 in 578. The mortality in British children is about 3–5% with nearly 10% of survivors developing neurological damage, principally deafness.[49] Conjugated *H. influenzae* vaccines were made available for general use in the UK following extensive experience in Finland, Canada, and the USA. The vaccine confers a high degree of protection and is safe, with side-effects limited to a local reaction or mild fever. The vaccines are immunogenic when given to infants at 2, 3, and 4 months and are conveniently given at the same time as the DPT vaccine. This programme, introduced in October 1992, was in addition to a catch-up programme for children up to the age of 4 years. A prospective study of bacterial meningitis carried out for three years (1991–3) during the introduction of the vaccine showed that the number of cases of *H. influenzae* meningitis in one region to have fallen by 87%.[50] Other studies have confirmed the success of the programme in reducing Hib invasive disease as successfully as programmes in the USA and Northern Europe.[51]

Poliomyelitis

Between the years 1985 and 1991, there were 21 confirmed cases of poliomyelitis in England and Wales: 13 cases were vaccine-associated (9 recipient, 4 contact), 5 were imported, and 3 were from an unknown source of infection.[52] Two polio vaccines are available:

(1) OPV: live oral vaccine (Sabin vaccine), and

(2) IPV: IM or SC injection of inactivated vaccine (Salk vaccine). In the UK, inactivated polio vaccine is used only for immunodeficient individuals and is also recommended for family contacts of such children.

OPV is a live attenuated vaccine which is administered by the oral route. Polio vaccination is normally given at 2, 3, and 4 months. A booster at is given at school entry (age 4–5 years) and again at 15–18 years of age.

Contraindications. The immunization should be postponed during an acute febrile illness particularly in a child with diarrhoea and vomiting.

Caution should be exercised in pregnancy with OPV, although there is no documented evidence that fetal damage has ever been caused. If the reasons for vaccination in pregnancy are compelling, then IPV or OPV should be given after the fourth month of pregnancy. If vaccination in early pregnancy is essential then the use of IPV is advised.

Both OPV and IPV may contain trace amounts of penicillin and strep-tomycin but these do not rule out their use except in the case of extreme hypersensitivity. Both vaccines contain neomycin in small amounts and OPV may contain polymyxin.

Adverse reactions. Very occasionally (approximately once in every 1–5 million doses), OPV will revert to its wild form in the vaccine and cause poliomyelitis in the child or a close contact. Contacts of a recently immunized baby should be advised of the need for strict personal hygiene, in particular, they should wash their hands after changing the baby's nappy. Joce[52] gave the risk of vaccine-associated paralysis as 1.46/million for the first dose, and 0.49/million for the second dose.

Unimmunized relatives should be offered a course of three doses of OPV at intervals of four weeks to coincide with the vaccination schedule of the infant. The risk is probably doubled in those over 50 years of age. For such people, and for those who are immunosuppressed or pregnant, IPV (Salk) polio vaccine is recommended. Booster doses are necessary every 10 years for travellers in endemic areas.

Polio immunization before foreign travel. This is easily forgotten when preparing a programme for the traveller but there is a serious risk of the infection in many countries. No adult should remain unvaccinated against this disease and where a live vaccine is contraindicated, the inactivated vaccine (IPV) should be used. The usual vaccine used is the live attenuated Sabin vaccine (OPV). Travellers infected with the HIV virus may receive OPV but if they are symptomatic IPV may be preferred.

The primary course for an adult is three oral doses of OPV at intervals of four weeks. If the individual is exposed to increased risk of infection then a booster dose should be given after 10 years. Booster doses are of importance to the traveller.

Oral polio vaccine and oral typhoid vaccine must not be given together and should be separated by at least two weeks.

Measles/mumps/rubella (MMR)

This vaccine was introduced in October 1988 with the aim of eliminating mumps, measles and rubella (and the congenital rubella syndrome) from Britain. The aim in relation to rubella is to achieve herd immunity rather than relying on promoting immunity in pregnant women. To achieve such a target, the vaccine uptake in children aged 1–2 years must be at least 90%, since there, is of course, a group of children who have not been immunized at the age of 2 years. Although most of these children will have been immunized during the UK national measles and rubella immunization campaign of November 1994, there will remain some susceptible individuals particularly in practices with a highly mobile population and a high proportion of recent immigrants. The campaign was successful in reducing the susceptibility of schoolchildren to measles from 10% to 3%, and to rubella from 20% to 6% in boys and from 11% to 2% in girls.[53]

Schoolgirl vaccination had fortunately reduced the proportion of pregnant women who are susceptible to rubella from approximately 10% before 1971 to 1.7% in 1989. By 1989, about 20 cases of congenital rubella syndrome were diagnosed each year. The infection rate in non-immune parous women is some three times greater than in nulliparous women.[54] The obvious reason for this is that parous women catch rubella from their children and so it was vital that this situation was remedied. There is no particular risk associated with 'double immunization' and the freeze-dried vaccine contains three attenuated live viruses. MMR is offered to children of both sexes in the second year of life.

The vaccine, live attenuated measles, mumps, and rubella, may be given to children of any age (over 12 months) and non-immune adults. It is usually given at age 12–18 months or at school entry.

Contraindications

1. acute febrile illness;
2. children with immunodeficient conditions (except HIV-positive children);
3. untreated malignant disease;
4. documented history of anaphylaxis following exposure to chicken or egg products;
5. history of sensitivity to neomycin or kanamycin;
6. another live vaccine injection during the previous 3 weeks;
7. pregnancy.

Children with a personal or close (first degree relative) family history of convulsions must be immunized as they are at high risk of convulsion should they catch measles. In the past it has been customary to recommend that these children should be given a simultaneous dose of human normal immunoglobulin but there is no evidence that this is necessary and indeed it may limit the effectiveness of the mumps and rubella components of the vaccine.

The risk of serious neurological reactions to measles vaccine is probably about 1/100 000 doses.

Adverse reactions

1. modified, uncommunicable measles, mumps, and rubella;
2. febrile convulsions;
3. pyrexia, either soon after immunization or within 5–10 days;
4. malaise, coryza, headache, parotid swelling, pruritus;
5. thrombocytopenic purpura (rare).

BCG (bacillus Calmette–Guérin)

The vaccine is a freeze-dried preparation of the Calmette–Guérin bacillus. Vaccination of children with BCG began in the early 1950s. The vaccine is over 70% effective and protection lasts for at least 15 years. Different health districts have different vaccination policies for tuberculosis. Most health districts continue to offer routine vaccination to all children aged 10–14 years who have been shown to be tuberculin-negative as a result of a Heaf or Mantoux test. However, health districts such as Oxfordshire, have discontinued routine vaccination of schoolchildren and vaccination is offered on a selective basis. In contrast, in London the City and Hackney health districts recommend immunization for all neonates, as the local prevalence of tuberculosis is among the highest in the country. The target is for 95% of secondary schoolchildren to be tuberculin-positive or given BCG. With the incidence of tuberculosis declining, schoolchildren are generally at decreasing risk. The incidence among Asian and African families, while decreasing, remains at a higher level than for the rest of the population. Most health districts selectively vaccinate new-born babies of families with a history of or at high risk of tuberculosis. Some minority ethnic groups object to racial origins being the basis for neonatal BCG vaccination and hence some health authorities prefer to offer the immunization to socially deprived families or to all neonates. Of 199 health districts in England and Wales, 15 have stopped their schools' programme and 31 have no policy for the immunization of neonates,[55] despite the fact that in eight of these districts over 3% of the population were of South Asian origin. It is important that each practice discusses with the local immunization co-ordinator the rationale for local policy and ensures, in the absence of clear guidelines, that children at risk are offered immunization.

The Mantoux and Heaf tests. *Mantoux test.* This involves the intradermal injection of a 1:1000 dilution protein purified derivative (PPD). The injecting dose is 0.1 ml. The Mantoux test is read between 72 and 96 hours after inoculation and a positive result is indicated by an indurated hard area of 6 mm or more in diameter.

Heaf test. This uses the Heaf 'gun' to produce a circle of six small punctures after tuberculin PPD solution has been applied to a small area of skin surface, usually in the inner forearm. Positive reactions in unimmunized individuals are those of grade 2 and above and in common with a positive Mantoux test indicate current or previous infection. A grade 3 or 4 reaction should be taken to indicate infection irrespective of previous BCG vaccination. As the true prevalence of tuberculosis amongst UK schoolchildren is very low, there will be a substantial number of false positive results and this should be borne in mind when the result is discussed with the parents. However, these individuals and their families and close contacts should be considered for investigation for tuberculosis and the result must be discussed with the community paediatrician or local director of public health. The Heaf gun must be disinfected before and after each testing session. Disposable head-apparatus is available and avoids the need to disinfect.

BCG administration route. The dose of BCG vaccine is 0.1 ml injected

Table 2.12 *BCG vaccination: contraindications and areas for caution*

- Acute febrile illness
- Tuberculin-positive individuals
- Those with Heaf grade I reactions, unless previously vaccinated, to be regarded as tuberculin-negative and, in the absence of contraindications, offered vaccination
- Preferable to avoid BCG vaccination in pregnancy, particularly in the early stages
- An interval of at least 3 weeks should be allowed before the administration of BCG and any other live vaccine, whichever is given first. No further immunization should be given for at least 3 months in the arm that has been used for BCG vaccination on account of the risk of regional lymphadenitis
- Generalized severe skin sepsis
- Immunodeficiency
- HIV infection, whether symptomatic or asymptomatic. This also applies to the new-born and young babies of HIV-positive mothers where the diagnosis of HIV infection in the infant is uncertain

---

intradermally (reduced to 0.05 ml intradermally for infants under 3 months of age). Injection must *not* be given subcutaneously. The site of inoculation should be at the insertion of the deltoid muscle as sites higher up may lead to keloid formation. The tip of the shoulder should be avoided and, for cosmetic reasons in girls, the upper and lateral surface of the thigh may be used. The injection must be intradermal whichever site is chosen.

The age of the vaccinee is variable (e.g. neonate or age 10–14 years if tuberculin-negative). Close contacts of infected individuals may be vaccinated at any age if they are tuberculin-negative. Tuberculin-negative travellers to endemic areas should be immunized at any age. It is interesting to note that BCG vaccination has consistently been shown to protect against leprosy. In fact some investigators have reported that it gives better protection against *Mycobacterium leprae* than against tuberculosis.[56] Table 2.12 shows contraindications and areas for caution.

A local reaction usually develops in children and adults some 2–6 weeks after immunization. The reaction is normal and takes the form of a papule which subsequently discharges, requiring no treatment. The lesion heals leaving a small scar.

Advice to parents. They should be informed that some 2–6 weeks following BCG vaccination a small papule will develop and will increase in size to about 7 mm diameter. The area may scale or crust and on occasion a shallow ulcer may appear. Bathing should not be prevented and occlusion should be avoided. If there is much weeping then a temporary dry dressing should be applied but removed as soon as possible. Impervious dressings delay healing and may contribute to a larger scar. They should only be allowed for very short periods (e.g. when swimming).

Adverse reactions. Deep, prolonged ulceration, sometimes associated with local lympadenopathy, may be the result of faulty injection technique. The vaccine has usually been given by subcutaneous rather than intradermal route in these cases. These children should be referred to the community paediatrician.

BCG vaccination of high-risk groups.[57] Health service staff, including medical students, locum doctors, agency staff, and contract ancillary workers should be Heaf-tested and vaccinated if necessary before working in areas of high patient risk. This protects both staff and patients; it is very unusual for hospital staff to acquire tuberculous disease from patients if they have had adequate protection before commencing employment. These recommendations also apply to staff in private hospitals, prisons, and old peoples' homes.

General practices who look after patients who have arrived from areas abroad where there is a high incidence of tuberculosis (especially South Asia and Vietnam) should ensure that the whole family has had the opportunity to be screened and that the health visitor has arranged follow-up.

Immunization of adults

Many adults are immunized as a result of foreign travel (see Chapter 15) but some immunizations are recommended for at-risk groups remaining in the UK. All adults should keep their tetanus immunization up to date and those in high-risk situations should receive hepatitis-B vaccine. These groups include health service workers likely to be exposed to blood products and clinical waste, public service workers, such as the police, fire-fighters, and refuse collectors, and all those whose lifestyle increases the risk of contracting the infection.

Rubella

Effective immunization of children should prevent women developing rubella in pregnancy. There is at present a cohort of susceptible young men who can transmit the infection and an increase in infection in this group in 1993 was accompanied by an increase in infections in pregnancy to 22 compared with only 2 cases in 1992. While we await the effects of immunization campaigns for all schoolchildren to work through, all women, irrespective of a history of immunization, should have their rubella status checked when they attend for contraceptive advice or for preconception counselling. Susceptible women should be offered immunization with advice to absolutely avoid pregnancy for a month afterwards. However, studies in the UK, Europe, and the USA have never identified any cases of congenital rubella syndrome due

Table 2.13 *Schedule for hepatitis B vaccination*

Standard schedule
- Two doses, one month apart, followed by a booster at 6 months

Accelerated schedule
- Three doses, at one month intervals, followed by a booster at 12 months

Doses
- Different preparations recommend different doses. See manufacturers' data sheets

Contraindications
- Acute or serious infection

---

to vaccination, in the first four weeks of pregnancy. Any woman who is discovered to be susceptible during pregnancy should be immunized once the child has been born.

Hepatitis B

The recombinant vaccines have been shown to be safe and efficient. Two doses one month apart, with the third at six months, have approximate conversion rates of around 95% (see Table 2.13). For intending travellers, vaccination is particularly of value for those intending to live abroad on an extended stay and is not usually necessary for short trips abroad unless to high-risk areas. The vaccine should not be given to individuals known to be hepatitis B surface antigen-positive or to patients with acute hepatitis. Hepatitis B vaccine may be given to HIV-positive individuals. Antibody screening prior to vaccination should be considered as vaccination may be unnecessary. Antibody titres should also be determined 2–4 months after immunization and non responders given a booster dose.

Immunization of infants born to women infected with hepatitis B. Babies born to mothers who are positive for hepatitis B e antigen have an 80% risk of perinatal infection with a 40% risk of cirrhosis or hepatocellular carcinoma later in life. It is recommended that these infants be vaccinated at birth.[58] This situation is particularly likely among women who have recently arrived in the UK and it is important that they should be screened for hepatitis B so that immunization can be organised.

Immunization of the elderly

Susceptibility to infection is greatest at the extremes of life and the regular contact that the practice team now has with every person over 75 provides an opportunity for appropriate immunizations to be given.

Tetanus

Deaths from tetanus have been reported amongst elderly gardeners and older people who risk tetanus-prone wounds should be up to date with their tetanus immunization.

Influenza

In the winter of 1989–90 there were 26 000 deaths in England and Wales, which were directly or indirectly attributed to the influenza A epidemic. Although epidemics are sporadic and not easily predicted, a substantial number of infections with influenza A (and/or B) occur every year. The risk factors for dying from influenza are age and chronic disease and over 80% of the excess deaths are in people aged 65 or over.[59] The vaccine is modified each year to ensure that it contains the strains most likely to be effective given the capacity of the influenza virus to vary antigenically from year to year. Older people (over 65) with the following conditions should be offered immunization:

- chronic pulmonary disease

- chronic heart disease

- chronic renal failure

- diabetes mellitus

- endocrine disorders associated with adrenal suppression

If, in addition, the practice looks after elderly patients (over 75) living in residential or long-stay accommodation, arrangements should be made to immunize them. The practice plans for the programme should be discussed ready to begin in September, remembering that a substantial income may result from a well-planned initiative. Susceptible patients should be identified using the age–sex register, disease index, or repeat prescription system. As always, a computer simplifies the administration of the programme. It is particularly important that debilitated and housebound patients are immunized as they are at a greatest risk. Immunization of these patients may conveniently be combined with home visits for other purposes by the doctors or nurses, providing there is a system in place which reminds them to take the vaccine with them. The composition of the inactivated influenza vaccine and recommendations for its use are issued annually in time for immunization programmes to be carried out.

When discussing the immunization with the patient it is helpful to inform them that well-designed studies have shown that only local side-effects result and that all side-effects are mild and transitory.[60]

Chemoprophylaxis against influenza A. Prophylactic administration of amantadine 100 mg per day is as effective as a vaccination against influenza A and may be started at the same time as the vaccination, to provide protection for the high-risk over-65s while the immunity develops.[61] The drug causes minor neurological side-effects in some patients and is contra-indicated in gastric ulceration and epilepsy. It should be used with caution in the presence of renal impairment where it can accumulate to toxic levels. Despite these side-effects and the emergence of resistant strains it is a useful adjunct to immunization, especially if an epidemic strain of influenza A is very different from those contained within the current vaccine.

Pneumococcal pneumonia

This affects about 1 per 1000 adults every year, although it is more common in the elderly. The vaccine available in the UK can induce immunity to 90% of the types of *Streptococcus pneumoniae* that cause systemic infections in the UK. The GP may consider administering the vaccine to elderly patients with chronic heart, lung, or liver disease or with diabetes mellitus. Patients who have had splenectomy or have sickle-cell disease should also be offered the vaccine as there are still unnecessary deaths reported from the failure to implement this policy.[62]

The vaccine comprises 25 μg of the purified polysaccharide from each of 23 serotypes of *Strep. pneumoniae*. It is given as a single dose, 0.5 ml by subcutaneous or intramuscular injection. Local pain and redness may occur and rarely fever and myalgia. Good immunity in the elderly lasts for at least five years: revaccination may lead to a severe local reaction and is not recommended routinely.[63]

Staying up to date

This section on immunization is up to date (Spring 1997). It is, however, essential that the reader also refers to the current editions of *Immunisation against infectious diseases* and *Health information for overseas travel*, both published by HMSO. The Chief Medical Officer also issues current guidance from time to time.

Antimicrobial chemoprophylaxis

The use of antimicrobial agents to prevent microbial diseases (chemo-prophylaxis) would seem an attractive means of preventing infection, par-ticularly when vaccination and other control measures cannot be applied. However, it is not always successful and is associated with several disad-vantages the most obvious of which are the financial implications and the risks of adverse reactions to the antibiotics used. Less obvious, but perhaps of greater hazard, is the selection of antibiotic-resistant pathogens both in the individual patient and the environment. Before embarking on prophylaxis, therefore, it is important to weigh up the advantages and disadvantages.

Chemoprophylaxis may be used to prevent infection arising either from out-side the body (exogenous) or from the patient's own body flora (endogenous).

Table 2.14 *Chemoprophylaxis*

Infection	Antimicrobial and dose
Malaria	See Chapter 15
Rheumatic fever	Phenoxymethylpenicillin 250 mg twice daily or sulphadiazine 1 g daily (500 mg for children)
Influenza A	Amantadine 100 mg daily
Pertussis	Erythromycin 125 mg qds for children up to age of 2 years
Meningococcal infection	Rifampicin 600 mg (10 mg/kg for child over 1 year; 5 mg/kg for infant) given twice daily for 2 days or ciprofloxacin, 500 mg as a single dose for adults (not licensed for this indication)
Haemophilus influenzae	Rifampicin 600 mg (20 mg/kg for children over 3 months) daily for 4 days
Diphtheria	Erythromycin 500 mg qds for 5 days
Urinary tract infections	See Chapter 10
Tuberculosis	Isoniazid 5 mg/kg (up to 1300 mg) daily
Pneumocystis carinii pneumonia	Co-trimoxazole 960 mg twice daily on 3 days each week or inhaled pentamidine monthly
Endocarditis	See Table 2.15

Most chemoprophylaxis used outside hospitals (Table 2.14) is directed at infection originating from exogenous sources—usually another human.

Malaria

Chemoprophylaxis for malaria is recommended for travellers to most parts of the subtropics and tropics. It is hampered by major problems of parasite resistance and drug toxicity.

Rheumatic fever

Chemoprophylaxis to prevent recurrences of rheumatic fever secondary to infections caused by *Strep. pyogenes* is a good example of 'ideal' chemoprophylaxis in that it is used to prevent infection with a single known organism with predictable susceptibility to a narrow spectrum antibiotic. Monthly injections of benzathine penicillin were used previously but this drug is no longer available in the UK and oral phenoxymethylpenicillin or sulphadiazine (for penicillin-allergic patients) are now recommended.

In children, chemoprophylaxis should be given for at least five years or until the child leaves school, whichever is the longer period. It may also be given to adults at increased risk of second attacks of rheumatic fever (hospital staff, young military recruits, or schoolteachers). How long prophylaxis should be continued in adults is, however, unknown.

Influenza

Amantadine may be given as chemoprophylaxis against influenza A strains. It is not effective against other strains of influenza virus or other viruses and is therefore only useful when there is a proven epidemic of influenza A in the community. It may be used after the recognition of an outbreak as an adjunct to vaccination, to protect during the interval before the vaccine-induced immunity develops in elderly or high-risk patients or in hospital staff and those with critical community roles.

Pertussis

Chemoprophylaxis with erythromycin can be used for non-immune children, especially babies, who have been in contact with pertussis and is sometimes effective in controlling pertussis outbreaks in closed communities.

Meningococcal meningitis

Chemoprophylaxis is indicated for two groups of contacts of patients with meningococcal septicaemia or meningococcal meningitis. The first group is preschool age and household contacts, including those sharing sleeping quarters in residential schools or military camps; and the second is individuals who have performed mouth-to-mouth resuscitation on a patient suffering from meningococcal disease.

Penicillin is inadequate for prophylaxis and rifampicin is recommended. Ciprofloxacin as a single dose of 500 mg or 750 mg seems a promising option in adults.

Haemophilus influenzae meningitis

The risk to child contacts of patients with invasive *H. influenzae* infections is of a similar order to that of contacts of meningococcal disease. Chemoprophylaxis with rifampicin is recommended for all household and daycare-centre contacts when children under the age of 5 years are exposed.

Diphtheria

Non-immune contacts of patients suffering from diphtheria should be offered chemoprophylaxis with erythromycin for 5 days.

Urinary tract infections

Chemoprophylaxis may be used in urinary tract infection (UTI) for one of two reasons: (1) either to prevent symptomatic recurrences in women with frequent or postcoital attacks of UTI; or (2) to prevent renal scarring in children with vesico-ureteric reflux and recurrent UTI (see Chapter 9). A low dose of trimethoprim or nitrofurantoin (50–100 mg nightly after emptying the bladder) is usually sufficient by eliminating uropathogens from the bowel and periurethral area.

Tuberculosis

In the UK, chemoprophylaxis against tuberculosis is reserved for infected contacts without clinical or radiological evidence of disease. In particular, childhood contacts of patients with open pulmonary tuberculosis who have positive tuberculin tests but normal radiographs, and for immunosuppressed patients with clinical or radiological evidence of previous tuberculosis. Isoniazid alone is usually given for 12 months.

Pneumocystis carinii pneumonia

This infection occurs in patients with abnormal cellular immunity, notable those with advanced HIV infection and children suffering from acute lymphocytic leukaemia. It is almost always a reactivation of latent infection and can be prevented in susceptible individuals by the long-term administration of co-trimoxazole. It is usually started in HIV-positive individuals once their CD4 (helper T cells) count has fallen below $250 \times 10^9/l$. In those who are allergic to co-trimoxazole, monthly inhalation of nebulized pentamidine is an acceptable alternative.

Bacterial endocarditis

Antibacterial prophylaxis is recommended when a procedure likely to be accompanied by a transient bacteraemia is performed in a patient known to be at risk of bacterial endocarditis, even though the efficacy of such chemoprophylaxis has never been determined. Those at risk include individuals with rheumatic or degenerative heart disease, ventricular septal defects, patent ductus, mitral valve prolapse (only when associated with a systolic murmur), bicuspid aortic valves, and those with prosthetic heart valves. The procedures that are considered likely to be associated with particular risk of bacteraemia are:

- Many dental procedures (particularly extraction, scaling and periodontal surgery)
- Genitourinary instrumentation;
- Gastrointestinal instrumentation (for those with prosthetic valves only)
- Tonsillectomy/adenoidectomy or instrumentation of the upper respiratory tract,
- Obstetric and gynaecological procedures (including intrauterine contraceptive device, IUCD, insertion) in those with prosthetic valves only.

Antibiotics should be started before the procedure in order that adequate blood concentrations are present at the time of bacteraemia; starting earlier merely leads to the rapid emergence of resistant strains within the mouth flora. The recommendations of the British Society of Antimicrobial Chemotherapy (BSAC)[64,65] have been widely adopted within the United Kingdom[66] (see also Table 2.15).

Table 2.15 *Infective endocarditis: antibiotic prophylaxis*

Dental procedures under local or no anaesthesia

1. Patients not allergic to penicillin and not given penicillin more than once in previous month:

   Amoxycillin 3 g single oral dose 1 hour before procedure (1.5 g for children 5–10 years old)

2. Patients who are penicillin-allergic or have received more than a single dose of penicillin in previous month:

   Clindamycin 600 mg single oral dose 1 hour before procedure (300 mg for children 5–10 years old)

The following patients should be referred to hospital:

1. Patients with prosthetic valves who require obstetric and gynaecological procedures (including insertion of IUCD).

2. Patients with prosthetic valves who require a general anaesthetic for dental procedures.

3. Patients who require a general anaesthetic and who are allergic to penicillin or who have had a penicillin more than once in the previous month.

4. Patients who have had a previous attack of endocarditis

Prosthetic joints

There is insufficient scientific evidence to support routine antibiotic chemo-prophylaxis for patients with prosthetic joints who are undergoing dental procedures and the working party of the BSAC has concluded that exposing such patients to the risk of severe reactions to antibiotics is unacceptable.[67]

Patients with absent or dysfunctional spleens[68]

Splenic macrophages play an important role in phagocytosis of bacteria and patients without spleens or with splenic dysfunction are at lifelong risk of fulminant infection. In addition to an immunization programme, including pneumococcal, Hib and influenza with meningococcal A and C vaccine for those who intend to travel, lifelong prophylactic antibiotics are recommended and should be offered to all patients. This will not be realistic in many instances, although this strategy has been used with success for patients with sickle-cell disease for many years. Phenoxymethylpenicillin or amoxycillin (with erythromycin as an alternative for those allergic to penicillin) are suitable choices. In any case, patients should be informed of the risk and keep antibiotics at home to start immediately if symptoms of infection such as temperature, aching, and shivering should develop. They should be instructed to seek immediate medical attention in these circumstances.

An exercise for the GP registrar

Carry out a survey in the practice or in the practices of the training scheme to answer the following questions.

- *Are patients with absent or dysfunctional spleens identifiable in the practices?*
- *Are these patients aware of their risk of overwhelming infection and do they inform health professionals when seen?*
- *Have these patients been immunised appropriately?*
- *Are these patients on antibiotic prophylaxis or do they have antibiotics at home for immediate use if necessary?*
- *Are all of the health professionals in the practice aware of the health risks when these patients travel?*
- *What is the practice policy agreed with the patient for the management of clinically apparent infection?*

After the survey is complete, carry out an audit with criteria based on the recommendations of a national working party.[68]

APPENDIX 1

Notifiable diseases

The Health Service and Public Health Act of 1968 requires that a doctor must notify the local medical officer for environmental health (now the Consultant, Communicable Disease Control—CCDC) of a patient with any one of the infectious diseases listed below. A fee is payable.

Anthrax	Meningococcal septicaemia
Cholera	Ophthalmia neonatorum
Diphtheria	Paratyphoid fever A or B
Dysentery (amoebic or bacillary)	Plague
	Polio
Encephalitis	Rabies
Food poisoning (actual or suspected)	Relapsing fever
	Scarlet fever
Infective jaundice	Tetanus
Lassa fever	Tuberculosis
Leptospirosis	Typhus
Malaria	Viral haemorrhagic fever
Marburg disease	Whooping cough
Meningitis	Yellow fever

In Scotland the law is different. It includes the same list *but minus*:

Encephalitis	Infective jaundice
Tetanus	Tuberculosis
but additionally:	

48

Continued fever

Erysipelas

Leptospiral jaundice

Membranous croup

Puerperal fever

Viral hepatitis

Northern Ireland is also different. The list is the same as for England and Wales *but minus*:

Food poisoning

Infective jaundice

but additionally:

Gastroenteritis

   (if under 2 years old)

Infective hepatitis

Leprosy

Malaria

APPENDIX 2

A protocol for the management of needlestick injury in general practice

1. Immediately following the injury the site should be washed thoroughly with soap and water. Free bleeding may be encouraged but the site should *not* be sucked.

2. The health care worker should be referred immediately to the doctor designated within the practice to deal with such injuries. This doctor should possess current information about post exposure prophylaxis in relation to hepatitis B and HIV infection and should be ready to initiate care. *Recommendations change as research findings are implemented and it is the employer's responsibility to ensure that policy is updated accordingly.* If necessary, the worker may be referred on to the doctor designated within the health authority to manage such injuries if the practice has decided that this will be the procedure. The name and telephone number of this individual should be immediately available in all practices.

3. The doctor responsible for managing the injury must then interview the source patient or the GP responsible for his/her care. The purpose is to determine the presence of risk factors for HIV or hepatitis B. If there are no risk factors the health care worker may be reassured.

4. If risk factors are present the source patient must be counselled and consent for screening for HIV and hepatitis B sought. Blood samples already obtained must not be tested without the consent of the source patient. If consent is withheld or the source patient cannot be identified, then the injury must be managed as if the blood were infected with HIV and/or hepatitis-B.

5. If the source patient is known to be infected with hepatitis B or risk factors are present, then post-exposure prophylaxis should be offered to the

health care worker within 24 hours of the injury. Blood should be taken first so that antibody status can be determined subsequently. Workers who have been previously immunized may be given a booster dose. Unimmunized workers may commence active immunization with hepatitis B vaccine and be passively immunized with hepatitis B immunoglobulin at the same time. This situation should be discussed with the local public health laboratory.

6. If the source patient is known to be infected with HIV or risk factors are present the worker must be counselled and an HIV test offered. Alternatively, blood may be taken and stored for future testing. Current advice is that prophylactic treatment should be given within 1–2 hours of exposure. Further management of this situation is properly carried out by the health worker's own GP in conjunction with the local HIV specialist team. Further HIV tests at 3 and 6 months would be advisable.

7. Full documentation of the circumstances of the injury is essential. Attention to confidentiality and the rights of both the source patient and the health care worker is of prime importance. Advice of specialist colleagues should be sought early and acted upon.

References

1. Stott N. The role of health promotion in primary health care. *Health Promotion* (1986) **1**: 49–53

2. Pill R, Peters T, Robling M. Factors associated with health behaviour among mothers of lower socio-economic status: A British example. *Soc Sci Med* (1993) **36**: 1137–44

3. Grist N. Foodborne infections and intoxications. *BMJ* (1990) **300**: 827–8

4. Harris J, Holm S. Is there a moral obligation not to infect others? *BMJ* (1995) **311**: 1215–17

5. Oakley A. Sexual health education interventions for young people: a methodological review. *BMJ* (1995) **310**: 158–62

6. Andersson-Ellström A, Forssman L, Milsom I. The relationship between knowledge about sexually transmitted diseases and actual sexual behaviour in a group of teenage girls. *Genito Med* (1996) **72**: 32–6

7. McGregor J. *et al.* Prevention of sexually transmitted diseases in women. *Obs Gyn Clinics N Am* (1989) **16**: 679–702

8. Kinnersley P. Attitudes of general practitioners towards their vaccination against hepatitis B. *BMJ* (1990) **300**: 238–9

9. McLauchlin J. Listeriosis: declining but may return *BMJ* (1992) **304**: 1583–4

10. Jackson M., Hutchison W. The prevalence and source of *Toxoplasma* infection in the environment. *Adv Parisit* (1989) **28**: 55–105

11. Gilbert R, Stanford M, Jackson H *et al.* Incidence of acute symptomatic

toxoplasma retinochoroiditis in south London according to country of birth. *BMJ* (1995) **310**: 1037–40

12. Hunter S. Storage of vaccines in general practice. *BMJ* (1989) **299**: 661

13. Thakker Y, Woods S. Storage of vaccines in the community; weak link in the cold chain? *BMJ* (1992) **304**: 756–8

14. Haworth E *et al.* Is the cold chain for vaccines maintained in general practice? *BMJ* (1993) **307**: 242–4

15 Jefferson N, Sleight G, Macfarlane A. Immunisation of children without a doctor present. *BMJ* (1987) **294**: 423–4

16 Liston A et al. Use of a contraindications checklist by practice nurses performing immunisations at a well child clinic. *J Roy Coll Gen Pract* (1989) **39**: 59–61

17. Nicoll A, Elliman D, Begg N. Immunisation: causes of failure and strategies and tactics for success. *BMJ* (1989) **299**: 808–12

18. *Immunisation against infectious disease.* London: HMSO (1996)

19. Fisher M. Treatment of acute anaphylaxis. *BMJ* (1995) **311**: 731–3

20. Rylance G, Bowen C, Rylance J. Measles and rubella immunisation: information and consent in children. *BMJ* (1995) **311**: 923–4

21. Kinder J *et al.* False contraindications to childhood immunisation. *Br J Gen Pract* (1992) **42**: 160–1

22. Begg N, Nicoll A. Myths in medicine. Immunisation. *BMJ* (1994) **309**: 1073–5

23. Hinman A, Orenstein W. Immunisation practice in developed countries. *Lancet* (1990) **335**: 707–10

24. Begg N, Gill O, White J. COVER (Cover of Vaccination Evaluated Rapidly): Description of the England and Wales Scheme. *Public Health* (1989) **103**: 81–9

25. White J *et al.* Vaccine coverage: recent trends and future prospects. *BMJ* (1992) **304**: 682–4

26. Jarman B *et al.* Uptake of immunisation in district health authorities in England. *BMJ* (1988) **296**: 1775–8.

27. Hart J T. The inverse care law. *Lancet* (1971) **1**: 405–8

28. Lynch M. Effect of practice and patient population characteristics on the uptake of childhood immunisations. *Brit J Gen Pract* (1995) **45**: 205–8

29. Li J, Taylor B. Comparison of immunisation rates in general practice and child health clinics. *BMJ* (1991) **303**: 1035–7

30. Bowling A, Jacobson B. Screening: the inadequacy of population registers. *BMJ* (1989) **298**: 545–6

31. Armstrong E A. The politics of inadequate registers. *BMJ* (1988) **299**: 73.

32. Pennington E, Wilcox R. Immunisation, practice records and the white paper. *J Roy Coll Gen Pract* (1988) **38**: 515–16

33. Peckham C. National immunisation study: factors influencing immunisation uptake in children. The Peckham report, London: *Action Research for the Crippled Child* (1989)

34. Kemple T. Study of children not immunised for measles. *BMJ* (1985) **290**: 1395–8

35. McGuire C. Accounting for public perceptions in the development of a childhood immunisation campaign. *Health Ed J* (1990) **49**: 105–7

36. Klein N, Morgan K, Wansbrough-Jones M. Parents' beliefs about vaccination: the continuing propagation of false contrindications. *BMJ* (1989) **298**: 1687

37. Jones K, Moon G. Multilevel assessment of immunisation uptake as a performance measure in general practice. *BMJ* (1991) **303**: 28–31

38. Morgan S *et al.* Knowledge of infectious diseases and immunisation among Asian and white parents. *Health Ed J* (1987) **46**: 177–8.

39. Simpson N, Lenton S, Randall R. Parental refusal to have children immunised: extent and reasons. **BMJ** (1995) **310**: 227–8

40. Feder G. Traveller gypsies and primary care. *J Roy Coll Gen Pract* (1989) **39**: 425–9

41. Ramsay M *et al.* Symptoms after accelerated immunisation. *BMJ* (1992) **304**: 1534–6

42. Hall R, Wiliams A. Special advisory service for immunisation. *Arch Dis Child* (1988) **63**: 1498–1500

43. Martin M. Diphtheria revisited. *Brit J Gen Pract* (1995) **45**: 394

44. Department of Health. *Diphtheria in the former USSR*. London: Department of Health (1993) (professional letter: PL/CMO(93)9)

45. Pichichero M. Pertussis and the pertussis vaccines. *Curr Op Infect Dis* (1993) **6**: 558–64

46. Ramsay M *et al.* Pertussis immunisation in children with a family or personal history of convulsions: a review of children referred for specialist advice. *Health Trends* (1994) **26**: 23–4

47. Miller D *et al.* Pertussis immunisation and serious acute neurological illnesses in children. *BMJ* (1993) **307**: 1171–6

48. Howard *et al.* Epidemiology of *Haemophilus influenzae* type b invasive disease in Wales. *BMJ* (1991) **303**: 441–4

49. Cartwright K. Vaccination against *Haemophlilus influenzae* b disease. *BMJ* (1992) **305**: 485–6

50. Urwin G, Yuan M, Feldman R. Prospective study of bacterial meningitis in North East Thames region, 1991–3, during introduction of *Haemophilus influenzae* vaccine. *BMJ* (1994) **309**: 412–14

51. Hargreaves R *et al.* Changing patterns of invasive *Haemophlilus influenzae* disease in England and Wales after introduction of the Hib vaccination programme. *BMJ* (1996) **312**: 160–1

52. Joce R et al. Paralytic polio in England and Wales, 1985–91. BMJ (1992) **305**: 79–82

53. Cutts F. Revaccination against measles and rubella. Side effects are outweighed by improved disease control. BMJ (1996) **312**: 589–10

54. Miller C L, Miller E, Sequeira P et al. Effect of selective vaccination on rubella susceptibility and infection in pregnancy. BMJ (1985) **294**: 1277–8

55. Joseph et al. BCG immunisation in England and Wales: a survey of policy and practice in schoolchildren and neonates. BMJ (1992) **305**: 495–8

56. Lienhardt C, Fine P. Controlling leprosy: multidrug treatment is not enough. BMJ (1992) **305**: 206–7

57. The subcommittee of the Joint Tuberculosis Committee of the British Thoracic Society. Guidelines on the vaccination of at risk groups in (April 1990). BMJ (1990) **300**: 995–9

58. Smith C, Parle M, Morris D. Implementation of government recommendations for immunising infants at risk of hepatitis B. BMJ (1994) **309**: 1339

59. Nicholson K. Influenza vaccination and the elderly. BMJ (1990) **301**: 617–18

60. Govaert T et al. Adverse reactions to influenza vaccines in elderly people: randomised double blind placebo controlled trial. BMJ (1993) **307**: 988–90

61. Nicholson K, Wiselka M. Amantadine for influenza A. BMJ (1991) **302**: 425–6

62. Deodhar H, Marshall R, Barnes J. Increased risk of sepsis after splenectomy. BMJ (1993) **307**: 1408–9

63. When to use the new pneumococcal vaccine. Drug Ther Bull (1990) **28**: 31–2

64. Working Party of the British Society for Antimicrobial Chemotherapy. The antibiotic prophylaxis of infective endocarditis. Lancet (1982) **ii**: 1323–6

65. Endocarditis Working Party of the British Society for Antimicrobial Chemotherapy. Antibiotic prophylaxis of infective endocarditis. Lancet (1990) **335**: 88–89

66. Simmons N A et al. Antibiotic prophylaxis and infective endocarditis. Lancet (1992) **339**: 1292–3

67. Simmons N A, Ball A P, Cawson R A et al. Case against antibiotic prophylaxis of patients with joint prostheses. Lancet (1992) **339**: 301

68. Working Party of the British Committee for Standards in Haematology: Clinical haematology task force. Guidelines for the prevention and treatment of infection in patients with an absent or dysfunctional spleen. BMJ (1996) **312**: 430–4

69. Waiijar U, Richmond S, Morrell P. Immunisation state of children born before term in the Northern region. BMJ (1989) **299**: 1013–14.

CHAPTER THREE

The response of the body to infection: symptoms, signs, and science

An understanding of the scientific basis of infection is an important component of developing sound clinical principles for its management in general practice. The commonest physiological response is fever and we have included the management of the feverish child here, an everyday situation in general practice which can cause anxiety for doctors and parents alike. The section on septic shock shows the effects of an uncontrolled bodily response to infection where the immune system has become hostile to the host; and the section on infection and immunodeficiency illustrates the effects on health when different components of the immune system fail. The chapter begins, however, with an account of the immunological basis of infection which is perhaps difficult in its science but rewarding, especially for those family doctors who did not encounter this topic as undergraduates!

Why do some people, but not others, become infected?

Infection can be defined as the process in which organisms invade the tissues or organs of the body and cause injury followed by reactive phenomena. This definition encompasses the three components of infection: invasion, injury, and some reaction on the part of the host. Humans are continually exposed to enormous numbers of microorganisms from the environment but only a small number of these are capable of satisfying the first two of these requirements, invasion and production of injury to the host tissues.

Invasion and injury

The initial step in invasion is binding of the organism to the surface tissues, a process termed 'adherence'. This is now recognized as an extremely complex process that is mediated by adhesins; these may be specific molecules on the viral or bacterial cell surface or adhesive organelles called fimbriae or pili that project from bacterial surfaces. Whichever adhesin is responsible, it often possesses some specificity for certain human cells and this explains the propensity of different strains of bacteria to cause disease at particular sites.

Once an organism is attached to a mucosal surface there are then two pathophysiological mechanisms by which it may cause infection. One is by the production by bacteria of toxins, proteins that adversely affect host cells, either locally or at a distance. Such toxins may be part of the structure of the bacterium (endotoxins); some of these are only released when the organism is lysed. More commonly, toxins are exotoxins that are released into the surroundings during growth of the bacterium. Some of these exotoxins (such as diphtheria, botulinum, and cholera toxins) are totally responsible for the manifestations of the disease process, whereas others (such as streptolysin O and other haemolysins) have less clear-cut roles in the disease process.

The other pathophysiological mechanism is the ability of the microbe to invade cells or penetrate tissues, a process that requires the organism to possess virulence factors that enable it to evade the normal host defence mechanisms. Only some of these virulence factors are clarified and they will be discussed below under the particular host defence mechanism that they are designed to overcome.

Host reactions: non-specific defences

The general function of the immune system is to recognize and combat any harmful infectious microbial agents with which the host comes into contact. The immune system has two major mechanisms that defend against infectious agents: (1) the non-specific or innate immune system; and (2) the specific or adaptive immune system. The non-specific host defence mechanisms are often the first response of the host to any encounter with an infectious agent.

Integrity of body surfaces and normal secretions

The first line of host defence against infectious agents is the natural barrier provided by the integrity of the body surfaces. Most organisms are unable to penetrate intact skin, which provides a very effective mechanical barrier to infection. The only organisms that do not require disruption of the skin integrity to enter the body are the larvae and intermediate forms of certain parasites (e.g. hookworm) and wart viruses. Any physical means that breaches this barrier will, of course, encourage infection by other microorganisms.

There are a number of normal secretions produced at body surfaces that play an important role in the prevention of infection. Cervical mucus, prostatic secretions, and tears all have potent antibacterial properties; some of this activity is due to lysozyme, an enzyme that kills bacteria by splitting a linkage in the bacterial cell wall. The acid pH of the gastric acid, the vaginal secretions, and urine are lethal to many bacteria and bile and pancreatic secretions also possess antimicrobial properties. Gastrointestinal peristalsis is an important line of defence and although there are some bacteria that are able to invade intact cells of the gastrointestinal tract, the virulence factors responsible are not yet understood. Among other physical defences are the mucus and cilia of the upper respiratory tract which combine to transport away from the lungs any particles that impact upon the mucosal surface.

Normal microflora

Many areas of the body are not sterile but contain microorganisms that have become adapted to exist in a symbiotic or commensal relationship with the host. This normal indigenous microflora is able to protect the host from invasion by pathogenic microbes either by competition for space or available nutrients, or by the production of substances that are toxic to other organisms. The commensal organisms that colonize normal human body surfaces vary from site to site. However, they are influenced to a certain extent by environmental and hormonal factors but, in general, they are quite predictable (Table 3.1). Alteration of the normal commensal flora can lead to overgrowth with pathogenic organisms or supra-infection with normally commensal organisms such as *Candida*.

Phagocytes

The function of the various phagocytic cells of the reticuloendothelial system is to engulf particles, including infectious agents, and then to destroy them. Phagocytes are all derived from the same stem cells, which can also differentiate into platelets or mast cells. The circulating phagocytes

Table 3.1 *Principal commensal organisms on healthy body surfaces*

Site	Organisms
Skin	**Bacteria** *Staphylococcus epidermidis* Corynebacteria *Propionibacterium acnes* **Fungi** *Malassezia furfur*
Mouth	**Bacteria** *Streptococcus* species *Fusobacterium* species Other anaerobic species
Bowel	**Bacteria** *Bacteroides* species *Peptococcus* species *Clostridium* species Other anaerobic species *Escherichia coli* *Klebsiella* and *Proteus* species
Vagina	**Bacteria** *Lactobacillus* species Döderlein's bacillus

are the polymorphonuclear granulocytes (neutrophils or eosinophils) and the monocyte. Each of these cells can leave the circulation and enter tissues during the inflammatory response. In addition, there are a number of phagocytic cells, derived from monocytes, that are permanently positioned to deal with infectious agents as they penetrate epithelial surfaces. Such cells are the macrophages of the lymph nodes, alveolar macrophages of the lung, the Küpffer cells of the liver sinusoids, and the synovial A cells of joints. Phagocytic cells attach to infecting microorganisms via a variety of surface receptors, engulf the organism into a phagosome and kill it by release of lysosomal enzymes into the phagosome. The surface receptors may be non-specific but phagocytosis is considerably enhanced by opsonization (see below) of the organism by complement or antibody.

Inflammation

The assessment and treatment of inflammation in a variety of body sites is a daily task for the general practitioner. Inflammation is the response of the body to infection or injury and has the function of increasing the immune response at the particular site. The response can be divided into three categories: (1) increased blood supply; (2) increased capillary permeability; and (3) migration of phagocytic cells into the tissues. The clinical appearances of redness, swelling, heat, and pain have been well described for centuries.

The attraction of phagocytic cells (both neutrophil polymorphs and monocytes) to the site of inflammation is termed chemotaxis and results from the production of certain molecules at the site. A particularly potent chemotactic substance is C5a, one of the activated components of the complement system (see below), which after production adheres to the endothelium of nearby capillaries. Once exposed to such a substance the phagocytic cells are induced to leave the circulation and to migrate to the site of production of the chemotactic molecule.

Other mediators of the inflammatory response include some cytokines and various prostaglandins, and other derivatives of arachidonic acid.

Cytokines

These are polypeptides that are produced by macrophages and lymphocytes during the initial exposure to an infectious agent. Developments in molecular biology have led to the recognition of a growing number of different cytokines; each usually has a variety of biological functions including the release of further cytokines. The best understood of these substances are interleukin-1, tumour necrosis factor, interferons, and various colony-stimulating factors. The interplay between these cytokines is far too complex to be given in detail but the net result of this so-called cytokine cascade is an increase in both the non-specific defences and the specific immune responses against pathogenic microorganisms.

The advances in recombinant DNA technology have led to the development of genetically engineered cytokines available in sufficient quantities for therapeutic intervention. Interferon-gamma and interleukin-2 have been used with limited success in the therapy of some malignancies and infections but toxicity has been a problem. Most success has been obtained from the colony-stimulating factors which have been used to increase the circulating monocyte and granulocyte counts in patients with leukaemias and after bone marrow transplantation.

Other developments have been aimed at blocking the harmful effects of an exuberant immune response, such as that seen in septic shock. Many of the physiological changes occurring in sepsis are mediated by tumour necrosis factor (TNF). Monoclonal antibodies against TNF are being developed and have been shown to protect experimental animals from many of the consequences of septicaemia. How beneficial similar preparations will be in humans is still undetermined.

Acute phase response

During infection the concentration of a number of proteins increases dramatically in the blood in response to various cytokines, particularly interleukin-1 and tumour necrosis factor. These substances are called the acute phase proteins. One of these acute phase proteins is C-reactive protein (CRP) which binds to molecules found on many bacteria and fungi (including the C-protein of pneumococci—hence the name). Once bound, CRP activates complement (see below) and also acts to promote phagocytosis by opsonization.

Natural killer cells

Natural killer (NK) cells comprise about 10% of the peripheral blood lymphocytes. They are not phagocytic but are important in controlling tumours and virus infections. These cells are able to recognize the changes produced on the surface of virally infected cells, then bind to these cells and lyse them.

Host reactions: specific immunity

Specific or adaptive immune responses differ from the non-specific responses in two important respects. First, the response is specific to each infectious agent, and second, the immune system possesses memory so that there is an accelerated response if the host is rechallenged with that infectious agent at a later date.

Antigens

These are substances that are capable of interacting with the products of the host's specific immune response. They are usually proteins, glycoproteins, or carbohydrates and are distinguished as immunogenic (capable of inducing a specific immune response) by their characteristic surface structure. Each antigen normally has several distinct areas of surface structure that can be recognized individually by the immune system. These individual areas are termed 'antigenic determinants' or 'epitopes': each antigen usually has its own particular set of epitopes.

Sometimes, an antigen is too small to be immunogenic by itself: if, however, it is bound to a tissue protein then its epitopes can be recognized and an immune response is initiated. Such antigens are called haptens.

Antibodies or immunoglobulins

These are glycoprotein molecules that combine specifically with antigens. They are manufactured by B lymphocytes. All immunoglobulins have a similar basic structure and are composed of four interlinked polypeptide chains: two shorter (light) chains and two longer (heavy) chains arranged in a Y-shape (Fig. 3.1). The basic structure of the heavy chains divides immunoglobulins into five classes, IgG, IgM, IgA, IgD, and IgE. IgG is the most abundant immunoglobulin in the body and can be further subdivided into four different subclasses, IgG1–4, on the basis of heavy chain structure. There are only two types of light chains found in all classes of immunoglobulins and the two light chains of an individual immunoglobulin are always of the same type.

The parts of each immunoglobulin molecule that recognize and bind to an epitope are the Fab (fragment of antigen-binding) sites. These Fab sites are situated at the ends of the arms of the Y (Fig. 3.1) and consist of variable regions of both the heavy and light chains that determine the unique

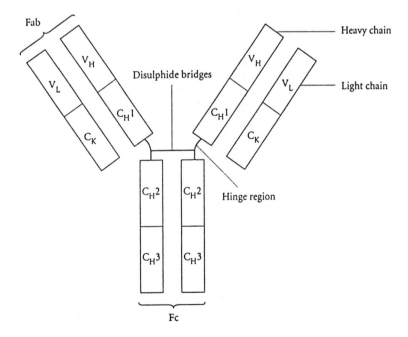

Fig 3.1 *Structure of basic antibody molecule. V_H, Variable domain of heavy chains; V_L, variable domain of light chains; C_H1, C_H2, C_H3, constant region domains of heavy chains; C_K (or C_λ), constant domain of light chains of kappa (K) or lambda (λ) type; F_{ab}, antigen-binding fragment of immunoglobulin molecule; F_c, crystallizable (or constant) fragment of immunoglobulin molecule.*

antigen-binding properties of that antibody. The stem of the Y-shape, made up of heavy chains only, is usually fairly constant for each class of immunoglobulin. It is termed the Fc (crystallizable fragment) site: it cannot bind antigens but serves to specify the particular biological functions of the antibody.

Biological functions of immunoglobulins.   The main biological functions of the 6 classes of immunoglobulins involve:

(1) *neutralization* of toxins (IgG, IgM),

(2) *opsonization,* which is the coating of antigen by antibody thus facilitating phagocytosis (IgG, IgM),

(3) *agglutination* of bacteria, enhancing phagocytosis (IgG, IgM),

(4) *lysis* of bacteria through activation of complement (IgG, IgM),

(5) *protection* of mucosal surfaces against bacterial adherance and toxins (IgA),

(6) *allergic response mechanisms* involving histamine release (IgE).

The complement system

The complement system consists of about 20 proteins that circulate in an inactive form but which can be activated to play a major role in the immune system. Activation of the system may occur by either of two independent pathways each of which is a cascade of reactions that leads to the formation of extremely potent biological products. Some of these act as opsonins, some induce the inflammatory response by binding to receptors on inflammatory cells, and the final product of either pathway is a complex of components that directly attack membranes to produce holes and cause cell lysis. Production of these powerful, and potentially dangerous, substances is extremely tightly regulated but specific details of the complement system are outside the scope of this Chapter. In general, however, the 'classical' pathway of activation is induced by the binding of antibody to antigen, whereas the 'alternative' pathway is antibody-independent and is initiated directly by molecules that have repeating chemical structures. Such molecules are found on the surface of a number of microorganisms.

The cellular basis of the specific immune response

The specific immune response depends on the recognition and elimination of foreign antigens by four major cell types; antigen-presenting cells, B lymphocytes (B cells), T lymphocytes (T cells), and macrophages.

Antigen-presenting cells.   There are a number of phagocytic cells in the body that act to enable lymphocytes to recognize free antigens. Some of these cells are macrophages (see below) but there are other specialized cells in lymph nodes and skin. Their primary function is to phagocytose antigens.

Once this occurs, part of the antigenic molecule is incorporated on the antigen-presenting cell surface membrane. Also on the surface membrane are the molecules that enable lymphocytes to recognize the cell as being of host origin ('self'). The presentation to the lymphocyte of the 'processed' antigen in conjunction with these 'self'-recognition molecules initiates the immune response.

B lymphocytes. All lymphocytes are derived from stem cells found in the bone marrow. Further differentiation then occurs. Certain lymphocytes were first discovered in chickens and were shown to differentiate in an special organ called the bursa of Fabricius: they were thus termed B lymphocytes (B cells). In humans, B cells differentiate in the bone marrow and then travel to peripheral lymphoid tissue. Other lymphocytes differentiate in the thymus and are termed T lymphocytes (T cells). During development both B and T cells acquire receptors specific for a single antigenic determinant and exposure to this epitope activates the cell.

B cells are responsible for the manufacture of antibody. Each individual B cell is capable of secreting only one specific antibody molecule and carries copies of this on its surface as an antigen receptor. The cell is activated to manufacture antibody by presentation of a specific antigen by an antigen-presenting cell and its binding to the surface-bound immunoglobulin of the B cell. Activation of B cells sometimes occurs without T-cell involvement but most antibody responses require close collaboration between T and B lymphocytes. This is achieved by a similar mechanism as described above—the presentation of processed antigen and host proteins to a particular T cell. The activated B cells then proliferate and differentiate into short-lived plasma cells, that produce the antibody, and longer-lived memory cells. The memory cells enable any subsequent exposure to the same antigen to lead to a more rapid, higher level, and longer-lasting antibody response (secondary antibody response).

T lymphocytes (T cells). These have numerous different functions which can be broadly classified into modulation of other cells in the immune response, production of cytokines, and direct killing of target cells. They comprise what is often referred to as the cell-mediated arm of the immune system and are important in defences against those pathogens that replicate intracellularly. The major pathogens in this category are listed in Table 3.2.

Regulation of the immune response is a result of the interplay between two subsets of T cells that differ in their surface markers. One group, the helper or inducer T cells express the CD4 surface antigen and the other, suppressor, T cells express the CD8 surface antigen (as, incidentally, do cytotoxic T cells). Helper cells not only augment antibody production by B cells but also secrete lymphokines, particularly interleukin-2 and gamma-interferon, that promote the function of macrophages, cytotoxic T cells and natural killer (NK) cells. These functions are depressed by suppressor T cells.

Table 3.2 *Major intracellular pathogens*

Viruses	**Fungi**
Herpesviruses	*Candida*
Measles	*Cryptococcus*
Bacteria	**Protozoa**
Listeria	*Toxoplasma*
Brucella	*Pneumocystis*
Salmonella	*Leishmania*
Mycobacteria	
Legionella	**Others**
	Chlamydia
	Rickettsia

Cytotoxic T cells recognize specific antigens on cell surfaces and then damage the cell surface leading to cellular lysis and death.

Macrophages.   These are mononuclear cells derived from monocytes. They are crucial in cell-mediated immunity. One of their functions (that of antigen presentation) is described above. Their second function is as effector cells. In order to kill intracellular organisms they need to become activated. This is achieved by lymphokines, particularly gamma-interferon, produced by T cells in response to antigen presentation. In the activated state macrophages will kill all intracellular organisms, not just the one that was presented to the T cell. In the activated state, macrophages also produce their own soluble mediators or cytokines which interact with and regulate the other cells involved in the specific immune response.

Fever and infection

Many infections are accompanied by a fever and many people view this as a serious symptom leading them to consult their GP. The basis for the rise in body temperature is described below, it is part of the host non-specific immune response to infection.

The ability of human beings to maintain a stable body temperature is dependent on successful functioning of the thermoregulatory centre in the hypothalamus. The neurones in this area are sensitive to changes in body temperature and are able to compensate for variations in heat production by adjusting the rate at which heat is lost from the body by sweating and vascular dilatation. In this manner the core temperature is regulated about a set point which is usually between 37.0°C and 37.5°C, regardless of geography or race. Body temperature does not remain absolutely constant throughout the day and everyone has evening temperatures up to a degree higher than those of the mornings. This daily rhythm is consistent for each individual and is independent of the environment. Fever is the persistent elevation of body temperature above the normal levels in an individual.

Pathogenesis of fever

It has been known for a long time that infections and other illnesses are accompanied by fever and that this involves a resetting of the hypothalamic thermostat to a higher level about which the regulation of heat production and loss continues normally. The complex pathogenic mechanisms involved are largely independent of the cause of the fever (Fig. 3.2). The common factor is that in response to a variety of infectious, immunological, and inflammatory stimuli (known collectively as exogenous pyrogens), antigen-presenting cells (monocytes and macrophages) produce a number of cytokines (see above). These cytokines have a wide range of effects on host metabolism and at least two of the compounds are now known to affect the hypothalamic temperature control centre (i.e. they act as endogenous pyrogens, (see Fig. 3.2)). One of these substances is interleukin-1 (IL-1) which is recognized as having a pivotal role in host defences (see above). IL-1 acts as a pyrogen by stimulating hypothalamic prostaglandin E_2 synthesis: this then acts on the vasomotor centre and leads to an increase in heat generation and prevention of heat loss, resulting in fever. A second cytokine is also pyrogenic. This is the

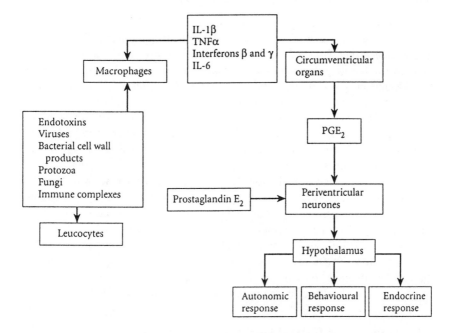

Fig 3.2 *Mechanisms causing fever. Circulating cytokines act on cells in the periventricular areas of the brain and induce the production of prostaglandins such as E_2 (PGE$_2$). PGE$_2$ acts on neurones whose axons innervate the hypothalamus and nearby areas that are involved in the autonomic, behavioural, and endocrine responses involved in fever.*

substance known as tumour necrosis factor (TNF) or cachectin. This also has profound metabolic effects (and probably accounts for the weight loss seen in certain infections). TNF is pyrogenic in two ways: it has a direct effect on prostaglandin E_2 release by the hypothalamus and also stimulates the release of IL-1. The situation is made even more complex by the fact that interferon-alpha (IFN-α), produced by cells in response to viral infections, is itself directly pyrogenic. Which, if any, of these substances is responsible for fever in a particular disease is not yet established but the lack of an acute phase response in certain virus infections might indicate that the fever is due to IFN-α rather than IL-1 or TNF.

The ability of aspirin and other anti-inflammatory agents, including paracetamol and ibuprofen, to act as antipyretics results from their blocking of prostaglandin production from arachidonic acid.

Since there are many factors which can stimulate the release of cytokines from macrophages, an elevated body temperature is, in itself, of very little value in determining the cause of an illness. In the past, emphasis has been placed on patterns of fever; diseases have been described as characteristically causing continuous, intermittent, hectic, or remittent fever. However, it is now generally recognized that such descriptions are of little value in individual patients as any one disease may produce many different temperature patterns.

The importance of fever in general practice

Fever is a common symptom and and many people, especially children, consult the doctor; as a result the average family practitioner will see several patients each day with pyrexia. Patients with fever are usually assessed clinically by the family doctor although the approach may vary.[1] This is shown in the differences in the use of thermometers in general practice.[2] In a study carried out by postal questionnaire in Surrey, 145 GPs were asked about the use of thermometers: 116 (80%) doctors replied of whom 7 did not have any method of taking a patient's temperature, 12 did not use thermometers, and 56 doctors used them infrequently. Most patients with fever are assessed clinically by the GP without recourse to investigation, with most patients improving within a few days of the initial consultation. However, patients often seem to be worried about fever, especially parents with febrile children.[3,4] Unfounded concern and misconceptions regarding the potential harmful effects of fever have given rise to the term 'fever phobia'.[5] A study of the impact of fever health education on clinic utilization[6] showed that well-designed audiovisual aids and a fever education programme can not only increase knowledge and improve parental confidence in managing fever at home but can also make a sizeable contribution to health cost savings by decreasing surgery attendance.

The treatment of fever: theory and practice

Fever as a sign of disease dates back to Hippocrates but until recently it was not thought to serve any useful purpose in the response to infection. Recent studies have changed this concept and provided evidence that moderate elevations of body temperature might be of definite value. Some of the most dramatic evidence of this comes from studies of the response to infection of cold-blooded animals such as lizards and fish. These animals, when infected, naturally seek out warmer environments to raise their body temperature. If they do so their survival is enhanced. The laboratory evidence of why this should be so suggests that many of the inflammatory and immunological responses in these animals (and also in mammals, including man) are improved by a moderate rise in temperature.

Now that there is evidence of a possible beneficial value of fever, it is questionnable whether the routine use of antipyretic treatment in febrile patients is warranted. The results from various studies have shown little or no increase in the length of symptoms following the treatment of infections in children and adults with antipyretics, but equally well they have not shown any consistent benefits. Some improvements have been noted in the comfort and behaviour of young children given paracetamol as antipyretic therapy for presumed viral infections but this was not marked.

Common sense would dictate that a patient should be treated with antipyretics (but never aspirin for children[7]) when the analgesic effect of the drug is required and that the increased metabolic consequences of a high fever in those with impaired cardiovascular systems should also be avoided by a reduction in fever. Otherwise there is little harm in allowing moderate fevers to persist.

While parents will undoubtedly feel happier assessing a child's temperature by use of a fever scan applied to the forehead or a clinical thermometer in the axilla it is less disturbing for small babies, and more reliable if the temperature is taken rectally. Kai[8] studied a group of parents in an inner city practice and reported great reluctance to use this method. The reluctance was based on fear of harming the child and on taboos connected with sexual abuse. The method was considered by many parents as appropriate for professionals only.

The technique for taking a rectal temperature is described by Keeley.[9] With the infant supine and lengthwise on a bed or couch the nappy is undone and both ankles are firmly held in one hand so as to flex and abduct the hips revealing the anus. With the other hand the examiner holds the thermometer, which has been well shaken down, between finger and thumb, 2–3 cm from the bulb. Lubricated with a little KY jelly and held at an angle of about 30 degrees to the horizontal, the bulb end lowest, the thermometer is gently inserted for a minute or two, with the flexed legs held firmly in the other hand. As Keeley points out the infant is familiar with this position having nappies changed and the procedure will cause little disturbance. Rectal temperatures of 36.5–37.5°C should be considered as normal. Proper cleaning of the thermometer is vital. It should of course be washed, dried, and disinfected. A spirit impregnated swab will suffice.

Correct management of fever in the home environment is of particular importance to the patient and in the case of a child, also to the parents. Kinmouth[10] compared the acceptability and effects on temperature of advice to unwrap children, or give paracetamol or warm sponging treatments in the management of feverish children at home. She concluded that to give paracetamol was more effective than sponging or unwrapping in controlling temperature in children at home and was more acceptable to parents. Warm sponging had an additive effect and reduced fever more quickly than paracetamol alone.

Febrile well-looking infants

The management of febrile infants in the first three months of life is difficult as they localize infections poorly and are at greater risk than older children for serious disseminated infection such as meningitis and septicaemia.[11] Rates of bacteraemia are reported by Long as 4–15%[12] and the risk of serious infection has been calculated to be more than 20 times greater than for older infants. Infants under 3 months of age present fewer diagnostic clues as to the aetiology of fever and particular care must be taken in assessment. It is of vital importance that clinicians listen to the mother of the child. Mothers *know* if a child is really ill and their history and opinion are an essential framework for assessing the diagnosis and deciding whether or not hospital admission is needed. It is a law of general practice that the parents' intuitions must be heard, and a second opinion sought if they insist their child is ill even in the absence of localizing signs. If the infant is toxic then referral is mandatory. If the GP is considering the use of antibiotics in an infant under 3 months it must be on the basis of a definitive diagnosis. As this includes ruling out otitis media, a urinary tract infection, skeletal or soft tissue infection, and gastrointestinal infections it is best to refer than to prescribe on incomplete evidence.[13] Non-toxic febrile infants must have detailed daily follow-up until they recover.

Management of a febrile child.   The care of a feverish child may pose a difficult and worrying time for parents. Readers may like to consider using a leaflet (see Appendix for an example) to form the basis for a practice leaflet to give to parents when they attend the surgery. Devising a leaflet with practice staff, and customizing it for the practice population, creates an opportunity to create a team approach to advice and management.

Management of convulsions with fever.   A workshop on the subject of child-hood convulsions with fever in July 1990[14] considered that it was important to distinguish 'convulsions with fever' and 'febrile convulsions'. Convulsions with fever include any convulsion in a child of any age with fever of any cause. The working group suggested that for the purpose of clinical management the term 'febrile convulsions' should be limited to 'a epileptic seizure occurring in a child aged from six months to five years, precipitated by fever arising from infection outside the nervous system in a child who is otherwise neurologically normal'. (A classification of convulsions is shown in Table 3.3.) The working group proposed that fanning, cold bathing, and tepid sponging were likely to cause discomfort and were not recommended. However, many parents

Table 3.3 *The classification of convulsions[17]*

Febrile convulsion
An event in infancy or childhood associated with fever but without
evidence of intracranial infection or defined cause. This is similar to the
National Institute of Health definition. Children with previous afebrile
seizures were excluded. Suspected seizures in the first 4 weeks of life were
excluded but convulsions during vaccination fevers were included

Complex febrile convulsion
Longer than 15 minutes, focal, or multiple (more than one convulsion per
episode of fever)

Recurrent febrile convulsion
More than one episode of fever associated with convulsions

Simple febrile convulsion
Not complex

Afebrile convulsion
Classification based on proposals of the International League Against
Epilepsy.[18] Children with more than one afebrile attack defined as having
epilepsy

---

and GPs disagree with this advice. The group recommended the use of an
antipyretic drug such as paracetamol. Adequate fluid intake is, of course, vital.
The anticonvulsant drug of choice is rectal diazepam but the routine use of
anticonvulsant drugs in children with recurrent convulsions and fever is not
recommended. It is important that parents should be reassured concerning
a child's development and neurological state following a febrile convulsion.
The risk of subsequent epilepsy following a single febrile convulsion when
there are no complex features is about 2.5%. In addition, Verity, in a
national cohort study,[15] concluded that the risk of epilepsy after febrile
convulsion was much lower than reported in many hospital studies and if
febrile convulsions cause brain damage that leads to later epilepsy this is a
rare occurrence.

The joint working group[14] discussed the question of when children with
fever and convulsions should be admitted to hospital. Some members
thought that all children should be admitted following a first convulsion
mainly because of the anxiety concerning the possibility of overlook-
ing meningitis. Most members thought that some selection was possible
and the following factors would certainly indicate admission after a first
convulsion:

- A complex convulsion: one lasting longer than 20 minutes with focal
  features, with incomplete recovery after one hour.

- A child aged less than 18 months.

- Early review by a doctor at home not possible.
- Home circumstances inadequate, or more than usual parental anxiety or parent's inability to cope.

Whatever the circumstances these children must be visited promptly and a full assessment carried out. Advice for the parents on how to cope while waiting for the doctor should be clear and straightforward and all reception and nursing staff should know how to advise about paracetamol and tepid sponging if they receive the telephone call. The GP should carry rectal diazepam in the emergency bag which is administered in a dose of 500 μg/kg for prolonged (over 15 minutes) or recurrent convulsions. A history of previous convulsions does not rule out the possibility of meningitis and GPs should bear this very much in mind.

Bacteraemia, septicaemia, and septic shock

Although the presentation of septicaemia may be dramatic other patients, especially the elderly, may be difficult to diagnose. Septic shock with its high mortality may follow; all GPs will see at least a few patients who will die in this way and an understanding of the underlying mechanisms will help in discussions with the family.

Bacteraemia means the presence of viable bacteria in the blood, as demonstrated by a positive blood culture, but it is not necessarily associated with any symptoms. Transient bacteraemias are quite common and can be associated with such trivial manipulations of infected sites as chewing or tooth-brushing. Bacteraemias are sometimes associated with rigors. These are true shaking chills with chattering of the teeth and shaking of the entire body: the term should not be synonymous with a feeling of cold and shivering.

Septicaemia

This is an imprecise term applied to a bacteraemia accompanied by symptoms, such as toxicity and hypotension, that imply that the bacteria are multiplying within the bloodstream. Despite developments in antibiotic therapy, septicaemia continues to be accompanied by a significant morbidity and mortality. Primary bacteraemia or septicaemia, again imprecisely, is bloodstream infection in which there is no obvious source of the infection elsewhere in the body, whereas a secondary septicaemia occurs in the presence of a localized source of the sepsis.

It is not possible to say which organisms are the most frequent causes of bacteraemia in the community since many episodes are transient and are either not reported or not investigated with blood cultures. It is likely, however, that the commonest organisms are the viridans streptococci from the mouth, which often enter the blood but rarely cause symptoms except in the setting of pre-existing heart valve abnormalities when endocarditis may result. The spectrum of organisms causing primary septicaemia in the community is much easier to delineate since almost all patients will be admitted to hospital and blood cultures will be taken. The common organisms depend on the age of the patient and the clinical setting. The occurrence of septicaemia in general reflects an interplay between a focus of infection from which bacteria can reach the bloodstream (common sites include the respiratory tract, urine, and biliary tract) and factors such as underlying disease or reduced host defences.

1. *Staphylococcus aureus* accounts for about 10% of cases and is often associated with the presence of a skin wound or abscess, bone or joint infections and sometimes with intravenous drug abuse. In about a quarter of cases no obvious source of infection is ever determined.

2. *Streptococcus pneumoniae* is a common cause of transient bacteraemia in patients with pneumococcal pneumonia, meningitis, otitis media, or sinusitis. Young adults may have pneumococcal septicaemia with no obvious site and occult pneumococcal bacteraemia is also a not uncommon cause of febrile convulsions in young children. Splenectomized patients and those with sickle-cell disease or other causes of splenic dysfunction are particularly prone to severe and fulminant pneumococcal septicaemias.

3. *Escherichia coli* is the most common organism causing septicaemia in the community. The infection usually arises from the urinary tract, biliary tract, pelvis, or gastrointestinal tract. Most cases occur in the elderly male with prostatism or persons with known biliary calculi.

4. The meningococcus can cause a transient bacteraemia but most cases are associated with an associated meningitis or a rapidly progressive septicaemia with a purpuric rash (see neurological infections, p. 214).

5. Non-typhoidal salmonella infections are usually seen as a consequence of recent diarrhoea and vomiting in either a very young child or an elderly person.

In those patients acquiring bacteraemia after admission to hospital, the portal of entry is usually associated with either a site of instrumentation, surgery, or a respiratory infection. The spectrum of organisms is influenced by the prior use of antibiotics, nosocomial colonization, and the immune status of the patient. Gram-negative aerobic bacteria, especially those resistant to multiple antibiotics are frequently isolated, particularly in the intensive care setting and in immunosuppressed patients.

Primary septicaemia usually presents as a severe illness with high fever, sweating, rigors, muscle pains, hyperventilation (and resultant respiratory alkalosis), headache, apprehension, and change in mental state. The elderly often have less florid signs and may merely present with confusion, immobility, and falls. With secondary septicaemia these symptoms are superimposed on those of the initiating infection (e.g. pneumonia, pyelonephritis, cellulitis, or wound infection). Commonly, there may be skin lesions that may suggest the primary focus of infection or give important clues to the aetiology. These include superficial pustular lesions which might suggest a staphylococcal or streptococcal or, usually in a young person with concomitant septic arthritis gonococcal aetiology. Classical petechial and ecchymotic skin and mucous membrane manifestations may occur with meningococcal septicaemia and occasionally also occur with other septicaemias and endocarditis. The rose spots of *Salmonella* bacteraemia are sparse macules over the trunk and abdomen. *Pseudomonas aeruginosa* septicaemia in immunosuppressed individuals typically causes lesions called ecthyma gangrenosum. These are round or oval, 1–5 cm in diameter and have a rim of erythema or induration. The central area is necrotic or possibly ulcerated.

Septic shock

As patients with septicaemia progress, hypotension and diminished organ perfusion develops—a condition associated with a high mortality. It is due to a complex series of enzymatic reactions triggered by microorganisms or microbial products in the bloodstream. The most important precipitant is endotoxin, a lipopolysaccharide component present on the surface of the Gram-negative cell wall. The endotoxin molecule comprises an outer chain of oligosaccharides which provide the diverse immunogenicity of the bacterium. Inside this is a core of hexose sugars of limited variation. Nearest to the cell wall is the lipid-A component which is similar in all Gram-negative bacteria and is responsible for the toxic activity. Gram-positive bacteria do not have endotoxin but they are capable of producing septic shock by the release of exotoxins which ultimately lead to similar inflammatory and metabolic disturbances.

Endotoxin activates a series of physiological cascades in a pathological manner. These include the systemic coagulation pathways, complement system, fibrinolysis, and bradykinin. At a local level there is inappropriate stimulation of cytokine functions, particularly that of tumour necrosis factor (TNF). Initially in sepsis, bradykinin and histamine release results in hypotension accompanied by peripheral vasodilatation. The heart rate and myocardial contractility increase so that in such septic shock the peripheries are well perfused (warm shock), there is hyperventilation and a raised cardiac output. Later, the peripheral resistance rises in response to increased noradrenaline release; intense vasoconstriction, pallor, cold peripheries, and oliguria occur (cold shock). The activation of the coagulation and fibrinolytic systems results in the syndrome of disseminated intravascular coagulation (DIC), which causes both thrombosis and clinical bleeding. The clinical features are petechiae, ecchymoses, peripheral gangrene; and collapse of the coronary, pulmonary, cerebral, and renal circulations.

The combination of acute febrile symptoms and shock requires urgent assessment and treatment for septicaemia and the patient requires immediate referral to hospital. The differential diagnosis may include pulmonary embolism, occult haemorrhage, myocardial infarction, and even adrenal insufficiency (in a patient with relatively minor infection).

Antibiotics must be given urgently to patients with suspected or proven septicaemia. The usual practice involves a very broad spectrum of cover but the choice of antibiotics must take account of the most likely organisms in the particular clinical setting. In practice the aerobic Gram-positive and Gram-negative spectrum and anaerobes are usually covered as completely as possible. Circulatory and respiratory support within an intensive therapy unit may also be needed.

Neither the use of corticosteroids nor opiate antagonists, such as naloxone, have been shown to improve survival in septic shock. Once septic shock has reached a certain critical point continued septicaemia is not necessary for perpetuation of a deteriorating downward spiral. One of the possible reasons why improvements in antibiotic therapy has not been associated with an increase in survival in severe sepsis is that antibiotics may release a bolus of endotoxin as they clear the bacteraemia. This endotoxin may act to fuel the fire of the inflammatory cascades. Immunotherapeutic approaches to counter the effect of endotoxin released from organisms killed by the initial antibiotic treatment have been tried. The introduction of an intravenous preparation of anti-endotoxin immunoglobulin (IgM) containing high titres of antibodies against lipid-A, has been associated with improved survival in septic shock caused by Gram-negative septicaemia, if it is given early in the course of the shock (before the irreversible stage is reached). It is, however, extremely expensive and there is as yet no rapid way of determining that sepsis is caused by Gram-negative rather that Gram-positive organisms (an anti-endotoxin would, of course, have no part to play in the treatment of the latter infections). Monoclonal antibodies to TNF, which would be expected to be equally effective in all forms of septic shock are currently being developed. Anti-TNF antibodies have the disadvantage, however, that TNF is only transiently present in the bloodstream and that it probably only one of several cytokine mediators of shock.

Infection and immunodeficiency

It is easy to understand why doctors despair about the problem of infection in the immunocompromised host as the literature abounds with reports of evermore exotic organisms causing disease in these patients. However, it is important to realize that notwithstanding the reports of rarities, most infections are caused by the same organisms that infect normal hosts and that it is usually only the frequency or severity of infection that is altered by the defect in immunity. Furthermore, it is very unusual for there to be a generalized susceptibility to infection and impairment of one of the three major defensive mechanisms described earlier, humoral immunity, phagocytosis, and cellular immunity, and is associated with a particular, well-recognized pattern of infective problems (Table 3.4). All GPs care for patients with impaired immunity from one or more of these causes and should be vigilant for the early signs of problems.

Table 3.4 *The principal infections in immunocompromised hosts*

Immune dysfunction	Condition	Resultant infections
Humoral immunity	Myelomatosis Chronic lymphatic leukaemia	*Streptococcus pneumoniae* *Haemophilus influenzae* *Neisseria meningitidis*
Cellular immunity	Lymphoma AIDS	*Listeria* *Cryptococcus* *Pneumocystis* Herpesviruses Mycobacteria Opportunistic pathogens
Neutropenia	Acute leukaemia	Staphylococcci Gram-negative bacilli *Candida*

Impaired humoral immunity

A variety of disorders interfere with the quantity or quality of B cells and the formation of immunoglobulins and the host is then unable to mount an effective antibody-mediated immune response. This is particularly crucial in the defence against encapsulated bacteria and Gram-negative bacteria. Humoral immune deficiencies are not generally associated with an increased frequency or severity of viral, fungal, or protozoal infections.

Some defects in humoral immunity are congenital: such primary immuno-deficiency disorders are associated with hypogammaglobulinaemia, either as an isolated problem or in conjunction with T-cell dysfunction. These patients typically develop chronic or recurrent infections of the middle ear, sinuses, and lungs, with or without bacteraemia.

Acquired deficiencies in immunoglobulin production occur in patients with B-cell disorders, such as multiple myeloma and chronic lymphatic leukaemia, and also in patients with protein-losing states such as burns or the nephrotic syndrome.

Patients with primary hypogammaglobulinaemia can be helped by regular replacement therapy with intravenous immunoglobulin preparations although this approach is not beneficial for those with myeloma and other B-cell disorders.

Neutropenia

This is often the result of haematological malignancy or the use of certain powerful cytotoxic drugs and patients in these categories are usually managed in hospital until the risk of neutropenia developing is very low. Therefore, the GP is much more likely to encounter neutropenia as an idiosyncratic side-effect of certain drugs. The list of these is formidable but among the most frequently implicated are gold salts, penicillamine, azothiaprine, carbimazole, and phenothiazines. Most GPs supervise patients on these drugs, particularly in the care of those with rheumatoid arthritis and chronic schizophrenia. Patients on these or other drugs with a potential for causing neutropenia should be regularly monitored using a reliable reminder system, the notes should be clearly marked and the development of neutropenia or symptoms suggestive of infection should be the signal for urgent investigation.

Defects in opsonization result in abnormal phagocytosis by neutrophils. Such a defect accompanies hypogammaglobulinaemia and complement deficiency and is also seen after splenectomy or in functional hyposplenism. These patients have frequent and often fulminant infections with encapsulated bacteria, particularly pneumococci and *Haemophilus influenzae*, and tend to have more severe attacks of falciparum malaria than those with intact spleens. Patients who have undergone splenectomy should be offered pneumococcal and *H. influenzae* type b (Hib) immunization and their records clearly marked; there is evidence that most of these patients have not been immunized. In a group of 263 unvaccinated splenectomized patients who died between 1975 and 1990, 22% had died from septicaemia or other infections.[16]

Impaired phagocytosis

The defect in immunity that is perhaps the most hazardous as regards the development of infection is a decrease in the phagocytic function of the neutrophils, particularly when it is due to a profound reduction in circulating granulocytes. This is usually secondary to drug therapy or malignancy. As the total neutrophil count falls below $1.0 \times 10^9/l$, the risk of acquiring an infection increases markedly and below 0.1×10^9 neutrophils/l this risk approaches certainty within a few days. Septicaemia, occurring out of the blue or secondary to localized oropharyngeal, skin, or perineal infection is characteristic. The sites of the infections are a reflection of the importance of the patient's own endogenous flora in the aetiology. Staphylococci, Gram-negative bacteria, and *Candida* are particularly common and the infections they cause tend to be prolonged, poorly responsive to therapy, and recurrent. Previous antibiotic therapy and exposure to a hospital environment may predispose to infection with the 'problem' Gram-negative bacteria such as *Ps. aeruginosa*, *Klebsiella*, or *Serratia* species.

Impaired cell-mediated immunity

The very young and the elderly have a physiological deficiency of cellular immunity and are more susceptible to infection with viral and non-viral intracellular pathogens than those in other age groups. This is also seen in during pregnancy when there are weaker cell-mediated immune responses, hence the increased susceptability to *Listeria* infection.

The pathological deficiencies of cellular immunity may be congenital or acquired. All the congenital ones are extremely rare and of little relevance to the GP. The acquired deficiencies are more commonly seen. They may result from malignancies, such as Hodgkin's disease, and certain other lymphomas, cytotoxic agents, or therapy with cyclosporin A, corticosteroids, or radiation. Transiently depressed cellular immunity also accompanies certain infections such as infectious mononucleosis and measles but the infection that has the most profound and persistent effects on cellular immunity is that caused by the human immunodeficiency viruses, which can ultimately result in the development of AIDS.

The organisms that cause infection in such patients include those such as *Pneumocystis* and *Nocardia* which do not usually cause disease in normal individuals and are therefore generally known as opportunistic pathogens. There is often nothing specific about the clinical presentation of infection due to an opportunistic organism and as therapy effective against the whole range of possible pathogens is unrealistic, the major burden on the doctor is the ensure that all possible efforts are made to make a specific diagnosis. General practitioners should refer patients with impaired immunity and non-specific symptoms and signs of infection for hospital investigation.

Complement deficiency

These deficiencies are rarely primary but occur relatively frequently in certain rheumatological disorders, particularly systemic lupus erythematosus (SLE). The consequences of the deficiency depend on whether the deficient complement component(s) is limited to the classical pathway or whether the alternative pathway is also impaired. The most common infection associated with deficiency of complement components is meningococcal disease, particularly that due to Group Y organisms.

APPENDIX

My child has a temperature: what should I do?

A basis for a practice leaflet: remember to adapt the contents to your own practice paying attention to readability and the needs of minority groups. The first section should display the practice details and the 24-hour telephone number.

Q: *Is a temperature serious?*

A: No, not necessarily; it is a symptom and not a disease.

All children have a high temperature at some time. The temperature of the body in adults and children is not constant and in children, in particular, can vary greatly from hour to hour, particularly if the child has a infection. The temperature is often higher in the evening or during the night just when parents are tired, anxious, and feel in need of help and advice. Many childhood illnesses produce a high and fluctuating temperature but this is *not* necessarily serious and may be caused by minor illness. A slight temperature is not uncommon following childhood immunization.

Q: *How do I manage my child with a high temperature?*

A: Here are a few do's and don'ts. Read them carefully.

If you have a thermometer take the child's temperature in the morning, midday, and before sleeping. If the temperature is 39 degrees centigrade or more repeat every two to three hours and write it down to show to the doctor or nurse. The temperature is probably best taken with the thermometer in the armpit with the arm held firmly for a couple of minutes. Temperature strips for the forehead are easy to use but can be unreliable. If you do not know how to take a temperature the health visitor can show you.

Do not wrap up your child tightly in thick clothing or bed-clothes and remove blankets from the bed. Do not add extra layers if the child is shivering.

If temperature reaches 38.5 degrees centigrade, tepid sponge head and body with cool not cold water. If you have an electric fan, place this several feet away; it will help rapid cooling. (Remember to keep fan away from any other small children.)

Give paracetamol (Calpol) in the dose suggested for the age of the child. The correct dose will be written on the bottle. Do *not* give aspirin in any form

Make sure that the child drinks large amounts of clear fluids. If the child is not willing, give small quantities every 15–30 minutes. Your doctor may have advised or prescribed some sachets of Dioralyte or a similar powder to which water is added. If so, follow the instructions carefully. Do not worry if child does not want to eat any solids over 48 hours or so. Fluids are much more important during this time. Some ill children, who reject most fluids, will happily drink a flat Cola (half water/half cola).

Breast- or bottle-fed infants will require additional clear fluid.
Look at nappy or pants frequently to make sure there is plenty of clear, light-coloured urine. If the urine is dark and there is very little then the child is not drinking enough.

Q: *When should I start to worry?*

A: Try to keep calm at all times. If you are first-time parents, or if you are coping by yourself, it is often a great help to seek the advice and support of more experienced family members or neighbours.

There is always a doctor available to give telephone advice or to visit should it be necessary. Sometimes you may be asked to bring the child to the surgery for urgent assessment if you have transport. No harm will result from bringing a feverish child out in the car. If your child has a high temperature in the evening it is far better to ring early rather than leaving it until the middle of the night when everything seems worse.

Most high temperatures return to near normal in 24–48 hours. You should inform us if your child runs a temperature of around 38 degrees centigrade for two days or more even if you are not unduly worried.

Q: *But when should I call the doctor?*

A: The decision to contact the doctor is sometimes a difficult one. If you are worried do phone for advice but in any case you should contact us if any of the following problems occur. (The surgery is open from 8 am to 7pm on weekdays and 8 am to 12 pm on Saturdays. The 24-hour emergency phone number is: 123 456)

Call us immediately *if:*
- The child has a convulsion (fit) or sustained jerking movements.
- The child is unable to swallow, particularly if he/she is dribbling an excessive amount of saliva.
- Any sudden dark rash, skin mottling, or rapid colour change appears.
- The child cannot easily move his/her head and neck, or it seems stiff, or the child is unable to lift his/her head off the pillow.
- The child is breathless, has very noisy breathing, seems to have difficulty breathing; or has severe prolonged coughing with distress.
- The child becomes unconscious (cannot be roused).
- The child becomes very lethargic, or floppy.

Call us soon (within 2–3 hours) if the temperature persists. Start fluids and paracetamol at once:

- in any child under 6 months.
- if the child has a high temperature and already has another chronic illness or condition such as diabetes, asthma, any malignancy, or is under hospital out-patient care.
- the child has had a previous convulsion or there is a close family history of convulsion.
- the temperature remains greater than 39 degrees centigrade

Call us soon (within 2–3 hours) if the following problems develop or persist. Start fluids and paracetamol at once:

- the child sleeps a great deal more than usual.
- there is inconsolable crying.
- any hallucinations (seeing things that are not there).
- if the child only passes a very small quantity of very dark urine, particularly if skin appears very dry and eyes seem sunken.
- if moving any limb causes pain.
- if the child cries when passing urine or the urine has a 'fishy' smell, or there is abdominal or back pain; this may mean a urine infection and will require very early treatment with antibiotics.
- The child complains of a headache or cries when the light is put on.
- The child develops earache

Between 8 am and 7 pm including weekends

If you have coped with a child with a temperature and you would like to discuss any problems or uncertainties telephone us for advice. The doctor or nurse may suggest that a surgery appointment or a home visit is necessary.

To summarize:
- Remember you can always ring the duty doctor for advice. Do not take a child with a temperature to the hospital accident and emergency department without contacting us first. It usually means a long wait and is not the best way to help your child.

- The **emergency telephone number is**: 1234–123456.

- In an **extreme emergency** and if, for any reason, you cannot contact the doctor, then an ambulance may be called by dialling 999.

Remember! Most temperatures are not serious
- Keep the child cool
- Give lots of clear fluids
- Give paracetamol in correct doses
- Keep a close watch for any change
- Telephone the doctor early if you are worried

References

1. Eskerud J *et al.* Fever in general practice II. Reasons for encounter, management and duration of fever conditions. *Family Pract* (1992) **9**: 425–32

2. Clarke S. The use of thermometers in general practice. *BMJ* (1992) **304**: 961–3.

3. Fletcher J L Jr, Creten D. Perceptions of fever among adults in a family practice setting. *J Fam Pract* (1986) **22**: 427–30

4. Kramer M S, Naimark L, Leduc D. Parental fever phobia and its correlates. *Paed* (1985) **75**: 1110–13.

5. Schmitt B. Fever phobia. Misconceptions of parents about fevers. *Am J Dis Child* (1980) **34**: 176–81.

6. Robinson J, Schwartz M *et al.* The impact of fever health education on clinic utilization *Am J Dis Child* (1989) **143**: 6 698–704

7. Glasgow J, Moore R. Reye's syndrome 30 years on. Possible marker of inherited metabolic disorders. *BMJ* (1993) **307**: 950–1

8. Kai J. Parents perceptions of taking babies rectal temperature. *BMJ* (1993) **307**: 660–2

9. Keeley D. Taking infants' temperatures. *BMJ* (1992) **304**: 931–2.

10. Kinmonth A, Fulton Y, Campbell M J. Management of feverish children at Home. *BMJ* (1992) **305**: 1134–6

11. Pantell R *et al.* Fever in the first six months of life. *Clin Ped* (1980) **9**: 77–82.

12. Long S. Approach to the febrile patient with no obvious focus of infection. *Paed Rev* (1984) **5**: 305–15.

13. Hewson P. Fever in early infancy. *Curr Op Infect Dis* (1993) **6**: 570–5

14. Joint Working Group of the Research Unit of the Royal College of Physicians and the British Paediatric Association. Guidelines for the management of convulsions with fever *BMJ* (1991) **303**: 634–6.

15. Verity C M. Risk of epilepsy after febrile convulsions: a national cohort study. *BMJ* (1991) **303**: 1373–6

16. Kinnersley P, Wilkinson C, Srinivasan J. Pneumococcal vaccination after splenectomy: survey of hospital and primary care records. *BMJ* (1993) **307**: 1398–9

17. Verity C M Risk of epilepsy after febrile convulsions: A national cohort study. *BMJ* (1991) **303**: 1373–6.

18. Commission on Classification and Terminology of the International League Against Epilepsy. Proposal for revised clinical and electroencephalographic classification of epileptic seizures. *Epilepsia* (1991) **22**: 489–501.

CHAPTER FOUR

The investigation of infection

Infection, potentially one of the most serious and life-threatening of presentations, is also a common complaint resulting in significant morbidity and loss of productivity. The general practitioner must, therefore, on the one hand recognize and manage infections such as meningitis or septicaemia which present acutely and often dramatically and on the other, cope with less serious complaints related to sore throats, ear infections, chest problems, urinary tract infections, and pelvic infections. One of the important tasks of general practice is to assess the severity of the complaint and decide which merit investigation, referral or treatment. In the context of a cash-limited health service, resources must be well used and each clinician should develop clear ideas about the criteria for investigation and referral.

Clinical decision-making

All surveys of the incidence and prevalence of problems presenting in primary care show infection, and particularly respiratory infection, to be a major part of the workload.[1-3] During the year 1991–2, 78% of the population consulted the GP at least once with 31% being seen for respiratory disease. The prevalence of acute respiratory infection was four times higher than any other disease of the respiratory tract.[4]

Infections present to the GP in a variety of ways. Apart from the symptoms and signs resulting from the body's general response, other symptoms may help to locate the body system principally affected. However, it remains a difficult task to identify those patients at risk of severe illness or even death when early symptoms and signs of infection are non-specific and the prevalence of life-threatening illness is low.[5] There is very little research on the predictive value of symptoms and signs in general practice making the decision to investigate a particular clinical presentation one based on experience and opinion rather than evidence.[6] In these circumstances, individual clinicians vary widely in their approaches.

In the absence of a wide literature, the authors of this chapter conducted a questionnaire survey to discover the general practice approach to the investigation of infection. We asked 120 GPs about their investigation of common infections and their use of antibiotics; 107 (89%) replied. The practices who participated were those that regularly taught undergraduates for St. Bartholomew's and the Royal London Hospital Medical School and are situated throughout the United Kingdom, along with 20 inner city practices who use the laboratory at the Homerton Hospital in Hackney, East London. They have provided background information, not available elsewhere, for this chapter.

Although GPs report that upper respiratory tract infection is the commonest infection that they see, and this is confirmed by studies of problems presenting in primary care,[6] they investigate infrequently before giving advice or treatment. Many GPs do not use antibiotics to treat certain classes of infections, even though they do not rule out bacterial infection by sending specimens to the laboratory. Many upper respiratory and gastrointestinal infections are judged to be viral and are treated symptomatically, tests only being carried out if the patient's condition worsens or the infection persists. Despite this widespread practice only a minority of the 107 GPs we surveyed claim to be able to distinguish viral from bacterial infection on clinical grounds. The GP has the potential to investigate patients with an infection in the same way as a clinician in a hospital out-patient or casualty department. In practice, this may not happen for reasons which relate to time, convenience, or a real or intuitive knowledge of the current prevalence of different infectious diseases in the practice population. The very common and irritating practice of hospital doctors re-investigating patients after hospital referral may also influence the decision.

Which patients, therefore, do GPs investigate and what sort of tests are likely to be requested? General practitioners use a wide range of tests to investigate infection in primary care; those most frequently performed are shown in Table 4.1. The proportion of the 107 doctors we questioned that are likely to use each investigation at some time is also shown. Our survey findings were confirmed in 1993 by a study in Bradford[7] which reported that mid-stream urine (MSU) test was by far the most frequently requested investigation (50% of all tests), followed by vaginal swabs (21%), and faecal samples (16%). All other investigations were requested at a rate of less than 2% of all requests. In this study, GPs were found to be more efficient users of the microbiology laboratory than hospital doctors, with 28% of the microbiology reports leading to a change in therapy. Most of the doctors in the authors' survey also used the examination of a full blood count and an ESR (erythrocyte sedimentation rate), in addition to culture or its alternatives when investigating some infections. This was particularly true of infection in elderly patients, which caused greater concern to the majority of the GPs that we surveyed, than any other group of patients presenting with infection.

The likelihood that a test may be requested reflects only in part the incidence of the relevant infection in general practice. The decision to investigate is based on the clinical presentation, including the severity, and the likely difference that the investigating clinician thinks that the result will make to the choice of therapy and outcome for the patient. Difficulty in obtaining a specimen, such as an endocervical swab or faeces, and problems

Table 4.1 *Investigations requested in general practice**

Investigation	Made use of (%)
Mid-stream urine (MSU)	99
High vaginal/endocervical swab	96
Wound/skin/abscess	87
Stool culture	87
Throat swab	65
Eye swab	47
Per-nasal swab	27
Blood cultures	19

* The authors' survey of 107 practitioners.

with transport to the laboratory also bear on the decision. Sometimes practical constraints lead to poor care. When the GP decides to manage a patient with a presumed infectious disease on the basis of probability and local knowledge of prevalence ('there's a lot of it about'!) it is important to remain vigilant for the clinical presentation and natural history that does not quite fit the usual pattern. The responses from the 107 GPs in the authors' survey correlated well with the experience of a microbiology laboratory in a busy inner city district general hospital. The test the GPs requested most frequently was MSU, although many doctors do not screen the urine for protein before they send it to the laboratory. High vaginal swabs, wound/abscess swabs, stool cultures, and throat swabs were all used to investigate patients although there were wide variations. Throat culture, for example, is characterized by high use by a few doctors, with others rarely requesting the investigation. Other investigations which are used infrequently include sputum culture, eye swabs, per-nasal swabs, skin scrapings, and paired blood samples to screen for viral infections. In general, the types of samples sent by GPs in order to investigate infections are simple and non-invasive with 90% comprised of either swabs or urine specimens.

Blood cultures are infrequently requested and may present a special problem to the GP. The reasons for this are practical, technical, and clinical. Unless there is a high demand for blood cultures the culture bottles required for them may be out of date before they are used. Once the culture is obtained it must be incubated at 37 °C or fragile organisms may not be sustained. Finally, it could be argued that patients who require blood cultures should be in hospital; they have already been identified as 'different' from other patients. It is sensible for the GP to discuss these patients with the microbiologist or infectious diseases specialist to plan management and follow-up whether the culture proves positive or negative.

When microbiological tests are sent to the laboratory a number of factors must be considered. What are the benefits and what are the costs to the patient, the practice, and the laboratory? For example, if a young woman presents with dysuria is it reasonable to:

- Do microscopy in the surgery?
- Do a strip test looking for protein?
- Start antibiotics on the basis of symptoms and history?
- Send urine to the laboratory and await results?
- Send specimen, prescribe antibiotics, and adjust therapy later?

All of these options may be used in practice although doctors have a preferred action which they usually justify on the basis of local patterns of practice. Similarly, although GPs report that upper respiratory tract infection is the commonest infection that they see, only a small number of enthusiasts regularly send throat swabs. Also, there is less consensus on the use of this investigation, in contrast to that which seems to prevail in the investigation of a urinary tract infection.

Viral infections

Although viral infections are very commonly seen in general practice they are, seldom formally diagnosed apart from a few notable exceptions, such as hepatitis, infectious mononucleosis, and HIV. Many laboratories do not have the facilities to offer viral diagnostic services to GPs and the procedures are in any case, usually too slow to influence patient management. The self-limiting nature of most viral illness and the lack of effective treatment also make investigation appear irrelevant. Developments in virology during the 1980s make the need for viral diagnostic tests more pressing. Many GPs will be involved in the care of immunosuppressed patients as a consequence of AIDS and the use of immunosuppressive drugs and cytotoxic agents. In these situations, the diagnosis of infection is important to enable the sensible use of antibiotics and informed discussion with the patient on prognosis and management. Recent advances have lead to the possibility of antiviral chemotherapy for several infections. Amantadine and acyclovir may be used in treating influenza A and herpes simplex virus, respectively, and ganciclovir is of use in immunosuppressed patients with cytomegalovirus disease. In fact, technology now allows reliable diagnosis of a wide range of viral infections with the results available within a few days of receiving the specimen (Table 4.2). These rapid tests are based on a variety of approaches; microbial antigens may be detected using polyclonal or monoclonal antibodies in enzyme immunoassays or immunofluorescence. The future development of the detection of viral DNA after amplification with the polymerase chain reaction (PCR) will also open up huge possibilities.[8]

Treating infection 'blind'

Table 4.3 shows the usual management of common symptoms by 107 GPs, on those occasions when they are considering the use of antibiotics. All of the actions in Table 4.3 may be justifiable in the context of some general

Table 4.2 *Availability of non-culture tests for rapid viral diagnosis*

Virus	Type of test
Respiratory	
Respiratory syncytial virus	Antigen detection
Gastrointestinal	
Rotavirus	Enzyme immunoassay
Hepatitis	
Hepatitis A	Detection of antihepatitis A virus IgM
Hepatitis B (acute)	Antigen and antibody detection
Herpesvirus	
Herpes simplex virus	Antigen detection
	DNA probe
Varicella zoster virus	Antigen detection
Cytomegalovirus	Antigen detection
Epstein–Barr virus (EBV)	Paul–Bunnell (detection of heterophile antibodies)
Human immunodeficiency	
HIV-1	Antigen detection

practice consultations, although the clinical certainties on which they are based are far from clear. Investigations which are convenient and possible for the patient may conflict with what might be considered ideal clinical practice. For the young woman with dysuria, optimal management would include performing a culture of a urine, but the threshold and significance differs in various clinical situations. A child with similar symptoms would certainly require a carefully taken MSU, since the documentation of a urinary tract infection in a child has greater implications than a simple urinary tract infection in a young woman.

The usefulness of tests

When a test is used to diagnose infection the clinician should consider the following questions:

1. Will the test give useful additional information in reaching a diagnosis?

2. Does the patient benefit from having the test performed?

3. What is the impact on the patient of a false positive or false negative result?

4. What is the effect on the patient of waiting for a result before initiating treatment?

The diagnosis of some infections increasingly depends on tests other than

Table 4.3 *Common symptoms and antibiotic use in general practice**

Symptom	Send specimen start antibiotics (%)	Send specimen, wait (%)	No specimen, start antibiotics (%)
Urinary tract infection	82	5	13
Sore throat	13	13	49
Vaginal discharge	55	32	12
Red eye	29	1	67
Infected leg ulcer	27	32	19
Wound	41	30	19
Cough	10	6	78
Ear discharge	35	6	56
Diarrhoea	2	63	20

* The approach adopted by 107 general practitioners in the authors' survey considering the use of an antibiotic for patients with common symptoms. Data were missing for 9 respondents. Other missing responses for each symptom are those respondents who claimed never to use an antibiotic for that *symptom.*

culture, all of which have a sensitivity of less than 100% thus leading to false negative results. Equally, these tests will have a specificity of less than 100% leading to false positives. An excellent diagnostic test has a sensitivity and specificity of 95% and many tests used in clinical diagnosis do not achieve this performance. It is important that the implications of sensitivity and specificity and the concepts of the positive and negative predictive value of a test are understood as it may be unwise to place reliance on the result of one test, particularly if the diagnosis has major implications for the patient.[9] These concepts are defined and explained in Table 4.4.

The positive predictive value (ppv) of a test varies with the prevalence of the disease in the population; as the prevalence falls so the ppv of a test falls with it and the negative predictive value (npv) rises. If the disease is uncommon then a large percentage of the positive results will be false positives. Testing for *Chlamydia trachomatis* infections using antigen detection tests is a good example. In the general practice setting, where the prevalence in asymptomatic women is less than 5%, a test with a sensitivity and specificity of 95% has a ppv of 50%. In other words, a positive antigen detection test may well be a false positive and should be repeated or confirmed by culture. A negative result is highly likely to be accurate in that the npv value is 99.7%. HIV testing in low prevalence populations is fraught with the same difficulties; a false positive result is more likely than a true positive in people tested for insurance medical examinations. The clinician must carefully consider

Table 4.4 *The sensitivity, specificity, positive, and negative predictive value of a test*

		Target disorder	
		Present	Absent
	Positive	a	b
Test result			
	Negative	c	d

- The sensitivity of a test is defined as the proportion of people with the target disorder who have a positive test result: a/(a + c)
- The specificity of a test is defined as the proportion of people who do not have the target disorder who have a negative test result: d/(b + d)
- The positive predictive value of a test is defined as the proportion of people with a positive test result who do have the target disorder: a/(a + b)
- The negative predictive value of a test is defined as the proportion of people with a negative test result who do not have the target disorder: d/(c + d)

these issues before ordering the test and decide how the result would be communicated when it may be a false positive and how to confirm the diagnosis. For bacteria and culturable viruses the reference test with which new tests are compared is culture. While the specificity of culture may reasonably be assumed, the sensitivity depends on the many factors which may compromise the recovery of an organism from a clinical specimen thus giving rise to a false negative. Recent improvements in technology have lead to the development of rapid tests for viral diagnosis which are more sensitive than the reference method. In situations where there is any doubt about which result is the true one, other methods (e.g. serological confirmation) should be carried out. Attention to collection of specimens and the techniques of the test will keep these problems to a minimum.

Investigations

The range and use of the common microbiological investigations requested by GPs, classified into those that are essential (given the type of patient and the presenting complaint), those that are desirable, and those that might be considered to be optional are shown in Table 4.5. Further discussion about the relevance of individual tests to everyday clinical practice, which is sometimes contentious, can be found in the Chapters on the corresponding body system.

Once the decision to take a specimen has been made, there are a number of logistical problems to be overcome. How does it get to the laboratory? Does the patient take it? Is there a collection service? Will the patient have

Table 4.5 *Guidelines for microbiological investigations used in general practice*

Specimen	Essential	Desirable	Optional
Mid-stream urine (MSU)	Children Pregnant women Men	Young women	
Throat	Ill children with systemic signs	Exudative tonsillitis	Any sore throat
Eye	Purulent discharge in neonate	Conjunctivitis	
Ear	Acute discharge	Chronic discharge	Discharge following antibiotics
High vaginal	New presentation of vaginal discharge	Recurrent thrush	
Endocervical	Acute pelvic inflammatory disease; possibility of sexually transmitted disease		
Faeces	Children with diarrhoea; Returning travellers with diarrhoea; Food-handlers with diarrhoea	Adults with diarrhoea	
Pus	Any site		
Blood cultures	Septicaemia, consider hospital admission		

presented before, or after, the collection has been made? Will it have to remain in the surgery overnight before the laboratory receives it? Should it be refrigerated, incubated, placed in bacterial or viral transport media? Local arrangements will largely determine the answers to these questions, but unless they are 'right' the validity of laboratory reports may be questioned and the interpretation of results suspect.

Finally, timeliness of reports is really what is relevant to their use in a clinical setting. Telephone reporting of potentially urgent results from the laboratory to hospital clinicians is usual practice and should be extended to GPs on a regular basis. Rapid receipt of results should improve as computer links with health centres and general practices increase, but will not replace the communication between GP and microbiologist which may be an important determinant in better out-patient care.

A general practice laboratory?

The question of whether a health centre or GP's surgery should maintain a practice laboratory is being considered increasingly. There are several reasons why it may be thought desirable to establish one. It has the potential to produce rapid results allowing for more informed and immediate decisions on patient management. It may, in the current climate of accounting for costs and expenditure, be less expensive than paying for laboratory investigations, and finally, it inevitably allows the GPs greater independence in making decisions about patient care.[10]

Arguments against local laboratories are equally cogent. Only a limited range of tests are available and none include culture and sensitivity testing which must clearly be the gold standard for most bacteriological investigations. Quality control has been shown to be difficult to maintain[11] and standardize. Also, considerations of health and safety standards, especially in view of the introduction of legislation on the Control of Substances Hazardous to Health (COSSH) in January 1990, are of considerable importance. This law replaced the Health and Safety Act of 1974 and makes the individual's employer personally and legally responsible for conditions of safety at work. The implications of such legislation in terms of handling biological fluids outside of properly controlled laboratory conditions must be formally and seriously addressed by GPs.[12] Many practitioners are not aware of their responsibilities under this legislation and practice nurses in one study were unaware of local external quality control procedures which would have ensured accuracy and safety.[11–13]

Preparation for introducing near-patient testing

If a general practice decides to embark on near-patient testing to improve the management of infection the following questions should be answered first:

Which tests will be undertaken and why?
- Which equipment is the best?
- How expensive will it be?

How will the equipment be maintained and repaired?
- What is the back-up when the system fails?

Will health and safety standards be initiated and maintained?

Personnel
- What skills are required?
- Who will undertake training and assessment?

Quality assurance?
- How will the accuracy and reliability of results be assured?

Reporting and interpretation of results
- Is the person reporting trained to interpret the results? If not, who takes responsibility?

Safety and infection control in general practice

Whether a practice carries out near-patient testing or not, there must be a policy to ensure that all staff exposed to body fluids, including those at risk of being bitten or scratched by patients, those who handle clinical waste, and those who take and handle specimens receive immunization against hepatitis B. All staff should be trained to avoid needlestick injuries[14] and a protocol for managing accidents should be available and regularly updated.[15] (See also Appendix 2, Chapter 2.)

Every practice must have a rigorous approach to the disposal of clinical waste. The use of sharps' containers and proper receptacles for dressings, etc., is mandatory and arrangements can be discussed with the health authority, the local authority, the local infection control nurse, or the hospital infection control officer. The GP will be legally liable if accidents result when proper arrangements have not been made. Surveys of the sterilization of equipment in general practice shows inappropriate use of chemical disinfectants and inadequate use of boiler sterilizers.[16] Practices should use an autoclave to sterilize instruments, such as vaginal speculae, or use disposables.[17,18] All instruments must first be scrupulously cleaned to remove all debris. Bowls used for washing instruments before sterilization should be cleaned with a hypochlorite or phenolic solution. It is the responsibility of the GP to ensure that these procedures are carried out to the highest standard.

Using the laboratory

Purchasing and providing in the health service

The reforms introduced into the health service in 1992 have led to changes in the relationship between the GP and the hospital laboratory service. There is an increasing awareness of cost and efficiency and an appreciation of the attitudes and behaviour required of both agencies in order to foster good standards of care for the patient. As always, the greatest improvement in the quality of care for the patient will result from the improved understanding of the role of both parties which comes from better communication. The ideal situation is described in Tables 4.6 and 4.7.

Table 4.6 *General practitioner requirements from the laboratory*

- Well-designed single request forms
- A safe method for the transport of specimens
- A safe policy and equipment for blood sampling
- A reference manual which includes sample requirements for each test, clinical indications for its use, and a guide to the interpretation of results. The sensitivity and specificity of non-culture methods used for the diagnosis of infection should be reported
- A laboratory newsheet describing new tests and their proper uses and any changes in the relevance of established tests to diagnosis. Local prevalences of community-acquired infections and patterns of antibiotic resistance might also be included
- A specimen collection service timed to reflect patterns of clinical practice
- An efficient and accurate system of reporting results with a failsafe mechanism for ensuring that potentially dangerous situations are dealt with appropriately
- A telephone helpline to discuss difficult clinical situations both in respect of diagnosis, test interpretation, and management including the use of appropriate antibiotics
- A commitment to participate in continuing medical education for the users of the laboratory. The exchange during these activities would be mutually beneficial

Table 4.7 *Laboratory requirements from the general practitioner*

- Request forms filled in completely and legibly to include clinical data
- Specimens in sealed containers and appropriately labelled
- Specimens correctly taken and stored in line with the laboratory recommendations
- The GP has reflected on the contribution of the test to diagnosis and management before requesting it
- The GP or a deputy is available to discuss important results with the medical microbiologist
- The GP will discuss the investigation of infection and the use of antibiotics in unusual or difficult clinical circumstances with the medical microbiologist

What to discuss with the microbiologist

General practitioners can gain a great deal from discussing clinical problems with the local microbiologist. The discussions also help the hospital specialist to gain some understanding of the nature of primary care and natural history of infection outside of hospital. When given the opportunity, GPs emphasize the following broad areas in which discussions with a microbiologist might be of benefit in helping in the management of patients in primary care.

Investigations

Problems concerning investigations fall into two main groups: (1) clinical advice relating to the investigation of specific patients; and (2) practical advice related to which specimens should be sent, under what conditions, and the anticipated length of time before results might be available.

1. *Clinical advice on investigations*
These queries relate most commonly to four categories of patients:

(i)   those with a pyrexia of unknown origin (PUO), often in a patient from abroad;

(ii) patients with persistent or recurrent infections (e.g. recurrent urinary tract infections in pregnancy);

(iii) ill patients in whom investigations to date have shown no abnormality;

(iv) situations in which screening might be of benefit.

There are no standard answers to any of these questions, but discussion between the GP and the microbiologist is likely to benefit by devising a plan to move the investigations forward in individual cases.

2. *Practical advice on investigations*
Discussions here are usually of a practical nature and may relate to the conditions under which specimens should be sent. Examples include investigation of pertussis, culture of which requires specialized media, and the need for specific media for viral isolation in certain clinical situations. The usefulness of skin scrapings for fungal culture occasionally leads to some debate and the requirement for repeated stool cultures, especially in food-handlers, are all the basis for discussion. Local microbiologists can help address a number of these problems, including turn-around times, with a local laboratory book which can also be a useful source on the latest guidance from the Public Health Laboratory Service (PHLS), for example, on good practice in screening and follow-up of food-handlers.

Antibiotic advice

General practitioners and microbiologists often discuss therapeutic options in a number of clinical situations. 'Best guess' therapy for simple urinary tract infection is helpfully guided by knowledge of local resistance patterns;

alternative therapy for patients with specific antibiotic allergies may be found, especially since most laboratories test more antibiotics than they routinely report; acceptable antibiotic therapy for pregnant or breast-feeding women is also a popular subject for discussion; and finally, antibiotic prophylaxis, most commonly for exposure to bacterial meningitis (*Neisseria meningitidis* and *Haemophilus influenzae*) is an important point of liaison between primary and secondary carers.

Interpretation of results

Many clinical microbiologists put comments on reports that are sent out to highlight the presence of unusual or unanticipated findings. This often relates to the finding of an unusual organism (e.g. *Pseudomonas aeruginosa* in a primary care setting) or a resistant organism (e.g. methicillin-resistant Staphylococcus aureus, MRSA). A subsequent conversation between the GP and microbiologist is often helpful in determining the significance of the finding and its appropriate management. *Corynebacterium diphtheriae*, which is isolated from a throat swab is usually non-toxigenic, but will require a great deal of discussion between the GP and the microbiologist to ensure that appropriate procedures are followed until toxin results are known. The significance of this and other culture results may again establish important communication links between GPs and microbiologists.

The general practitioner and infection control

The final area in which the GP often finds discussion useful relates to infection control. Issues relating not only to prophylaxis but to reporting of notifiable diseases (see Appendix 1, Chapter 2) and to the management of potential contacts, often in conjunction with the Consultant in Communicable Disease Control, require close liaison. Finally, practical issues relating to decontamination of equipment, sterilization, and surgery policies for sharps and spillages may be beneficially discussed with the local infection control nurse or microbiologist. If the reader is not fortunate in his/her relationship with the local microbiologist an invitation to the practice, or to speak at the local postgraduate centre might alter the situation and release a valuable resource for the management of infection in the primary care setting.

References

1. Fleming D M, Norbury C, Crombie D. Annual and seasonal variation in the incidence of common diseases. Twenty-three years experience of the Weekly Returns Service of the Royal College of General Practitioners. *RCGP Occasional Paper* 53. London (1991)

2. Davey P *et al*. Repeat consultations after antibiotic prescribing for respiratory infection: a study in one general practice. *Brit J Gen Pract* (1994) **44**: 509–13

3. Eskerud J R, *et al*. Fever in general practice: Frequency and diagnoses. *Family Pract* (1992) **9**: 263–9

4. McCormick A, Fleming D, Charlton J. *Morbidity statistics from general practice. Fourth national study* (1991–1992) OPCS London: HMSO 1995 (ISBN 0 11 691610 9)

5. Holme C. Incidence and prevalence of non-specific symptoms and behavioural changes in infants under the age of two years. *Brit J Gen Pract* (1995) **45**: 65–9

6. Owen P. Clinical practice and medical research: bridging the divide between the two cultures. *Brit J Gen Pract* (1995) **45**: 557–60

7. Tompkins D S, Shannon A. Clinical value of microbiological investigations in general practice. *Brit J Gen Pract* (1993) 43: 155–8

8. Cheun Lee P, Hallsworth P. Rapid viral diagnosis in perspective. *BMJ* (1990) **300**: 1413–18

9. Sackett D, Haynes R B, Guyatt G, Tugwell P. *Clinical epidemiology: a basic science for clinical medicine.* Boston/Toronto/London: Little, Brown and Company. (1991)

10. Hilton S *et al.* Near patient testing in general practice: a review. *Brit J Gen Pract* (1990) **40**: 32–6

11. Hilton S. Near patient testing in general practice: attitudes of general practitioners and practice nurses, and quality assurance procedures carried out. *Brit J Gen Pract* (1994) **44**: 577–80

12. *Guidelines for implementation of near-patient testing.* Association of Clinical Biochemists. London: Royal Society of Chemistry. (1993)

13. Cooke R, Hodgson E. General practitioners and health and safety at work. *BMJ* (1992) **305**: 1044.

14. Anderson D *et al.* Preventing needlestick injuries. *BMJ* (1991) **302**: 769–70

15. Lockie C, Murray S, Southgate L. Management of needlestick injuries. (letter) *Brit J Gen Pract* (1991) **41**: 432

16. Foy C et al. HIV and measures to control infection in general practice. *BMJ* (1990) **300**: 1048–9

17. British Medical Association. A code of practice for sterilisation of instruments and control of cross infection. London: *BMA* 1989

18. Hoffman P *et al.* Control of infection in general practice: a survey and recommendations. *BMJ* (1990) **297**: 34–6

CHAPTER FIVE

The treatment of infection

This chapter turns to the question of treatment of infection and in particular the use of antibiotics. In the period 1977–87, about 50 million prescriptions for antimicrobial agents were written in the UK representing 12.5% of all prescriptions.[1] Over the period 1980–91 there was an overall increase of 45.8% in England for the number of prescriptions for antibiotics with the greatest rise in prescriptions for quinolones.[2] The decision to treat a patient with antibiotic therapy should not be entered into lightly. Reaching for the prescription pad to offer a patient antibiotic therapy unnecessarily must be one of the commonest ways that harm is done to patients in modern general practice. The harm to the patient is usually merely at the level of inconvenience but very occasionally it may become life-threatening. In addition, a great deal of money is wasted; the Audit Commission have estimated that £275 million could be saved from the NHS drugs' bill if overprescribing was reduced and it cites antibiotics as one of the principal reasons.[3] Although it is well recognized that clinicians prescribe antibiotics for complicated reasons and not simply because they believe that it is the appropriate therapeutic option,[4] it is important that they have insight into their own behaviour and that management plans reflect a mature consideration of the interplay of clinical, interpersonal, and societal factors that affect all prescribing decisions. In this chapter, the art and science of antibiotic therapy will be considered and readers encouraged to reflect on the balance achieved within their own practice.

The basis for prescribing antibiotics

Prescribing patterns in the treatment of infections vary greatly between countries, regions, and doctors. Each decision to prescribe is influenced by a multitude of factors some of which may not be readily identifiable by the prescribing doctor but which derive from clinical experience, medical education, and many other areas of influence. While some factors lead to rational and sensible prescribing others lead to apparently irrational behaviour. From time to time most GPs adopt a prescribing policy which may appear to be inappropriate but which is suitable in the particular circumstances.

Howie[56] has made a considerable contribution to understanding the influences that affect the ways in which GP use diagnostic terms and manage respiratory illness in general practice. In 1976[7] he showed that variations in social and psychological history had a major effect on the decision to prescribe. In another study[8] he showed that the use of antibiotics for episodes of acute respiratory illness in children was related to use of psychotropic drugs by their mothers. The time of highest antibiotic use of the children coincided with the time of lowest psychotropic drug use in their mothers. He suggested that the child's presentation was a presentation of the mother's anxiety and that prescribing antibiotics merely compounded the problem.

A New Zealand study[9] found that antibiotics were prescribed at more consultations (14.9%) than any other drugs. Figures from the health service indicate that one-quarter of all antibiotic prescriptions in general practice are written for patients under six years old. Over 24 million prescriptions for antibiotics were written for patients in the United States with acute otitis media in 1985 (National Centre for Health Statistics; data obtained from the National Ambulatory Medical Care Survey 1985). The usage of antibiotics far exceeds the prevalence of bacterial infection in childhood; clearly overprescribing exists.

A survey of oral antibiotic prescriptions for all age groups was carried out in a semi-urban general practice and lead to the construction of a practice formulary.[10] Antibiotic prescribing was reviewed after it had been used for a year and showed that there was a reduction in antibiotic costs without an increase in the number of patient consultations, home visits, or referrals to hospital. While most prescriptions in general practice are for respiratory tract symptoms there is also cause for concern in the treatment of genitourinary and skin infections. The GP is by no means the only offender, hospital doctors should also plead guilty!

Most bacterial infections in general practice are, however, due to organisms that are sensitive to well-tried, well-established antibiotics; these should be used as a first-line choice. General practitioners should be aware of the factors influencing choice and attempt to create and maintain an established antibiotic policy or practice formulary that encourages logical, simple, and economic prescribing. The wide variety of considerations which must be born in mind are shown in Table 5.1.

Therapy decisions

Many of these influences on the decision to prescribe an antibiotic are not 'clinical'. The thoughtful physician in general practice or hospital will already have a built in awareness of their contribution to the quality of diagnosis and management. Clinical tunnel vision frequently results in non-compliance or iatrogenic morbidity. Motivation to give the best treatment involves holistic awareness.

The reader might like to consider the suggestions in Table 5.2 to adopt as practice policy. Any one of the issues would form the basis for a practice clinical meeting or a tutorial with the trainee.

Table 5.1 *Factors influencing the prescribing of antibiotics*

Clinical
Assessment of probability of bacterial/viral cause
Swab or specimen microbiology (if available)
Knowledge of local prevalence of disease
Duration of infection
Site
Severity of infection
Differential diagnosis includes severe illness (e.g. meningococcal)
Concurrent disease
Possible drug interaction

The patient
Age and weight
Pregnancy
Breast-feeding
Malabsorption
Renal function
Hepatic function
Compliance
Social circumstances (e.g. living alone)
Mental state
History of drug sensitivity or allergy
Possible photosensitivity

The family
Parental skills
Health of other members of the family, particularly parent or carer
'Hidden agenda' of accompanying adult/carer
Patient or family expectations

The doctor
Doctor–patient relationship (negotiating treatment)
'Defensive' medicine
Peer group example or pressure
Length of consultation available
Clinical competence and confidence
Status: principal/trainee/locum
Cost to the NHS
Practice formulary
Recent Postgraduate Education meeting or visit from pharmaceutical
    representative
Hospital prescription to be continued.
Multiple management/poor communication/poor records

The context of the consultation
Temporary resident
Impending holiday
Availability of appropriate treatment
Distance from pharmacy
Accessibility of laboratory service
'Friday evening' surgery
Cost to the patient

Table 5.2 *Suggested practice policy on prescribing antibiotics*

- Prescribe generically
- Identify infecting organism and prescribe accordingly
- Do not prescribe expensive or new antibiotics when simpler well-tried treatment is available.
- Critically appraise drug company literature
- Develop and use a practice formulary
- Avoid multiple drugs and 'more is better' attitude
- Be aware of the implications of:
  - Local antibiotic sensitivity patterns
  - Prescribing in pregnancy
  - Drug interactions
  - Correct and appropriate anti-infective treatment in the chronically ill and at the extremes of life
  - Failure to obtain agreement and consent
  - Poor record-keeping

Each time a doctor decides to prescribe in the treatment of infection he/she must appreciate that a 'successful' doctor–patient encounter is patient-centred on a variety of topics, including the acceptability of treatment. Cockburn *et al.*[11] investigated the process and content of general practice consultations during which antibiotics were prescribed. Analysis of videotapes of consultations lead them to conclude that:

General practitioners did not provide adequate details of some important aspects of prescribed antibiotic regimens. Given the large quantities of antibiotic agents that are prescribed in general practice, this has major implications: outcomes may be poor; wastage undoubtedly occurs and repeat prescriptions may be needed. Moreover, according to the measures that were used in this study, doctors and patients are still far from being the equal partners that is implied in the mutually reciprocal relationship, which both doctors and patients say is important.

The 'Six Ws' of antibiotic prescribing

The complicated nature of the transaction leading to the prescription of an antibiotic has been reviewed in the previous sections. The reader might find it convenient to remember the following summary of the issues that should be reviewed during the consultation.

1. Who?

Before antibiotics are prescribed, the individual patient, his/her history (including allergies and current medication), vulnerability, and social circumstance need to be assessed. The very young, elderly, and patients who are on immunosuppressive therapy (of whom there are increasing numbers in the community) would clearly lower the decision threshold for treatment in uncertain cases. Patients with a fever who are living on their own in whom one might like to 'wait and see' may require early intervention because circumstances do not readily permit an expectant approach. A student alone in a flat with an attack of influenza is a familiar example of this problem.

2. Why?

The therapeutic basis for prescribing antibiotics rest on the assumption that a bacterial infection is present which is likely to be amenable to available antibiotic treatment. Patients are often confused by this and may assume that any infection (viral, protozoal, fungal, or bacterial) can be usefully treated with antibacterial agents. This view is entirely under-standable amongst the lay public, especially when it is fuelled by such confusions in daily newspapers which at one and the same time call *Staphylococcus aureus* (e.g. MRSA) or α-haemolytic streptococcus both a virus and a bacteria (*Sic*)! For clinicians, however, there should be reasonable clinical evidence that a bacterial infection is present before antibiotics are prescribed. In general practice this may not necessarily mean that positive culture results have been received—they rarely will have been—but that the clinical situation is such that it is likely or very likely that bacterial infection is present. If there is doubt and the patient is 'safe', then investigations should be sent and treatment withheld until culture results are known.

3. Where?

The site of an infection often determines the choice of the antibiotic, its dose, and the route of administration. The principal need is to obtain an adequate concentration of antibiotic at the site of infection to deal with the infecting organisms. This requires an appreciation of the basic pharmacokinetics of the antibiotic especially with respect to its penetration into various tissues, including devitalized tissues. Some antibiotics (e.g aminoglycosides) are inactivated by purulent material and are not very effective, for example, in the treatment of abscesses.

4. When?

Antibiotics should ideally be started after specimens have been collected and/or as soon as possible once the decision to use them has been made. The single critical exception to this in general practice is when bacterial meningitis is suspected. Under these circumstances, intramuscular (IM) or intravenous (IV) antibiotics should be given without waiting for a lumbar puncture to be performed and the patient should be referred urgently to hospital.

5. Way?

In general practice most antibiotics are given by the oral route. The important exception is again bacterial meningitis when intramuscular or intravenous antibiotics *must* be used. There is no place for oral therapy here. Occasionally, in an attempt to avoid hospital admission some GPs may start a patient with a chest infection or pneumonia with an IV or IM dose of antibiotics. Such patients obviously require careful selection and frequent review. Finally, topical antibiotics have a limited role in general practice. They are most frequently and appropriately used in conjunctivitis and sometimes in acne. Almost as frequently, but less appropriately, they are also used in ear drops where they may give rise to problems with colonization by difficult and resistant organisms. Aminoglycoside-containing preparations should never be used in the presence of a perforated tympanic membrane.

6. Which?

This is the last question which should be asked in attempting to decide about antibiotic therapy, but unfortunately it is often the first. Ideally, before choosing an antibiotic for the treatment of infection the identity of the infecting organism should be known. The decision in general practice, however, will often be on the basis of an empirical best guess since treatment will of necessity often be commenced before culture results are available. Under these circumstances the choice will depend on the likely focus of infection and a knowledge both of the colonizing flora and the likely pathogens to infect the area. Considerations of patient allergy, preference (up to a point), likely penetration into the site, and potential side-effects will all be involved in the choice. Thus, prescribing erythromycin for a urinary tract infection even in a penicillin-allergic patient is not sensible since it is unlikely to be active against common urinary pathogens (i.e. coliforms) and, moreover, it does not achieve therapeutic levels within urine. Once specific culture results and antibiotic sensitivity results are known appropriate adjustments to therapy should be made.

Compliance with therapy: oral antibiotics

Many studies have shown that about 30% of patients fail to follow advice: this is as true of compliance with antibiotic therapy as any other treatments. This situation can only be improved by awareness and understanding of the reasons which stem from factors within the patient, the doctor, the relationship between them, and the nature of the therapy (Table 5.3). Many of the reasons for non-compliance stem from poor communication

Table 5.3 *Factors contributing to poor compliance with treatment*

The patient
- Age, intelligence, and mental state
- Expectations of therapy
- Degree of illness
- Past experience
- Patient's perception of severity of illness
- Rejection of diagnosis

The doctor
- Available time
- Consultation skills: does the patient feel understood? Was the explanation adequate?
- Doctor's understanding of patient factors
- Doctor appears competent to the patient

The therapy
- Acceptability of preparation (e.g. tablet size, taste of liquid)
- Possible drug interaction
- Drug allergy or sensitivity
- Unpleasant side-effects
- Misinformation: friends, neighbours, etc.
- Polypharmacy, or patient on several unrelated treatments
- Recommended length of course

The doctor–patient interaction
- The consultation outcome is dependent on a good interaction and quality of information transfer, usefully assessed by audio or videotape of consultation

Social context
- Prescription cost
- Elderly person living alone
- Recalcitrant child or infant
- Carer difficulties
- Distance from pharmacy

---

between doctor and patient leading the patient to doubt the doctor's clinical competence or concern or both.

Problems resulting from inappropriate use of antibiotics

There is evidence of inappropriate antibiotic use in both hospital and the community; misuse may have consequences for the patient in that drugs may be given when infection is not in fact present, infections may be inadequately treated, and unnecessary side-effects may result. There are in addition wider environmental issues relating to the emergence of resistant organisms and to escalating costs.

The emergence of resistance to antibiotics

Antimicrobial agents exert strong selection pressures on populations of bacteria, favouring the survival of those organisms that are resistant to them. The mechanisms that render a bacterium resistant are the result of changes in its genetic material. This genetic variability may occur by a variety of mechanisms:

1. Single point mutation of a pair of nucleotide bases within the bacterial chromosomal DNA.
2. Spread of circular extra-chromosomal DNA molecules called plasmids. These are widespread within bacteria and predate the introduction of antibiotics. Plasmids are self-replicating.
3. Portions of DNA that are not self-replicating but which can move either from one part of the bacterial chromosomal or plasmid DNA to another or between the two. These portions of DNA are called transposons. Some transposons can move from one bacterium to another independent of the chromosome or a plasmid. Plasmids or transposons can encode multiple antibiotic resistance mechanisms and hence can transfer resistance to several antibiotics under the selection pressure from a single agent.

There are several mechanisms of antibiotic resistance described in bacteria. The first, and most common, is enzymatic inactivation of the antibiotic. This is the chief means by which bacteria are resistant to the beta-lactam antibiotics (the penicillins and cephalosporins particularly), but also plays a part in the inactivation of aminoglycosides, macrolides, and chloramphenicol. Resistance also occurs by means of changes in the permeability of bacterial membranes (preventing diffusion of antibiotics to their intracellular sites of action), alteration of target sites (e.g. penicillin-binding proteins or ribosomal targets) so that the antibiotics no longer bind to them, and active pumping of antibiotic out of the cell. Each of these mechanisms can be mediated by genetic material on chromosomal or plasmid DNA.

Whatever the mechanism, and nature is endlessly inventive, the net result is that every decision to prescribe antibiotics should include attention to the possibility of resistance and newer antibiotics should be reserved for those infections that cannot be dealt with by well-tried simple first-line choices. An example of the speed of evolution of common bacteria is shown by the fact that the prevalence of intermediate or full resistance of pneumococci to penicillin increased from 1.5% in 1990 to 3.9% in 1995, and resistance to erythromycin increased from 2.8% to 8.6%.[12] A dialogue with the local microbiologist about local patterns of resistance should be the norm for every modern general practice.

Antibiotic costs

While clinical considerations are given priority in deciding antibiotic therapy, cost must always be considered. The most expensive is not always the best! Appendix 1 shows the relative costs based on a seven-day course at the usual dosage of antibiotics prescribed in general practice. As the absolute costs are more likely to vary over time than relative costs the table gives the costs in terms of 'currency units' calculated from figures in the *British National Formulary* (BNF), March 1997. The most expensive (azithromycin) has been given a currency unit of 100 and this results in the least expensive (tetracycline) being given a currency unit of 3 (i.e. azithromycin is 33 times more expensive than tetracycline).

Every GP can guard against lapsing into bad habits in prescribing antibiotics by active participation in continuing medical education, the use of the BNF, discussing the introduction of a practice formulary and engaging in medical audit.

Audit of antibiotic prescribing

Without audit, change is neither sensible or measurable. Changing the clinical policies and attitudes of any group of doctors working together is, however, far from easy. One of the great strengths and weaknesses of general medical practice is the individuality of doctors. Some GPs see audit as imposing conformity rather than encouraging rationality and resent any limits on their clinical freedom. There are large differences between the range, amounts, and costs of antibiotic prescribing between doctors caring for similar groups of patients. If there is to be any correct approach to the management of infection in general practice some of these doctors must change their prescribing habits! Only medical audit conducted among peers in local settings will answer the question of who should change and in what direction.

The introduction of audit in a group practice setting requires sensitivity to the differing interests, ages, and clinical motivation of all members. A catalyst is necessary, and may arise in a variety of ways, for example:

- One member of the practice with a particular interest and motivation may initiate change
- General dissatisfaction with irregularities in current prescribing
- Concern over prescribing costs
- Hospital, local, or regional prescribing policies
- Reading of current medical literature
- Information received from Prescription Pricing Authority Information Services (PACT Level 3)

Wyatt *et al.*[13] described an audit of the prescription of oral antibiotics in Northern Ireland. They concluded that although the survey found reasonable, conservative prescribing, the trend towards increased use of occasional agents had both clinical and cost implications which could be addressed by the use of a prescribing formulary. After the introduction and evaluation of the effects of a formulary the group reported a disappointing effect on prescribing in that doctors continued to introduce non-formulary and more expensive antimicrobials even though they were not justified on clinical grounds.[14] The authors concluded that beneficial and sustained effects could be ensured only with quarterly review of PACT and peer review. This is supported by a Swedish educational programme conducted over five years with regular audit and feedback which led to the desirable outcomes of reduced prescribing of antibiotics, an increased use of penicillin V and a decrease in the use of broad spectrum agents.[15] Needham et al.[11] reported the introduction and audit of a general practice antibiotic formulary in a semi-urban general practice. They commented, 'This study has shown that introducing a formulary to practice leads to savings in drug costs and a more unified approach to prescribing without any apparent detriment to the patients in terms of greater numbers of consultations, home visits or hospital referrals'.

In this chapter we have discussed the influences on the prescribing of antibiotics and we would urge the reader to develop the discussion within the practice so that it becomes a habit to view one's prescribing with a critical eye. A personal or practice formulary is a natural result of this process, or at the very least the regular use of the BNF becomes second nature.

Anti-infective agents

The remainder of this chapter describes commonly used and important anti-infective agents (old and new) that are encountered in general practice. Some are reserved for severe infections managed within the hospital setting but are included because they will be discussed in discharge letters and for some at least the pattern of use may change, particularly in immunocompromised patients. In any event changes in the range of care which will be undertaken in general practice and the likely increase in primary care beds will lead to an extended range of drugs being supervised by GPs. An understanding of the mechanism of action of these agents deepens the understanding of the clinician using them and avoids a 'cook-book' approach to therapy.

Antibiotic agents

These are of course, the most commonly prescribed anti-infective agents used in general practice. Given that many infections managed in general practice are treated in the absence of a proven microbiological diagnosis, the GP should become comfortable with one or two agents from each class so that 'best guess' empirical therapy in particular clinical circumstances can be recommended. The reader is referred again to the 'Six Ws' before prescribing an antibiotic agent and reminded of the problems of resistant organisms and unnecessary costs which result from an irresponsible approach.

A basis for a practice review of antibiotic prescribing

Appendix 2 at the end of this chapter shows antibiotics which could be used for the treatment of bacterial infections in general practice.

In many common situations, such as patients with a sore throat or diarrhoea, the use of any antibiotic may be unnecessary, and for the most part a practice formulary will comprise a minority of the agents included in Appendix 2. The decision to include expensive new drugs for occasional use should be taken only after full consideration of the alternatives and their use should be closely audited. The reader, along with the practice team is invited to review the list of agents we have included and to evaluate them against the 'Six Ws' and the relative costs.

More detailed descriptions of the agents we have included follow with some explanation of their modes of action and their limitations. We present them in the same order as that adopted by the BNF which should be found on the desk of every British GP!

Penicillins

Structure and mode of action. The basic structure of the penicillins is shown in Fig. 5.1. They all consist of a beta-lactam ring attached to a five-membered sulphur-containing ring and a side chain. The beta-lactam ring is essential for the antibacterial activity; the antibiotic inhibits bacterial cell wall synthesis. The cell walls of bacteria are kept rigid by a component called peptidoglycan which is synthesized by the organism in a complex series of steps. The final stages in this synthesis are dependent on a number of enzymes known as penicillin-binding proteins (PBPs) which are situated within the bacterial cell wall. The penicillins (and indeed all beta-lactam) antibiotics work by binding to certain essential PBPs and inhibiting the incorporation of new peptidoglycan into the cell wall leading to lysis and death of the organism.

Development of resistant microorganisms. Microorganisms are able to resist the effects of different beta-lactam antibiotics in a variety of ways. In some, the PBPs are structurally different so that the antibiotic is unable to bind to the site of action. In others, it is the inability of the antibiotic molecule to penetrate to its site of action. The most common mechanism, however, is the production by the bacterium of enzymes that can destroy the beta-lactam

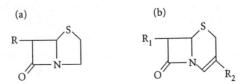

Fig 5.1 Basic structurs of (a) penem (penicillins) and (b) cephem (cephalosporins) R, R_1, R_2; side chains.

antibiotics. These enzymes are called beta-lactamases and there is are a large number of different types each with its own substrate-specificity. The genetic information enabling a bacterium to produce a beta-lactamase may be on the chromosome or on plasmids and the latter can be transferred between bacteria by conjugation, thus spreading the resistance from one organism to another (or even from one species to another).

Absorption, distribution, and excretion. The gastrointestinal absorption of the various penicillins differs markedly depending on their stability to gastric acid and whether they are ingested with food, which tends to delay and reduce absorption. Their excretion is rapid and is principally via the kidney—either by tubular secretion or by glomerular filtration or both—although a minor degree of metabolism in the liver does occur. The half-life of most penicillins is one hour or less unless the patient has renal impairment. Only in severe degrees of renal failure (a creatinine clearance of <10 ml/min), however, does the dosage of most penicillins need reduction. The tubular secretion of the penicillins can be markedly decreased by probenecid, thus producing higher plasma concentrations.

The tissue distribution of most penicillins is moderate with therapeutic levels in tissues such as the lung, kidney, bone, and soft tissues. Penetration into the cerebrospinal fluid (CSF), eye, and prostate is negligible in the absence of inflammation. As a result of low fat solubility, penicillins do not penetrate intracellularly. They do, however, readily cross the placenta and are also excreted in breast milk. Pharmacokinetics in children are similar to those in adults.

Hypersensitivity reactions. The penicillins are rarely associated with any severe toxicity. The chief adverse effects are hypersensitivity reactions, ranging from potentially fatal IgE-mediated anaphylaxis or interstitial nephritis to serum sickness-like illnesses and minor skin rashes. Anaphylaxis is uncommon, occurring in less than 1 per 1000 patients, with a slightly higher rate in atopic individuals. Much more commonly, allergic reactions to penicillin are idiopathic and produce rashes that resemble that of measles. Usually, such reactions are minor but occasionally these can progress to exfoliation or to the Stevens–Johnson syndrome. If any form of true allergic reaction occurs then the further administration of any penicillin derivative should be avoided unless formal skin testing for penicillin allergy can be performed. It is important that the fact of penicillin allergy be properly established and the patient's records marked accordingly. Too many patients believe themselves to be allergic on the basis of ill-defined episodes and others remain ignorant of the fact that they might be in danger from administration of the drug. This does not apply to the maculopapular rash that commonly occurs when ampicillin or amoxycillin is given to patients with infectious mononucleosis or lymphatic leukaemia; this is not due to true penicillin allergy. Other rare forms of toxicity with penicillins are neutropenia, haemolytic anaemia, and hypokalaemia.

Any of the oral penicillins can cause gastrointestinal upsets but this is especially likely with the broadspectrum agents such as ampicillin. More severe diarrhoea may be due to pseudomembranous colitis in association with *Clostridium difficile* infection.

Penicillins V and G

The natural penicillins are active against many Gram-positive bacteria (with the exception of staphylococci, which are now almost always resistant in the community as well as in the hospital), *Neisseria*, spirochaetes, and many of the Gram-negative anaerobic bacteria found in the oropharynx. Benzyl penicillin (penicillin G) is usually given parenterally in doses 0.5–1.0 mega-unit (1 Mu = 600 mg) every 4–6 hours; much higher doses may be needed in endocarditis or meningitis. It should be carried in the emergency bag for immediate treatment of meningococcal meningitis. Penicillin V is the preferable oral penicillin and in adults the routine dose is 250–500 mg, 6-hourly.

Antistaphylococcal penicillins

The isoxazolyl penicillin flucloxacillin is resistant to staphylococcal beta-lactamases but has less activity than penicillin against other Gram-positive bacteria and is inactive against Gram-negative organisms. Its only indication, therefore, is for staphylococcal infections. There are staphylococci that are resistant to the antibiotic as a result of altered penicillin-binding proteins; these strains are termed methicillin-resistant *Staph. aureus* (MRSA). Methicillin is another antistaphylococcal penicillin that is not used in the UK.

Aminopenicillins

Spectrum of activity. Ampicillin and amoxycillin have a broader spectrum of activity than penicillin but are not stable to the beta-lactamases of staphylococci or Gram-negative bacteria. Against Gram-positive bacteria they have similar or slightly less activity than penicillin although they are more active against *Enterococcus faecalis* (faecal streptococci).

Resistance is now common in many (up to 50% or more) of domiciliary *Escherichia coli* and 10–20% of *Haemophilus influenzae*, reducing their utility in community-acquired urinary and respiratory infections. Amoxycillin is significantly better absorbed than ampicillin after oral administration, although there are a number of esters of ampicillin (bacampicillin, pivampicillin, and talampicillin) that are better absorbed. The standard dose of all these compounds is usually 250 mg or 500 mg, given 2–4 times daily. A single 3 g dose of amoxycillin is used for cystitis.

Cephalosporins

Structure and spectrum of activity. Cephalosporins are semisynthetic beta-lactams (see Fig. 5.1) derived from a natural antibiotic obtained from a fungus originally isolated in 1945 in seawater near a sewage outlet. Structurally, they resemble penicillins except that the molecules contain a six-membered ring rather than the five-membered ring of the penicillins. Their mechanism of activity is also similar to that of the penicillins and the most important bacterial mechanism of resistance is again the production of beta-lactamases. The cephalosporins are classified on the basis of their spectrum of antibacterial activity into so-called generations. None has any useful activity against faecal streptococci, *Listeria*, *Legionella*, or *Campylobacter* species.

Only a small number of the many available cephalosporins are absorbed orally. Their pharmacokinetics are essentially the same as penicillins, with limited tissue distribution and primarily renal excretion. They cross the placenta. Some of the third-generation agents penetrate into the CSF sufficiently well for them to be useful in the treatment of meningitis. Oral cephalosporins provide a useful alternative to penicillins for a number of community-acquired infections but are infrequently drugs of first choice in general practice.

Adverse reactions and allergy to cephalosporins.   Adverse reactions are uncommon and often trivial. Hypersensitivity reactions usually consist of macular rashes although anaphylaxis can occur. Allergic reactions to cephalosporins do occur in penicillin-allergic patients and although the incidence is much lower than the 10% often quoted, if possible a non-beta-lactam agent should be used instead. Occasional, nephrotoxicity, thrombocytopenia, haemolysis, and bleeding, due to hypoprothrombinaemia, have been reported. Diarrhoea can result from administration of those cephalosporins with a broad spectrum of antibacterial activity.

First-generation agents. These cephalosporins have good activity against Gram-positive cocci and relatively modest activity against some Gram-negative bacteria such as *E. coli*. The oral first generation agents are cephradine, cephalexin, and cefadroxil: their use is limited to soft-tissue and urinary infections—none has useful activity against *H. influenzae*. They are usually administered as 500 mg oral doses every 6 hours, but the longer half-life of cefadroxil enables twice-daily administration.

Second-generation agents. These cephalosporins are more beta-lactamase stable and hence somewhat more potent against *E. coli*, *Klebsiella* species, and some *Proteus* strains. Most, but not the cephamycins (see below), also have good activity against *H. influenzae* (including most ampicillin-resistant strains) and *Neisseria* species. They include cefamandole, cefuroxime, cefaclor, and two cephamycins (molecules with a 7-methoxy group), cefoxitin, and cefotetan. These latter compounds have the added advantage of activity against many anaerobic bacteria, especially *Bacteroides fragilis*. Cefaclor and the orally administered ester, cefuroxime axetil, are each suitable for the treatment of otitis media and chest infections as well as the infections for which first-generation cephalosporins are used. The doses normally employed are 500 mg or 1 g given every 8–12 hours.

Third-generation agents. These cephalosporins are much more active than others against Gram-negative bacteria but are less active than first-generation agents against Gram-positive cocci. The third-generation agents that can be given orally are cefixime, ceftibuten, and cefetamet. They each have very good activity against most Gram-negative and many Gram-positive bacteria but no useful activity against *Staph. aureus*, most anaerobes, or *Ps. aeruginosa*. Their main uses are in otitis media, other respiratory tract infections, and urinary tract infections, particularly those that fail to respond to other antibiotics. Cefixime and ceftibuten have the advantage of a half-life that enables once-daily dosage. Cefixime absorption is only 50% or less and there is quite a high incidence of diarrhoea after its use; ceftibuten is better absorbed.

Beta-lactamase inhibitors

Some beta-lactam compounds have little intrinsic antimicrobial activity but are capable of binding to beta-lactamases and inactivating them. They thus protect other beta-lactam antibiotics from hydrolysis by these enzymes. The three beta-lactamase inhibitors presently available are marketed in fixed combinations with beta-lactam antibiotics.

Clavulanic acid

This beta-lactamase inhibitor is available in the UK as a 1:2 combination with amoxycillin (as co-amoxiclav) for either oral or parenteral use and in a 1:15 combination with ticarcillin for parenteral usage.

The addition of clavulanate to amoxycillin makes the latter effective against beta-lactamase producing staphylococci, *H. influenzae, E. coli,* and some anaerobes. It is usually given as 250–500 mg amoxycillin/125–250 mg clavulanate doses every 8 hours.

Sulbactam

This is a similar compound to clavulanic acid but is available for parenteral administration only in combination with ampicillin. It has good *in vitro* activity against most organisms responsible for mixed intra-abdominal or pelvic infections.

Tazobactam

This beta-lactamase inhibitor is available in combination with piperacillin for parenteral use only.

Tetracyclines

Mode of action, spectrum of activity, absorption, and excretion. The tetra-cyclines interfere with microbial protein synthesis at the ribosomal level and have bacteriostatic activity against a wide range of Gram-positive and Gram-negative bacteria as well as organisms such as *Mycoplasma, Chlamydia, Rickettsia,* and ureaplasmas which lack a cell wall. Their use has declined, however, largely as a result of the spread of resistance among many common bacterial pathogens and the development of safer antibiotics.

Most tetracyclines are absorbed from the stomach or upper small bowel after oral administration. They are best given in the fasting state: the concurrent administration of calcium, magnesium, aluminium or iron salts, and dairy products reduces absorption. The tetracyclines are lipid-soluble and penetrate well into most tissues: this is particularly true for minocycline and doxycycline. Tetracyclines also cross the placenta and are excreted in breast milk.

Most of the tetracyclines are excreted mainly via the urine (by glomerular filtration) and to a lesser extent in the bile. Minocycline is one exception: it has a low renal clearance and is probably metabolized to a large extent. Doxycycline is also different. Its principal excretion is as a conjugate in the faeces and there is no accumulation in patients with renal insufficiency. The half-lives of most tetracyclines are 6–12 hours but those of minocycline and doxycycline are 16–18 hours.

Side-effects and contraindications.   The most frequent adverse reactions seen with the tetracyclines are gastrointestinal. They are irritant and cause nausea and vomiting. More seriously, oesophageal ulceration can occur if they are taken without adequate fluid last thing at night. The patient should be warned about this. Diarrhoea is also quite common and may be due to active infection with *Cl. difficile* (pseudomembranous colitis).

The tetracyclines have a number of other important untoward effects. They are deposited in developing teeth and cause a permanent yellow-brown discoloration. The degree of this is dependent on the age of the child and the duration of the tetracycline administration but in general these antibiotics should not be given to pregnant women or to children up to the age of eight (the period when calcification of the permanent dentition is occurring). The tetracyclines also exacerbate uraemia by inhibiting protein synthesis and increasing amino acid metabolism. Mild phototoxicity can occur with doxycycline and severe hepatotoxicity can occur following administration of large doses of intravenous tetracycline, especially in pregnancy. Minocycline is associated with vestibular disturbances occurring 2–3 days after it is first administered, especially in women. The problem disappears a few days after the drug is stopped.

Aminoglycosides

Although the aminoglycosides are an important group of antibiotics they are hardly used in general practice because they are not absorbed from the gut and have to be given parenterally. However, some are used topically, principally in treating external ear infections where the ototoxic risk must be remembered. The members of the group are streptomycin, gentamicin, netilmicin, tobramycin, neomycin, kanamycin, and amikacin. They are used predominantly in hospitals to treat serious infections caused by enteric Gram-negative bacteria and are also effective against some staphylococci. Their mode of action is by bactericidal interference with protein synthesis. Resistance can be the result of changes in the target site or from the acquisition of plasmids encoding for inactivating enzymes. There are a number of these enzymes which each act on different aminoglycosides to a variable extent.

Aminoglycosides have a spectrum of serious adverse effects which are shared by all members of the group to some degree. The chief toxicities are dose-related ototoxicity, which can affect both the auditory and vestibular functions, and nephrotoxicity. Damage to the eighth nerve is caused by irreversible damage to the sensory hair cells: hearing loss begins with the high frequency sounds and is related to total aminoglycoside administration.

Erythromycin and other macrolides

Mode of action, spectrum of activity, absorption, and excretion. Until recently there was only one macrolide readily available in the UK, erythromycin. New compounds have now been introduced which overcome many of the shortcomings of this antibiotic. All macrolides act by inhibition of protein synthesis and their bacteriostatic activity encompasses many Gram-positive cocci, selected Gram-negative species (such as gonococci, *Campylobacter*, and *Bordetella* species), and atypical pathogens such as mycoplasma and chlamydia. Many *H. influenzae* strains are resistant.

Erythromycin is largely inactivated in the acid of the stomach and the drug must be given orally either in an acid-resistant enteric-coated form or as a variety of different acid-stable salts. There is a lack of metabolism of the acid-stable estolate and stearate salts and so the levels of the active erythromycin base are very similar whatever preparation is used. The usual dosage is 250–500 mg, 6-hourly for adults. Erythromycin can also be administered (rather painfully) intravenously.

Erythromycin is principally excreted in the bile and it penetrates satisfactorily to all sites except the brain and CSF. Its toxicity is not very severe but gastrointestinal problems, especially epigastric discomfort, nausea, vomiting, and diarrhoea are quite frequent. Occasionally, dose-related cholestatic jaundice can follow oral erythromycin salts.

The newer macrolide antibiotics include clarithromycin and azithromycin. Clarithromycin has better activity than erythromycin against *H. influenzae* (largely as a result of a microbiologically active metabolite), only needs to be given twice daily and has a much lower incidence of gastrointestinal side-effects. Azithromycin also has good activity against *H. influenzae* but its striking property is an ability to concentrate to a very high degree intracellularly. This leads to a very long half-life and many simple infections can be cured by either a single dose (a single dose of 1 g is very effective therapy for chlamydial genitourinary infections) or two to three days daily administration of the drug. Both of the new macrolides also have activity against *Mycobacterium avium-intracellulare*, an atypical mycobacterial infection particularly common in AIDS patients, and have been used successfully. There is also a strong indication that clarithromycin might be a drug of choice for therapy of *Helicobacter pylori* gastritis (see p. 262).

Clindamycin

This agent has a similar mode of action as erythromycin and also has similar activity against most Gram-positive bacteria. Most Gram-negative bacteria, including meningococci, and enterococci are resistant. Clindamycin has good activity against many penicillin-resistant anaerobic bacteria such as *B. fragilis*. It is well absorbed after oral administration and penetrates extremely well into many fluids and tissues, including bone. The usual oral dose is 150–300 mg given every 6 hours and 900 mg 3 times a day or 600 mg 4 times a day intravenously. Although clindamycin crosses the placenta and is excreted in breast milk, it does not cross the blood–brain barrier even when the meninges are inflamed. A minority of the drug is excreted in the urine, the majority being metabolized in the liver and excreted via the bile. Clindamycin is available as a vaginal cream for the treatment of bacterial vaginosis but is an expensive alternative to metronidazole.

A major problem with clindamycin is the high incidence of diarrhoea which occurs in about 10% of those given the drug, either orally or parenterally. Somewhat less than half of the patients with diarrhoea have the serious syndrome called pseudomembranous colitis or antibiotic-associated colitis. This is due to toxin production by strains of *Cl. difficile*. Although this syndrome can follow therapy with almost any antibiotic, the frequency with which it occurs after clindamycin has limited the use of clindamycin, especially in elderly patients.

Other less important adverse effects are skin rashes and transient elevation of liver enzymes.

Other antibiotics

Chloramphenicol

This antibiotic has a broad spectrum of activity against many Gram-positive and Gram-negative bacteria, including anaerobes, rickettsia, chlamydia, and mycoplasmas. Chloramphenicol inhibits protein synthesis in bacteria: this is usually a static effect although against some pathogens (including *H. influenzae*) it is bactericidal. Its potential for serious toxicity and the development of safer alternatives means, however, that chloramphenicol is now only used systemically for certain well-defined indications.

Its only use in general practice is as a topical agent in eye and less frequently, external ear infections.

Fusidic acid

This antibiotic is restricted to the treatment of infection due to penicillin-resistent staphylococci. Its use in general practice is as a topical preparation for the skin or eye.

Sulphonamides and trimethoprim

Mode of action and spectrum of activity.   The sulphonamides were the first effective chemotherapeutic agents to be developed and although they were extremely useful initially, resistant strains of bacteria became commonplace and the usefulness of these drugs diminished dramatically. The development of trimethoprim and its use in a fixed combination with sulphamethoxazole (as co-trimoxazole) led to an increased usage although recently the need for the combination in most bacterial infections has been questioned and trimethoprim is usually given as monotherapy.

Sulphonamides are structural analogues of para-aminobenzoic acid and competitively inhibit the enzyme that enables many bacteria to utilize this compound for the synthesis of folic acid. This synthetic pathway does not occur in mammalian cells which have to obtain preformed folic acid in the diet. Although many streptococci, *H. influenzae*, *Nocardia*, and some Gram-negative enteric bacteria and meningococci remain sensitive to sulphonamides many others are now resistant as a result of mutations or plasmid transfer.

Sulphonamides used for the treatment of systemic infections are readily absorbed after oral administration, distributed throughout the body, metabolized to inactive forms in the liver and excreted as both parent drug and metabolite through the kidneys. They readily traverse the placenta and small amounts are found in human milk.

Adverse reactions.   Hypersensitivity reactions are relatively common from sulphonamides and range from a variety of simple rashes, including erythema nodosum and photosensitivity, to severe erythema multiforme and the Stevens–Johnson syndrome. The earlier compounds tended to be relatively insoluble and to crystallize within the renal tubules but this is not seen with modern sulphonamides. Alkalinization of the urine is no longer necessary. Haematological problems also occur: haemolytic anaemia (sometimes associated with deficiency of glucose-6-phosphate dehydrogenase), agranulocytosis, and aplastic anaemia can all result. Finally, sulphonamides should not be given during the final weeks of pregnancy or to the neonate since they can displace bilirubin from protein-binding and lead to kernicterus in the child.

Trimethoprim

Mode of action.   Trimethoprim is a dihydrofolate reductase inhibitor. This enzyme catalyses the step in folic acid synthesis after that blocked by sulphonamides. Initially, it was introduced only in combination with sulphamethoxazole as co-trimoxazole (see below), in order to produce synergistic activity against a variety of bacteria, but trimethoprim is now widely used as single therapy.

The antibacterial spectrum of trimethoprim includes most aerobic Gram-negative and Gram-positive bacteria. Some bacteria, such as Gram-negative anaerobes and *Ps. aeruginosa*, are intrinsically resistant; other organisms acquire resistance as a consequence of alterations in their dihydrofolate reductase enzymes.

Trimethoprim is usually administered as 100 mg tablets orally and penetrates well into many tissues, including prostatic fluid, sputum, and CSF. Most of the drug is rapidly excreted unchanged in the urine by tubular secretion; the remainder is metabolized to inactive forms. Small amounts are excreted in breast milk.

Trimethoprim has a small effect on human dihydrofolate reductase which can be clinically important in the elderly and other individuals with pre-existing folate deficiency. It should not be used in pregnancy. In such cases, bone marrow suppression and megaloblastic changes can result. These adverse effects can be prevented or treated by administration of folinic acid (which does not affect the antibacterial efficacy of the trimethoprim).

Co-trimoxazole

The combination of trimethoprim and sulphamethoxazole was introduced to take advantage of the synergistic interaction between the two drugs, a synergy that was thought to reflect their action on sequential steps in bacterial folate metabolism. The true mechanism of synergy is now recognized as being due to effects of both drugs upon dihydrofolate reductase. The synergistic activity is maximal when the two drugs are in a ratio of 20:1 (sulphona-mide:trimethoprim). The antibacterial spectrum of the combination is similar to that of the individual drugs although synergy means that bacteria that are resistant to sulphonamides and moderately resistant to trimethoprim can still be sensitive to the combination. Co-trimoxazole is also active against several protozoa, including malaria parasites and *Pneumocystis carinii.*

The sulphonamide in the combination (sulphamethoxazole) and the formulation of the tablets (80 mg trimethoprim and 400 mg sulphamethoxazole) was chosen to achieve peak serum concentrations of sulphamethoxazole 20 times higher than those of trimethoprim (in order to obtain optimal synergy). The differences in tissue penetration and urinary excretion of the two drugs mean, however, that such a ratio is rarely obtained outside the serum.

The toxicity of cotrimoxazole is essentially that of the two components. Patients with AIDS are particularly prone to adverse reactions to co-trimoxazole and frequently develop fever and rash when this therapy is used for pneumocystis infections. Although it has been widely used in general practice for otitis media and urinary tract infections, it is now rarely indicated and is not recommended for inclusion in a practice formulary with the only exception to its exclusion being for patients with AIDS.

Quinolones

The older members of this class of antimicrobial agents (nalidixic acid and cinoxacin) only had limited activity against common Gram-negative bacteria and were used for urinary tract infections alone. Recently, there have been a number of developments, particularly the introduction of fluorinated

4-quinolones, which have resulted in agents with broad antimicrobial activity and the ability to treat a wide range of infections.

Mode of action.   Quinolones inhibit the bacterial enzyme DNA gyrase and this prevents the introduction of negative supercoils into the DNA: without this supercoiling, bacterial DNA transcription and replication cannot occur and the organism rapidly dies. Resistance does not develop rapidly, probably as a consequence of the fact that it is not yet shown to be plasmid-mediated.

The quinolones are generally well tolerated. Most adverse reactions consist of mild gastrointestinal intolerance, headaches, dizziness, and skin rashes. All the agents can cause cartilage erosions and arthropathy in the weight-bearing joints of immature animals. Although this has not been reported in man, these drugs are not recommended for use in children or pregnant women.

The quinolones can be divided into a number of groups based on their spectrum of activity and pharmacokinetic properties.

Nalidixic acid

The earliest quinolones (nalidixic acid, cinoxacin) have limited intrinsic activity against most common Gram-negative enteric bacteria but Gram-positive organisms and *Pseudomonas* species are resistant. They achieve very high concentrations in the urine. Nalidixic acid can cause benign intracranial hypertension and overdosage has been followed by convulsions.

Norfloxacin

This agent is about 100 times more active against Gram-negative bacteria than nalidixic acid and is also active against *H. influenzae* and gonococci. Its activity against *Ps. aeruginosa* and staphylococci is limited and there is no useful activity against anaerobes and most streptococci. Concentration of the drug in the serum are inadequate for the treatment of most systemic infections but it achieves excellent urinary concentrations. Norfloxacin is also excreted in significant amounts in the faeces.

Ciprofloxacin

The latest fluorinated quinolones have similar antibacterial activity to norfloxacin but are even more potent especially against *Ps. aeruginosa*. There is also useful activity against some *Chlamydia* and *Mycoplasma* strains. The inactivity against *Streptococcus pneumoniae* remains an Achilles' heel. These compounds are rapidly and well absorbed and have an extremely high volume of distribution (a measurement of their penetration into body fluids, tissues, and cells). Hepatic metabolism does not occur or is very limited and excretion is predominantly renal. Excretion via the intestinal mucosa is also important and there is remarkably little drug accumulation in all but terminal renal failure. These compounds are effective in infections outside the urinary tract. Oral and intravenous preparations are available for ciprofloxacin.

Nitrofurantoin

This agent is a synthetic compound that does not achieve antibacterial concentrations in the plasma but is concentrated in the urine. The organisms commonly causing urinary infections, including *E. faecalis*, are sensitive to the drug and it can therefore be used for the treatment or prevention of most simple urinary tract infections. Quite how nitrofurantoin works is not known but it is probably via the effect of metabolites upon bacterial DNA.

The urine should not be alkalinized as this reduces the antibacterial efficacy of nitrofurantoin. In renal failure less of the drug is excreted so that the efficacy is reduced and the slight accumulation in plasma may increase the chances of toxicity.

Side-effects of nitrofurantoin. The most common side-effects of nitrofurantoin are nausea, vomiting, and anorexia due to gastrointestinal irritation. The macrocrystalline form of nitrofurantoin is associated with less gastrointestinal problems. A variety of hypersensitivity reactions occur with any form of nitrofurantoin. Acute pneumonitis, starting within hours or days of initiation of therapy is more likely to occur in the elderly. It causes fever, rigors, cough, shortness of breath, and chest pain: eosinophilia and pulmonary infiltrates are found. It usually settles with cessation of therapy but more serious chronic pulmonary fibrosis is seen rarely, particularly after several months of therapy. Nitrofurantoin colours the urine brown.

Antimycobacterial agents

The principles of treating mycobacterial infection rest on the use of multiple drug regimes over an extended period of time. This is true both for 'straight-forward' pulmonary disease caused by *Mycobacterium tuberculosis*, in which therapy with three agents for two months followed by a further four months of treatment with two agents is recommended, and for atypical *Mycobacteria* disease. With the increase in the incidence of tuberculosis and the treatment of the infection carried out as an out-patient, many GPs will work with chest physicians in supervising and prescribing for these patients.

Isoniazid

This inhibits the synthesis of a cell wall component unique to mycobacteria. It kills dividing mycobacteria but is only static for resting bacteria. It is well absorbed after oral or intramuscular administration and it readily penetrates throughout the body. The drug is metabolized and most is rapidly excreted as metabolites in the urine. The initial metabolite is the result of acetylation and the rate of this is genetically controlled. Fast acetylators have much lower serum concentrations of those who are slow acetylators. Slow acetylation is found in about half of Western Europeans, a higher proportion of Scandinavians, and a very low percentage of Orientals. Acetylator status is not of any therapeutic importance but slow acetylators may accumulate toxic concentrations of the drug if their renal function is impaired. Isoniazid is commonly used in treatment regimes for *M. tuberculosis* in combination with rifampicin and pyrazinamide.

Adverse reactions. These include hepatitis, rashes, fever, and peripheral neuritis. The latter occurs quite frequently in those given more than 5 mg per kg (body weight) isoniazid daily and can be prevented by prophylactic pyridoxine. The hepatotoxicity is more common in the elderly and those with alcoholic liver disease. Patients on isoniazid should be warned to stop therapy and seek medical advice if they develop symptoms suggestive of hepatitis (i.e. anorexia, nausea, fatigue and jaundice).

The most important isoniazid drug interaction is with phenytoin and concentrations of the latter need monitoring when isoniazid is concurrently administered.

Ethambutol

This is well absorbed and distributed through the body. It is bacteriostatic for mycobacteria and is usually given in combination with other antituberculous therapy only until the sensitivity of the organism to other therapy is confirmed. At high dosage the most serious toxicity is retrobulbar neuritis, leading to decreased visual acuity and red-green colour blindness. Hence, those on ethambutol should be warned to report any optic symptoms. The dose is 15 mg/kg/day.

Pyrazinamide

This has become one of the first-line therapies for tuberculosis as a result of its bactericidal action and low toxicity. The most serious side-effect is hepatotoxicity and liver function should be checked every few weeks while the patient is on therapy.

Rifampicin

Although rifampicin (called rifampin in the United States) is primarily used for the treatment of mycobacterial diseases, it is increasingly being used for the treatment or prophylaxis of infections caused by a variety of other bacteria. Rifampicin inhibits bacterial RNA synthesis and is bactericidal. Resistance occurs if there is mutation of the target enzyme. Rifampicin is very active against *M. tuberculosis* and *M. leprae* but is less predictably active against the atypical mycobacteria. It also has good activity against most Gram-positive bacteria (including staphylococci) and against *H. influenzae* and meningococci.

Rifampicin is well absorbed and widely distributed throughout the body, including the CSF: as a result of the excellent penetration the patient should be warned that various body fluids and the faeces will turn orange-red. Rifampicin is metabolized in the liver and excreted in the bile—an enterohepatic circulation then ensues. The half-life is prolonged in patients with hepatic disease but there is no accumulation in renal failure.

Most patients given rifampicin develop minimal elevation of the serum transaminase levels, although this mild hepatotoxicity generally settles even if the drug is continued. Occasionally, however, more severe liver damage occurs. This can be assumed if there is elevation of the serum bilirubin and such a change is an indication to stop therapy. Other side-effects are rashes, thrombocytopenia, and an immunologically mediated 'flu-like' syndrome that follows intermittent (less than twice-weekly) rifampicin dosing.

Drug interactions. Rifampicin is a potent inducer of liver microsomal enzymes and this results in increased metabolism, reduced plasma concentrations, and less efficacy of a number of concomitantly administered drugs. Included in these are oral contraceptives and anticoagulants.

Antifungal agents

Antifungal agents have become increasingly important in general practice; patients are presenting with a wider spectrum of disease (e.g. oral/oesophageal candidiasis) and recent developments have led to the availability of less toxic, oral, and more accessible agents.

Imidazoles

The imidazoles inhibit the synthesis of the cytoplasmic membranes of some fungi, particularly yeasts. There are four imidazoles available: clotrimazole, econazole, miconazole, and ketoconazole: only the latter is now used for therapy of systemic infections. The cutaneous or vaginal preparations of clotrimazole, econazole, and miconazole are all absorbed to a very small degree and all can cause local stinging, itching, or burning. Ketoconazole absorption after oral administration is always variable but sufficient to treat some systemic yeast infections: absorption is diminished further by co-administration of H_2 blockers such as cimetidine.

Imidazoles can upset steroid pathways in patients and a number of endocrine problems can result. Gynaecomastia and loss of libido in men and menstrual abnormalities in women have been reported as a result of ketoconazole administration. Ketoconazole-induced hepatitis is rare but can progress rapidly and is potentially lethal. Patients need to be alerted to this and have liver function checked regularly.

Triazoles

These compounds are closely related to the imidazoles and act in a similar way on fungal sterol metabolism. They have less effect on human sterol pathways and do not have many of the drawbacks of ketoconazole. Many compounds are under development but only two, fluconazole and itraconazole, have been introduced as yet. Itraconazole is structurally very similar to ketoconazole but achieves somewhat higher tissue levels and is better tolerated. It has important activity against *Aspergillus* infection. Fluconazole is very different: it is water-soluble, almost completely absorbed from the gut and penetrates very well into the CSF. Fluconazole does not appear to cause any endocrine disturbances in humans. Since it can be administered by the oral, topical, or intravenous routes it has become an important drug in the treatment and prophylaxis of cryptococcal meningitis and in oropharyngeal candidiasis in patients with AIDS. It is also highly effective in the treatment of vaginal candidiasis which has failed to respond to local, topical treatment.

Terbinafine

This is an orally and topically active allylamine, which does not interfere with steroid hormone production in the host, thus reducing the interactions with other medications. It has a broad spectrum of activity against the dermatophytes and yeasts and has been shown to be at least as effective as griseofulvin in cutaneous dermatophytes.

Griseofulvin

This has fungistatic activity only against dermatophytes and after oral administration is concentrated in keratinized tissues. Hence, newly keratinized tissues are protected from fungal attack but treatment with griseofulvin must be continued for several weeks or months until uninfected tissue replaces that infected by dermatophytes. Griseofulvin is thus a useful agent for the treatment of dermatophytic infections of the hair and nails, where topical agents cannot be used.

The most frequent adverse effect of griseofulvin is headache but this normally abates with continuing therapy. Fatigue and a variety of minor gastrointestinal symptoms have also been recorded. Griseofulvin is an enzyme inducer and hence may lead to accelerated metabolism (and hence reduced efficacy) of drugs such as warfarin and some oral contraceptives.

Nystatin

Nystatin is a polyene antifungal antibiotic that is used topically for therapy of candidiasis of the skin, mouth, vagina, and gastrointestinal tract. It is a bitter solution that is not absorbed. Adverse effects are very uncommon.

Antiviral agents

The development of antiviral agents over the last two decades now allows the treatment of specific viral infections, many of which present in general practice. As with bacteria, the presence of selective drug pressure has already lead to the emergence of resistant virus populations.[16]

Idoxuridine (IDU)

This resembles thymidine and has inhibitory activity against some herpes-viruses. It is, however, toxic when given parenterally and it is only used topically for herpes simplex infections of the eye and skin. For cutaneous use it needs to be dissolved in dimethylsulphoxide, a powerful solvent, which can cause skin maceration. IDU use has largely been superseded by acyclovir.

Acyclovir

Mode of action. Acyclovir is a synthetic analogue of guanine, a purine base that is a constituent of DNA. Acyclovir inhibits DNA synthesis but in order to have an antiviral action it first needs to be triphosphorylated. The first step in this metabolic pathway is catalysed by a viral enzyme, thymidine kinase. This enzyme is only present in cells infected by certain herpesviruses and therefore acyclovir has a very high therapeutic ratio—in uninfected cells very little acyclovir is phosphorylated and hence the effect on human DNA is minimal.

Acyclovir is essentially only effective against herpesviruses. It is particularly active against herpes simplex viruses but its activity against varicella zoster virus is about 10-fold less. There is very little useful antiviral activity against cytomegalovirus and other herpesviruses. There are topical preparations for the skin and the eye, and both intravenous and oral formulations. When given intravenously it must be administered by infusion over an hour or so. The bioavailability is only 20%. The standard 200 mg tablets are sufficient for herpes simplex virus infections, but individual doses of 800 mg need to be given to inhibit varicella zoster virus. Higher doses do not produce higher blood levels. Acyclovir is widely distributed in the body and is largely excreted in the urine.

Very few adverse effects have been recorded. Occasionally, nausea, rashes, or phlebitis have followed intravenous therapy and encephalopathy is very rare.

Valaciclovir

This oral prodrug of acyclovir produces higher plasma concentrations than the parent drug after oral administration. A dose of 1 g three times daily is better than acyclovir at limiting the pain associated with herpes zoster. A dose of 500 mg twice daily is used in genital herpes.

Famciclovir

This is an oral prodrug of penciclovir, another synthetic nucleoside with a very similar mechanism of action and spectrum of antiviral activity to acyclovir. Famciclovir has the advantage of only needing to be administered two or three times daily. It is licensed at present for herpes zoster and genital herpes: for the former a dose of 250 mg three times daily seems at least as effective as acyclovir. The same dose is used for primary genital herpes and 125 mg twice daily for recurrences.

Ganciclovir

Ganciclovir is structurally similar to acyclovir but can not be given orally and is considerably more toxic. Its use is limited to therapy for sight-threatening or potentially lethal cytomegalovirus infections in immunocompromised patients, particularly those with AIDS. It needs to be given daily by intravenous injection and commonly results in bone marrow suppression or cerebral, liver, or kidney dysfunction. It is also mutagenic and teratogenic in experimental animals.

Patients on ganciclovir need close supervision and it is likely that this may increasingly be undertaken within general practice as part of shared care for AIDs patients.

Amantadine

This is only effective against influenza A virus strains. It is well absorbed and is then excreted unchanged in the urine. Some accumulation occurs in the elderly and others with renal impairment.

The problem with amantadine is that although it is useful both as prophylaxis and therapy of influenza A infections, it is not always easy to distinguish this infection from other respiratory viral infections except in the epidemic situation.

Accumulation of amantadine can cause neurological toxicity ranging from insomnia and lack of concentration to convulsions and hallucinations. Those with pre-existing neurological problems and those with renal impairment need closely monitoring. Amantadine should not be given in pregnancy.

Anti-HIV drugs

The mainstay of treatment for HIV infections is zidovudine, a thymidine analogue that inhibits replication of HIV. There are a number of newer compounds, including didanosine (ddI), zalcitabine (ddC), stavudine (d4T), lamivudine (3TC), ritonavir, indinavir and saquinavir.[17] In this rapidly changing field, GPs need to liaise with local HIV specialists.

Conclusion

The first five chapters of this book have dealt with principles and relationships that determine the management of the patient with infection in general practice. However, the presentation of infectious conditions usually relates to a particular part or system of the body. It is therefore necessary to explore these body systems before returning to an holistic approach to the patient with infection.

APPENDIX 1

The Approximate Relative Costs of a Seven Day Course of a Selection of Antibiotics

Antibiotic	Dosage	Relative cost
Azithromycin	*Six Tabs of 250 mg	100
Clarithromycin	250 mg bd	83
Ciprofloxacin	250 mg bd	75
Cefaclor	250 mg tds	71
Co-amoxiclav	250 mg tds	66
Doxycycline	200 mg stat. + 100 mg od	31
Flucloxacillin	250 mg qds	15
Erythromycin	250 mg qds	8
Metronidazole	400 mg tds	7
Amoxycillin	250 mg tds	5
Ampicillin	250 mg qds	5
Trimethoprim	200 mg bd	4
Phenoxymethylpenicillin	250 mg qds	3
Tetracycline	250 mg qds	3

* Six Tabs = Full course

APPENDIX 2

Developing a practice formulary for antibiotic prescribing*

Condition and organisms	Antibiotics. Select an appropriate agent according to organism isolated	Comments*
Upper respiratory tract infections Tonsillitis, *Strep. pyogenes*	Phenoxymethyl-penicillin, erythromycin	70% of sore throats are viral. Amoxycillin is no better than penicillin and has more side-effects. It causes rashes in patients with infectious mononucleosis
Recurrent tonsillitis	Co-amoxiclav or oral cephalosporin	Justified in proven recurrent streptococcal throat infections
Otitis media; *Strep. pneumoniae, H. influenzae, Staph. aureus,* group A streptococci, *M. catarrhalis,* anaerobes	Amoxycillin, trimethoprim, co-amoxiclav, cefaclor, cefixime	*H. influenzae* may be resistant to amoxycillin. Erythromycin has poor activity against *H. influenzae* and should not be used for otitis media

Otitis externa;
Staph. aureus, Proteus, and other Gram-negative organisms, *Aspergillus niger, Candida albicans* — Usually topical treatment with antiseptic, antibiotic, or compound anti-infective cortico-steroid preparations — Aural toilet aimed at keeping the ear dry is the most important part of treatment. Topical preparations containing aminoglycosides or quinolones should be used for <7 days because of the risk of ototoxicity, local reaction, or overgrowth with resistant bacteria or fungi. They should not be used at all if there is a perforated eardrum

Malignant otitis externa;
Ps. aeruginosa — Ciprofloxacin — More likely in diabetic patients and may cause progressive and life-threatening illness. These patients must be referred urgently

Sinusitis;
Strep. pneumoniae, H. influenzae, M. catarrhalis, anaerobes including *Bacteroides* and micro-aerophilic streptococci — Amoxycillin, co-amoxiclav, doxycycline, clarithromycin — Doxycycline should not be prescribed for children. It may cause acute indigestion in adults unless swallowed whole with plenty of water during a meal

Lower respiratory tract infections
Bronchitis: exacerbation of chronic obstructive airway disease in mild to moderate cases;
Strep. pneumoniae, H. influenzae, M. catarrhalis — Ampicillin, amoxycillin, erythromycin — Amoxycillin is better absorbed than ampicillin in the presence of food. Toxicity is rare with aminopenicillins. Most *Moraxella* spp. and many *Haemophilus* spp. are now resistant to aminopenicillins. Trimethoprim has poor action against *Moraxella*. Nausea, vomiting, and abdominal pain are frequent side-effects of erythromycin

Bronchitis: end-stage disease and bronchiectasis; *Ps. aeruginosa,* atypical organisms, Gram-negative enterobacteria — Co-amoxiclav, cefaclor, cefixime, azithromycin, clarithromycin, ciprofloxacin — This range of antibiotics is used for more complicated cases often involving atypical or less common pathogens

Acute pneumonia in the normal host;
Strep. pneumoniae, H. influenzae, Staph. aureus, M. pneumoniae, Legionella pneumophila, Chlamydia pneumoniae, C. psittaci, Coxiella burnetti — Penicillin, ampicillin/amoxycillin, erythromycin, clarithromycin, co-amoxiclav, flucloxacillin — First choice treatment must cover *Strep. pneumoniae*. British Thoracic Society recommendation for blind treatment of uncomplicated cases is ampicillin and/or erythromycin. Antibiotic with an antistaphylococcal activity is indicated during an influenza epidemic

Gastrointestinal infections
Helicobacter pylori in proven peptic ulcer disease — 'Triple' or 'double' therapy using antibiotics selected from amoxycillin, tetracycline, clarithromycin, and metronidazole — The regimes used for eradication of *H. pylori* also include ulcer-healing drugs and are subject to intense research and development while effective and efficient regimes are determined

| Severe infectious diarrhoea; *Shigella, Salmonella, Campylobacter jejuni* | Ciprofloxacin, ofloxacin, erythromycin | Antibiotics for *Salmonella* are necessary only for extremes of age, underlying debility or in the immunocompromised patient. Many *Shigella* spp. are highly resistant to antibiotics. Quinolones are not suitable for children. Erythromycin may be useful for proven *Campylobacter* infections but the illness is usually self-limiting |

Urinary tract infections

Acute cystitis; Gram-negative bacteria including *E. coli, Proteus, Klebsiella, Enterococcus faecalis, Staph. saprophyticus, Ps. aeruginosa*	Trimethoprim, co-amoxiclav, oral cephalosporin, nitrofurantoin, ciprofloxacin	Current local sensitivities should be known. Ampicillin resistance is now >50% of Gram-negative isolates in some practices. *Ps. aeruginosa* does not commonly cause UTI in healthy people
Prophylaxis against recurrent UTIs	Trimethoprim, nitro-furantoin, cephalosporin, norfloxacin	Regime tailored to circumstances of the patient and discussed with microbiologist and/or renal specialist
Chronic bacterial prostatitis; *E. coli, Proteus, Pseudomonas, Klebsiella*	Norfloxacin, ofloxacin	Care of these patients will often be shared with a specialist

Female genital tract infections

| Vaginitis; *Candida albicans. Trichomonas vaginalis, Gardnerella vaginalis* with picture typical of bacterial vaginosis | Topical antifungals: clotrimazole. Oral antifungals: fluconazole, metronidazole, topical clindamycin | It is important to rule out the possibility of upper genital tract infection which may coexist |
| Upper genital tract infection and cervicitis; *Chlamydia trachomatis, N. gonorrhoeae, Bacteroides*, Gram-negative bacteria | Azithromycin with co-amoxiclav. Ciprofloxacin with metronidazole. Injection of cephalosporin with doxycycline | Untreated upper genital tract infection can lead to infertility and chronic ill health. The regimes we have included are for pelvic inflammatory disease. Women with systemic symptoms should be referred for definitive diagnosis and partners should also be treated |

Skin and soft tissue infections

| Impetigo; *Staph. aureus*, group A streptococci | Topical treatment: neomycin, tetracycline, fusidic acid, mupirocin. Oral therapy: fluclox-acillin, phenoxymethyl-penicillin | Topical antibiotics should be used for <14 days because of sensitization. Systemic antibiotics may be necessary in oral therapy |
| Staphylococcal nasal carriers | Neomycin and chlorhexidine, mupirocin | |

---

* The authors of this chapter suggest you photocopy these pages and use them as a basis for developing a practice policy which includes reasons for accepting or rejecting our listed antibiotics.

References

1. Department of Health and Social Security. Prescriptions dispensed by pharmacy and appliance contractors, England 1977–87. *Statistical Bulletin* (1989) 4/2/89

2. Davey P *et al.* Growth in the use of antibiotics in the community in England and Scotland in 1980–93, *BMJ* (1996) **312**: 613

3. Audit Commission. *A prescription for improvement: towards more rational prescribing in general practice.* London: HMSO 1994

4. Britten N. Patients' demands for prescriptions in primary care. Editorial. *BMJ* (1995) **310**: 1084–5

5. Howie J G R. A new look at respiratory illness in general practice: A reclassification of respiratory illness based on antibiotic prescribing. *J Roy Coll Gen Pract* (1973) **123**: 895–904

6. Howie J G R. Further observation on diagnosis and management of general practice respiratory illness using simulated patient consultations. *BMJ* (1974) **111**: 540–3

7. Howie J G R. Clinical judgement and antibiotic use in general practice. *BMJ* (1976) **111**: 1061–4

8. Howie J G R, Bigg A R. Family trends in psychotropic and antibiotic prescribing in general practice. *BMJ* (1980) **280**: 836–8

9. Simpson J B. Pharmaceutical prescribing by Canterbury general practitioners. *NZ Fam Physician* (1984) **11**: 164–8.

10. Needham A, Brown M, Freeborn S. Introduction and audit of a general practice antibiotic formulary. *J Roy Coll Gen Pract* (1988) **38**: 166–7

11. Cockburn J, Reid A I, Sanson-Fisher R W. The process and content of general practice consultations that involve prescription of antibiotic agents. *Med J Aust* (1987) **147**: 321–4

12. Johnson A, Speller D, George R *et al.* Prevalence of antibiotic resistance and serotypes in pneumococci in England and Wales; results of observational surveys in 1990 and 1995. *BMJ* (1996) **312**: 1454–6

13. Wyatt T D *et al.* Antibiotic prescribing: the need for a policy in general practice. *BMJ* (1989) **300**: 441–4

14. Wyatt T D *et al.* Short lived effects of a formulary on anti-infective prescribing: the need for continuing peer review? *Family Pract* (1992) **9**: 461–5

15. Mölstad S *et al.* Antibiotics prescription in primary care: A 5-year follow-up of an educational programme. *Family Pract* (1994) **11**: 282–6

16. Field A K, Biron K K. 'The end of innocence' revisited: resistance of herpesviruses to antiviral drugs. *Clin Microbiol Rev* (1994) **7**: 1–13

17. Drugs and Therapeutics Bulletin. Major advances in the treatment of HIV-1 infection. *Drug Ther Bull* (1997) **35**: 25–29

CHAPTER SIX

Infections of the head and neck

Although the major part of this chapter will be devoted to sections on the ear, nose, and throat, and the eyes, we begin by remembering the proximity of these parts of the body and the common pathogens that affect them all. If we use abbreviation 'TENS' (throat, ears and eyes, nose, and sinuses), it serves as an *aide-mémoire* for the 10 major colonizing and infecting organisms of the area (Table 6.1). Most of these bacterial organisms can both colonize and cause infection and part of the clinical and microbiological skill involved in making a diagnosis is related to deciding when a colonizing organism has become an infecting one. The issue is further complicated if the bacterial infection is secondary to a viral infection.

Infections of the ear, nose, throat, and sinuses

Patients present very frequently in general practice with infections of the upper respiratory tract, ears, and sinuses.[1] Each year an average family doctor will see about 600 patients with an upper respiratory tract infection and a 100 cases of 'tonsillitis'. Only one in five of people who are affected consult the doctor and 40% of these consultations are for children under 5 years of age. Although many of these infections are benign and self-limiting and can be attributed to a viral aetiology, it is well recognized that it

Table 6.1 *Bacterial organisms that may infect the ear, nose, and throat*

Beta-haemolytic streptococci (groups A, C, G)
Corynebacterium (*diphtheriae, haemolyticum, ulcerans*)
Bordetella pertussis
Mycoplasma pneumoniae
Neisseria gonorrhoeae
Moraxella catarrhalis
Streptococcus pneumoniae
Haemophilus influenzae
Staphylococcus aureus
Pseudomonas aeruginosa

can be very difficult to distinguish, on clinical grounds, between viral and bacterial infection in certain sites of the head and neck. Added to this is the well-established association between primary viral and secondary bacterial infections. Even with a diagnosis as straightforward as 'a cold', 0.5% of episodes will be complicated by secondary bacterial sinusitis and 2% with otitis media.[2] In addition, the prodromes of some systemic illnesses such as measles and meningitis begin with upper respiratory complaints. Finally, those infections that do have a bacterial origin may be difficult to diagnose since the colonizing flora of the area is frequently the same as that involved in the infection. This chapter will explore some of these issues and will consider in some detail how ear, nose, and throat (ENT) infections may present and be managed in general practice.

The common cold (coryza)

Epidemiology and impact on general practice

Coryzal symptoms are a very frequent occurrence; the weekly incidence of common cold is between 100 and 250 per 100 000 individuals.[4] Young children may have between 8 and 12 colds per year, whilst adults tend to experience only 2 or 3. Parents of younger children often complain of having frequent colds which probably reflects the introduction of new viral strains into the household as contact with other children increases.

Many adults do not bother presenting to their GP since they recognize that the illness is self-limiting and benign. Infants and young children may be brought to the doctor more frequently, partly to obtain prescriptions for symptomatic relief but also for parental reassurance, especially if symptoms of otitis media or a persistent cough are present. The approach that the doctor adopts to these consultations is an important part of the fabric of the relationship with the family which may develop over many years. It is essential to discover if there is any reason for a lack of confidence in managing minor illness in small children. An unsupported or depressed mother, family dysfunction, or a previous cot death are all examples of the many factors that can undermine parents' confidence and lead them to seek advice. Some parents simply lack information and it is important to spend time explaining about the natural history and home management of upper respiratory tract infections, giving written advice suited to the level of understanding, ethnic background, and first language if necessary. The doctor should also confirm that no one in the house is smoking in the same room as the child, check that the family have a positive relationship with the health visitor, and that the child is fully immunized. In order to increase confidence for next time, the arrangements in the practice that ensure accessibility, availability and continuity should be outlined and the practice leaflet given to the parent to take home. An invitation to return if they are worried or new symptoms develop and the opportunity to report progress in a telephone follow-up also increase security. Parents who are made to feel unwelcome or stupid in these circumstances and who lack confidence in the arrangements to contact the doctor are much more likely to call at night or to take the child to the local hospital accident and emergency department. Throughout this complicated transaction it is important for the clinician to remember that a major reason for parental anxiety is that occasionally babies who have a minor 'cold' become ill very quickly and die. As we work to increase parental confidence and independence we must also listen carefully to the mother who insists that her child is very ill and examine and follow-up that baby with great care. In any case, when the complications of a cold such as lower respiratory tract infections or sinusitis develop then the GP may need to intervene with appropriate investigations and antibiotics.

Aetiology

Colds are caused by a variety of different viruses, most notably rhino-, adeno-, corona-, myxo-, and paramyxoviruses. Many of these have multiple strains allowing for exposure to viruses not previously encountered. They may cause a simple coryzal presentation or they may be part of the prodrome of other viral illnesses, notably of measles.

Clinical features

Symptoms of coryza or the common cold are a universal experience. A mild sore throat with laryngitis may be the first complaint, followed by nasal discharge, sneezing, and occasionally a cough. Fever is unusual and should suggest a different diagnosis. Symptoms usually persist for up to a week, but unless complications arise, are self-limiting. After a short incubation period of 48–72 hours, there may be a mildly infected pharynx and a nasal discharge. Children may also have a red tympanic membrane and loss of the light reflex, but pain is not a prominent feature of viral otitis media. There are no physical signs in the chest although exacerbations of asthma and a reduction in peak flow may occur in susceptible individuals.[3]

Diagnosis and investigations

Diagnosis of the common cold is clinical and usually made by the patient. Measles is also a clinical diagnosis but a history of recent contact may be of help in the coryzal stage of the prodromal illness.

Treatment

This is symptomatic and may involve a nasal decongestant, especially at night, and analgesia such as paracetamol and aspirin in adults. Antibiotics are not indicated for simple colds. Complications and infection with bacterial pathogens will be considered below. Patients with asthma should be advised to increase their prophylactic steroids and bronchodilators if they feel a cold coming: many patients have learned to do this for themselves!

The catarrhal child, viral infections, and asthma

Some children suffer repeatedly from a stuffy nose, night cough, and earache but do not exhibit convincing signs of infection on examination. Many of these children have an allergic basis for their complaints, some develop glue ear and some of them have asthma. Decongestants are of little relevance and antibiotics should only be used for acute otitis media meeting the criteria. It is important to make the definitive diagnosis of asthma as correct treatment will control the symptoms.

In addition, some studies have reported an association between upper respiratory viral infections, particularly rhinovirus infections, and exacerbations of asthma in schoolchildren,[5] although further research is needed to establish a causal link. Most parents quickly become aware of the risk of worsening asthma after the start of a cold and increase prophylaxis and symptomatic treatment accordingly. The GP should discuss this aspect of care at the regular review and ensure that the family are clear about the safe limits before they should seek medical advice.

Sore throat, laryngitis, tonsillitis, and peritonsillar abscess (quinsy)

Epidemiology and impact on general practice

Complaints of sore throats are among the most common seen in general practice, with an incidence of at least 80/1000 patients per year (weekly returns 1991).[4] Despite the huge workload for GPs and the discomfort and occasional danger for patients which results, the investigation of the complaint and the use of antibiotics remain controversial.[6,7]

Aetiology

The major bacterial agent of concern is the group A streptococcus. Although a number of other TENS agents can cause pharyngitis and tonsillitis, including *Haemophilus influenzae*, *Mycoplasma pneumoniae*, *Neisseria gonorrhoeae*, group C and G streptococci, and *Corynebacterium diphtheriae*, it is the group A streptococcus (GAS) which causes the most controversy. Severe disease due to GAS has been declining over the past 40 years but reports from the USA in the late 1980s show a rise in the incidence of acute rheumatic fever and severe invasive disease associated with the reappearance of highly virulent M types 1, 3, and 18, which were responsible for much of the severe disease seen earlier in the century.[8] This is viewed as an important and ominous change in the epidemiology of GAS disease and is likely to be reflected in similar cases appearing in the UK.[9]

Rarely, a mixture of organisms consisting of a fusiform bacillus and a spiral organism, *Borrelia vincenti*, are also involved in the aetiology of sore throats, causing anaerobic pharyngitis, eponymously called Vincent's angina. In this context, *Fusobacterium necrophorum* can cause a postanginal septicaemia (Lemierre's disease) that is preceded by an exudative tonsillitis and which is associated with jugular vein septic thrombophlebitis and spread of the organism to distant sites such as the lung and joints.

Among the viruses, which are responsible for about 70% of sore throats seen in general practice, coxsackievirus, adenovirus, influenza, parainfluenza, herpes simplex, Epstein–Barr virus, and cytomegalovirus have all been implicated in pharyngitis.

Clinical features

These are conditions which may present as part of the coryzal complex of complaints, as separate, unique symptoms or as part of a systemic illness. They may usefully be considered as a spectrum of complaints with a related anatomy and similar aetiological agents. Symptoms range from hoarseness and mild pharyngeal irritation to severe pain which may compromise the intake of food and drink as swallowing becomes increasingly difficult. The patient may also complain of fever, headache, muscle and joint pains, of a rash, or of tender 'swollen glands'.

The degree of pharyngeal, tonsillar, or palatal infection can be variable, as can the presence of exudates, ulcers, or vesicles. If a quinsy or peritonsillar abscess develops this may appear as a large red swelling of the soft palate with the tonsil pushed down and to the side. The patient usually has a fever and may appear toxic. Tender lymph nodes in the submandibular and deep cervical region may be found. Very rarely, a membrane may be visible and should alert the physician to the possibility of diphtheria. There may be an accompanying rash and/or conjunctivitis and signs of acute otitis media which is the commonest complication of tonsillitis. It is, of course, usual to examine the tympanic membranes to exclude otitis media in patients who present with a sore throat. Most sore throats and laryngitis, irrespective of the causative agent, are self-limiting and not associated with complications if left untreated.

Diagnosis and investigations

The diagnosis of viral or bacterial aetiology on clinical grounds alone is only moderately reliable with a positive predictive value for GAS reported in one study as 0.52.[10] In a review of studies of the effectiveness of clinical diagnosis of GAS tonsillopharyngitis, Pichichero[11] concludes that for most patients the clinical diagnosis is unreliable except for a subset of children (20%) and adults (65%) who present with sore throat as part of viral upper respiratory infection. They have accompanying rhinorrhea, cough and hoarseness, and an absence of fever, tonsillopharyngeal erythema or exudate, and cervical lymphadenitis. He proposes that these patients do not require further investigation or antibiotic treatment. The clinical history and examination is principally directed at identifying these people and establishing the severity of the infection. The conversation with the patient will determine their worries and expectations of treatment and their level of understanding of upper respiratory tract infections (URTIs) and enable a jointly agreed plan of action.

When a throat swab is sent to the microbiology laboratory, investigations are directed towards detection of haemolytic streptococci (A, C, and G), and it is the GAS that is of particular concern. Many laboratories still routinely culture for *C. diphtheriae* and a Gram-film is used to detect the presence of Vincent's organisms since these organisms are difficult to culture. Specialized media is usually required to grow the fastidious and delicate *N. gonorrhoeae* and hence should be specifically requested. The requirement for microbiological investigations in cases of pharyngitis is, however, controversial in general practice and will be discussed further below.

Group A streptococci is grown from approximately 30% of older children and adults who have cultures taken because they complain of sore throats. Of these approximately 50% will be carriers. If it is essential to prove that the growth of group A streptococci from a throat swab implicates the organism as a pathogen rather than as a colonizing organism, then antistreptococcal antibodies can be measured, commonly antistreptolysin O titre (ASOT) and anti-DNAase antibodies. A rise in these antibodies suggests significant infection and patients may be at risk from the non-suppurative complications of GAS infection (i.e. rheumatic fever and acute glomerulonephritis). The rest will be carriers and the sore throats in these patients may be due to a different agent.

There are currently a number of tests that are available for rapid diagnosis of GAS in the surgery. These include ELISA and latex tests, but while they are of high specificity they are less sensitive than culture.[12,13] In these circumstances a positive result is likely to be reliable whereas a negative result may be a false negative.

Plasma levels of C-reactive protein rise rapidly in response to infection with a greater response to bacterial rather than viral sore throats and kits are available for use on capillary blood in general practice and are a useful adjunct to clinical assessment.[10] As near-patient rapid tests become more reliable they will be used more widely in primary care, but clinicians who wish to make a definitive diagnosis of the presence of GAS in a patient with a sore throat should use culture at present.

Is it important to identify group A streptococcus in patients with sore throats?
It is widely known in UK general practice that about 70% of sore throats are viral. This observation is frequently used to justify a nihilistic approach to investigation and treatment. However, about one-third *are* due to a treatable bacterial infection.[14] Is it therefore, reasonable for all patients to be managed as if they had viral infections?

If pharyngitis is due to GAS, then the treatment of choice is penicillin V or erythromycin for 10 days. The arguments for therapy are threefold:

(1) to prevent the suppurative complications of GAS infection such as otitis media and acute sinusitis;

(2) to prevent the non-suppurative complications (i.e. acute rheumatic fever) but not post-streptococcal glomerulonephritis;

(3) to prevent spread of the disease.

Studies have confirmed that UK general practitioners make very little use of throat swabs in the management of sore throats.[15] In the US, it is common practice for patients who present with a sore throat to have a throat swab taken and for the results of the swab to determine whether antibiotic therapy is to be commenced. This approach allows accurate and appropriate prescribing of a cheap and effective antibiotic (i.e. penicillin V). In the UK, practice is much more variable and often depends on whether the patient appears 'toxic' with severe symptoms and signs.

So what is the relationship between culturing and treatment in the management of GAS infection. The answer must be that in the ideal world anyone presenting with a sore throat would have a throat swab investigated, except in the context of a streptococcal outbreak when treatment without culture is appropriate. In the real world, however, the benefit of culture must be compared to the costs. This will include not only transport and laboratory costs, but the cost to the patient on the one hand of having a swab taken, awaiting results, and then having to return to the surgery for a prescription if the result is positive; and on the other, of being unnecessarily treated with antibiotics either because cultures were negative or because the sore throat had a different aetiology.

It must therefore be reasonable to ask whether it matters whether we identify and treat pharyngitis due to GAS. Although there is no good evidence that antibiotic therapy actually decreases symptoms in what is usually a benign, self-limiting illness, given the aims of treatment stated above, the answer almost certainly is *yes*. This is because the suppurative complications include otitis media and acute sinusitis and there is now ample evidence that treatment with penicillin can prevent 98% of expected cases of rheumatic fever associated with GAS pharyngitis.[16] Although this has now become a rare disease (0.6/100 000 children/year in 1985), there is evidence that rheumatic fever is on the increase again in the USA. While several factors such as the introduction of penicillin, a general reduction in the frequency of carriage of GAS in the population, better living conditions, and a reduction in the virulence of rheumatogenic streptococci, may have contributed to the fall in incidence in the USA and Western Europe,[17] the reduced prescription of antibiotics as a routine treatment for sore throats has been suggested as a factor in recent outbreaks of rheumatic fever in the USA.[18] Moreover, group A streptococcal septicaemia has had a fixed mortality of 25%, despite appropriate antibiotic therapy, although

Table 6.2 *Questions for discussion in forming a practice policy on how to diagnose sore throats*

---

1. Will near-patient tests be used to diagnose group A streptococci (GAS) infection

2. When should a throat swab be taken?

3. Is it appropriate for antibiotic therapy to be commenced without a throat swab being sent?

4. If GAS is grown, how is infection to be distinguished from carriage?

5. Is one throat swab sufficient to diagnose or exclude GAS?

6. Should therapy be commenced prior to the results of culture being known? If so, when?

7. Does specific antibiotic therapy influence the natural outcome of the disease?

8. Should contacts be investigated and/or treated?

---

the relationship to pharyngeal carriage and infection in these patients has not been well defined. It is therefore an organism to be respected and we would advise that GPs consider and discuss all of the arguments and questions presented above, both within the practice and with the local microbiologist before deciding a practice policy in relation to the management of sore throats.

Table 6.2 summarizes the issues that should be considered when practice policy on the relevance of throat swabs is decided. (It might also usefully form the basis for a tutorial with the registrar.)

Treatment

Several studies have shown that if a GP thinks that tonsillitis is present antibiotics are more likely to be prescribed than if the clinical condition is thought to represent just a simple sore throat. Recent studies in Dutch general practice confirm that over half the patients consulting with acute tonsillitis would be treated with penicillin.[1] Nonetheless, it is well documented that clinical judgement alone is a poor arbiter of the presence of GAS and certainly cannot satisfactorily determine its significance. The practice of expensive and unnecessary antibiotics being prescribed when simpler, cheaper, and safer agents (penicillin V or erythromycin) is also widespread.[19] There is never any justification for using broad spectrum antibiotics to treat the uncomplicated sore throat as the prescription is aimed at GAS which is virtually always sensitive to either penicillin V or erythromycin. It is worth remembering that the prescription of ampicillin for a sore throat, especially in young adults, can be complicated by the

Table 6.3 *for the debate: Diagnosis and management of sore throat**

Identify patients with sore throat and runny nose, cough, and hoarseness who do not have fever, erythema of tonsils and pharynx, an exudate, or cervical lymphadenitis (65% of adults, 20% of children)

No further investigation or antibiotic treatment recommended. Explain viral aetiology and self management to the patient

Of the remaining patients identify those with mild to moderate symptoms and no suppurative complications

Observe (take swab), and review plan as necessary

The remaining patients have moderate to severe symptoms and/or suppurative complications

Send a throat swab or perform near-patient test. Start penicillin immediately or await culture on basis of clinical need. Stop penicillin if culture negative

* This is the authors' approach to diagnosis and management.

development of a rash if the pharyngitis is part of the presentation of infectious mononucleosis. If infection is shown to be due to Vincent's organisms then treatment with penicillin or with metronidazole will be of benefit.

Some parents prefer to rely on homeopathic medicines for children with frequently recurring URTIs including sore throats. A recent randomized controlled trial of this approach for children with recurrent URTIs did not reduce symptoms, or the use of antibiotics.[20]

This whole area has proved one of the most difficult for the authors of this book to resolve between themselves and there have been several heated debates. Our different backgrounds in hospital and general practice and the conflicting literature makes it difficult to present the reader with certainties. The authors, on balance, recommend the approach presented by Pichichero,[11] which identifies those individuals who do not need further investigation or treatment on the basis of the clinical picture, and we prefer to send throat swabs for those patients in the remaining group with clinically severe or recurrent infection, in the knowledge that some milder infections will have a bacterial cause (Table 6.3). Teenagers and young adults with severe purulent tonsillitis should also have investigations for infectious mononucleosis carried out when they present (see below). In those in whom suppurative complications have already supervened, it is reasonable to culture and treat before results are known. If culture results come back as negative (a pharyngeal swab taken by vigorously swabbing the tonsils and pharynx should be positive in 90% of cases of GAS) then antibiotics should be stopped. In patients in whom the organism is cultured, antibiotics should be commenced and continued for a full 10 days.[1,16] It is common in general practice to give short courses which may then result in ineffective treatment and relapse. Delay in treating GAS pharyngitis of up to 9 days may still prevent rheumatic fever.

The final consideration is whether it is worth screening family contacts. Acquisition rates of up to 25% have been recorded in some families. Clearly symptomatic family members require investigation and treatment if cultures are positive. Asymptomatic carriage may be sought in certain situations which include overcrowding, a family member with rheumatic fever, or known local cases of rheumatic fever.

Future research in diagnosis and management of sore throats. In the age of evidence-based practice it is striking how many of the questions about sore throats remain unanswered or have been studied in the USA in settings which may not generalize well to the UK. Research in UK practice could usefully be directed at how symptoms and signs perform in diagnosis in the British primary care setting; the most cost-effective way to identify patients with GAS infections; randomized controlled trials of penicillin in those with documented GAS infection (rather than carriage) to see what the benefits of treatment are in relation to the reduction of symptoms, time lost from work or education, side-effects of medication, and the prevention of otitis media and sinusitis. Finally, studies to determine whether any benefits would be regarded as important enough by patients to justify taking antibiotics would complete the picture. The numbers required to demonstrate a 50% reduction in the attack rate of rheumatic fever with penicillin are so large as to make such studies impracticable.

Infectious mononucleosis

Epidemiology and impact on general practice

Infectious mononucleosis[21] (glandular fever) is caused by the Epstein–Barr virus (EBV) which is a common herpesvirus which succeeds in infecting more than 90% of the population. While the infection can occur at all ages, many infections in children are asymptomatic with the majority of clinical cases occurring in adolescents. In the 1980s, 75% of the cases reported to the weekly returns of the Royal College of General Practitioners were in the 15–44 age group; 1 in 50 cases of tonsillitis in the age group were due to the infection.[4] Most people are immune by the age of 25 and are not susceptible to re-infection. The virus persists in the salivary glands and is shed in saliva for months after clinical recovery. The infection is spread by exchange of saliva as in kissing and the incubation period is between 3 and 7 weeks.

Aetiology and clinical features

The virus infects B lymphocytes stimulating them to produce antibody. This provokes a vigorous immunological response in which T lymphocytes proliferate to suppress and destroy the infected B lymphocytes. This battle results in most of the infected cells being eliminated but a small proportion persist leading to lifelong latent infection. The presence of large numbers of T cells in the blood is the explanation for the 'atypical mononuclear cells' which are reported during the infection. The classic syndrome of infectious mononucleosis is fever, sore throat, and adenopathy. Headache, myalgia, and anorexia are also relatively common. On examination, the patient may have a severely infected throat with oedema and a purulent exudate over the fauces and tonsils which rarely can cause an obstruction to breathing. There is widespread swelling of lymph glands and about half of the patients have splenomegaly. Hepatomegaly occurs in about 12% of cases with overt jaundice in 9%.

Diagnosis, investigation, and treatment

While the clinical features may be strongly suggestive the laboratory diagnosis is by examination of the peripheral blood for an absolute lymphocytosis with a large number of 'atypical' mononuclear cells and the presence of heterophile antibodies by the locally available test.

In most cases, the illness is self-limiting and best treated symptomatically. There is no evidence from controlled studies that antivirals, such as acyclovir, are of use in uncomplicated infections and evidence for the minor beneficial effects of corticosteroids on symptoms is outweighed by concerns about their potential to have an adverse effect on the biology of the infection.[22] Patients should be told to avoid contact sports for at least a month as there is an increased risk of rupturing the spleen. Post-viral fatigue may be a problem and a graded return to full activities may be necessary.

Occasional complications of acute EBV infection include airway obstruction, haemolytic anaemia, thrombocytopenia, aplastic anaemia, encephalitis, myocarditis and pericarditis, and hepatitis.

Influenza

The term 'influenza' is often misused and applied vaguely. It describes a collection of symptoms related to infection of the respiratory tract accompanied by various degrees of malaise. More accurately, it is the clinical condition resulting from infection with influenza viruses.

Epidemiology and aetiology

Three major classes of influenza virus are recognized; A, B, and C. Influenza C is a relatively minor cause of respiratory problems but A and B strains are major causes of morbidity and mortality, particularly in the very young and in the elderly. Each strain tends to occur in well-circumscribed epidemics during the winter months. Following a new strain of virus, spread is virtually world-wide within one or two years. A shift in the glycoprotein structure of the virus leads to a new surface glycoprotein against which much of the human population has no antibody. Major shifts in structure lead to pandemics. The viral strain causing the Asian influenza epidemic of 1957 and the Hong Kong influenza strain of 1968 are examples.

Influenza is spread primarily by respiratory droplets. Spread occurs rapidly, particularly within institutions such as boarding schools, military camps, and nursing homes. Mortality is primarily in the elderly and in the very young and is usually as a result of a severe viral pneumonia or a secondary bacterial infection.

Clinical features

The onset of influenza is usually abrupt with fever, myalgia, headache, and a harsh, dry cough. The duration of symptoms varies according to the particular strain and may be from 2–7 days. A presumptive diagnosis is usually easy during an epidemic but can be more difficult with sporadic infection. The GP must take a careful history and remember to include any information about recent overseas travel as other infections are easily missed during the high workload of an influenza epidemic.

While the clinical course of influenza is usually short, primary complications may occur in the respiratory tract, producing a primary viral pneumonia. Rapid death, even in healthy young adults, and patients at both extremes of age who are particularly vulnerable, may occur.

Aspirin and salicylates must not be used for children as they may precipitate Reye's syndrome. This is found in association with influenza B and, more rarely, influenza A infections. This rare syndrome presents when, during the course of an influenzal illness, a child becomes particularly ill; vomiting and confusion may follow leading to seizures and coma.

A further complication of influenza is superinfection by bacterial organisms such as *Staphylococcus aureus*, *Streptococcus pneumoniae*, and *H. influenzae*. Bacterial superinfection may also occur as a secondary process 10 days after the acute onset of the viral illness. This is often due to *Staph. aureus*.

Diagnosis and investigations

The influenza virus can isolated from respiratory secretions during the initial phase of an influenzal illness. Some virus laboratories can perform direct immunofluorescence on respiratory secretions thereby achieving rapid diagnosis. Retrospective serological diagnosis can be made by examination of paired sera at two-week intervals. If bacterial superinfection is a concern sputum should be sent to the microbiology laboratory for culture.

Treatment

In mild influenza infections supportive measures only are necessary. Bed rest, fluids, and paracetamol may be of benefit. The drug available for treatment of viral pneumonia is amantadine, although the antiviral activity of amantadine is limited to influenza A. Although amantadine does not have a place in the routine early treatment of influenza A a case can be made for its use in an institutional environment and for at-risk groups such as the elderly or those with chronic disease.[22] The use of amantadine is limited, to some extent, by its various toxic effects on the central nervous system, such as confusion, dizziness and insomnia although these problems are uncommon in normal dosage and only tend to occur if renal function is impaired.

If secondary bacterial pneumonia occurs appropriate antibiotic therapy is flucloxacillin or co-amoxiclav which are active against *Staph. aureus*. In an outbreak of influenza in an institutional setting, especially with vulnerable patients, early intervention with antibiotics should always be considered.

Prevention

The prevention of influenza and the circumstances in which prophylaxis with amantadine or antibiotics should be considered are discussed in detail in Chapter 2.

Epiglottitis and bacterial tracheitis

Epiglottitis is a rare condition but it is important because it can rapidly progress to become a medical emergency. It is characterized by a progressive cellulitis of the epiglottis and its surrounding tissues which usually presents in young children under the age of 6 years, although it has recently been described in detail in adults.

General practitioners will most commonly see epiglottitis among children although each GP may encounter a case only once or twice in clinical practice. With the introduction of Hib vaccine this disease will become even rarer. Nevertheless, all GPs must know how to approach the situation. The major differential diagnoses will be croup and, much less commonly, bacterial tracheitis. Whilst the conditions may be distinguished on clinical grounds, definitive diagnosis may have to await proper inspection of the epiglottis under controlled conditions in hospital. Both epiglottitis and bacterial tracheitis are emergencies and require urgent hospital admission. When a child is to be admitted as an emergency the GP should prepare the parents for the fact that there may be a need to intubate or perform a tracheotomy after admission. Where diagnostic difficulties may be greater, however, is in the adult population since the diagnosis is much rarer and therefore must first be remembered before it can be considered. In this population the diagnosis is more likely to be confused with retropharyngeal or peritonsillar abscesses (quinsy) which may also cause upper airway obstruction.

Aetiology

Haemophilus influenzae type b (Hib) is the most common bacterial agent isolated in patients with epiglottitis. It is responsible for most cases of infection in young children and for just over a quarter of adult cases. Now that children are routinely immunized with Hib vaccine we can expect a dramatic reduction in the number of cases due to this organism. Other bacteria which have been implicated include *Strep. pneumoniae*, *Staph. aureus*, *H. parainfluenzae*, and viridans streptococci. Viruses have not been shown to cause this disease.

Bacterial tracheitis is, as its name suggests, a bacterial infection which occurs as a result of superinfection following a viral illness. Whilst both influenza and parainfluenza viruses have been reported in the literature, parainfluenza 1, 2, and 3 have been associated with the illness with much greater frequency. The most frequently isolated bacterial pathogen is *Staph. aureus*, followed by *H. influenzae*, and *Strep. pneumoniae*. Other streptococci and Gram-negative organisms have also been implicated.

Clinical features

Characteristically, in epiglottitis the young patient, more commonly a male, has had an 8 to 12-hour history of fever, sore throat, and complains of difficulty in swallowing. The child's parents may notice marked drooling associated with the dysphagia and the patient may find it more comfortable to sit leaning forward. Inspiratory stridor and a hoarse voice are common findings. There are reports of illnesses which are so fulminant that the patient progresses from being completely well to having total airway obstruction in less than one hour. In croup, with which this illness may be confused, the history is less acute, often with a preceding upper respiratory tract infection in slightly younger children and the epiglottis is normal.

Bacterial tracheitis is an uncommon infection of the upper airways presenting in young children who are usually less than 3 years of age. It can occasionally cause problems in older children with approximately 10% of children being between the ages of 8 and 13 years. It is characterized by an acute presentation preceded by a prodromal URTI, with subsequent subglottic swelling and purulent tracheal secretions but with an entirely normal epiglottis. There may be severe respiratory distress and, as in epiglottitis, croup may be the initial diagnosis.

Under no circumstances should the GP attempt to visualize the epiglottis or take a swab if the diagnosis of epiglottitis is being considered. The patient should be referred to hospital where, on controlled, direct examination of the throat the characteristic 'cherry red' epiglottis will be seen. Care must be taken during visualization and it is essential that measures are used to secure the airway since such a manoeuvre could precipitate total obstruction of the larynx.

Diagnosis and investigations

The diagnosis of epiglottitis is clinical and constitutes one of the life-threatening emergencies seen in children in UK general practice. In the hospital setting, the risks of delay in obtaining X-rays and their lack of sensitivity have been documented. Up to 25% of cases may have evidence of pneumonia and lateral neck X-rays may demonstrate 'the thumb sign' associated with acute epiglottitis. A peripheral leucocytosis is usually present and cultures of blood and from the epiglottis may grow the implicated organism. Most cases of childhood epiglottitis will have a bacteraemia but only rarely is meningitis found in association with epiglottitis.

If an X-ray of the neck is performed in a case of bacterial tracheitis (and the same circumspection should be used as for epiglottitis), it will show subglottic narrowing. A significant number of chest X-rays will show lung-shadowing with chest infiltrates. The total peripheral white cell count may be normal, but there is often a left-shift with an increased neutrophil count on the differential.

Treatment

Both epiglottitis and bacterial tracheitis should be regarded as emergencies. The GP may be required to insert 2–3 wide-bore needles below the cricoid cartilage as a life-saving resuscitative measure before hospital admission. Primary therapy is initially supportive and the maintenance of an airway should be the major consideration. Whilst there has been some debate in the past over the advisability of conservative management with observation of the airway versus early elective intubation, studies have shown that mortality with epiglottitis varies between 6% and 25% in those patients who have been observed. If epiglottitis is confirmed by visualization of the swollen 'cherry-red' epiglottis intubation or tracheostomy should be performed.

In bacterial tracheitis, the epiglottis will be normal but there will be severe subglottic swelling and copious secretions. Once the airway has been secured cultures from the blood, epiglottis, and tracheal secretions should be obtained.

Epiglottitis. Medical therapy must be directed in the first instance against *H. influenzae*. Intravenous chloramphenicol has been the mainstay of antibiotic therapy in the past, because it is active against beta-lactamase-producing *H. influenzae*. However, intravenous cephalosporins such as cefuroxime (200 mg/kg/day) or cefotaxime (150 mg/kg/day) are also beta-lactamase-stable, do not require measurement of levels, extend the spectrum of activity against the other pathogens associated with epiglottitis, and are now considered by many to be first-line therapy. Treatment should be continued for 7–10 days, but the patient may be extubated once the fever has settled and the swelling of the epiglottis has resolved.

The second important question to be addressed with respect to epiglottitis is the requirement for prophylaxis for contacts. The American Paediatric Association has recommended prophylaxis with rifampicin for invasive *H. influenzae* since 1986. In 1991, similar recommendations have been made in the UK. The recommendation for invasive disease in which there is a child apart from the index case under the age of 4 years in the household requires that rifampicin (adult dose: 20 mg/kg/day) be given to all members of the household for 4 days. Parents should, however, be warned to observe young children with care since secondary cases may still occur, despite prophylaxis.

Bacterial tracheitis. Therapy may be initially guided by results of the Gram-film. If this is unhelpful then empirical therapy with an agent such an cefuroxime should be given until specific therapy based on definitive culture and antibiotic sensitivity results is advised.

Case history

The 12-year-old sister of a 4-year-old boy telephoned the doctor at 9.30 pm. "Mummy can't get to the 'phone, come at once, Steven is very ill he is burning up, not breathing properly and there is a whole lot of water coming from his mouth."

This history alerted the doctor to the diagnosis of epiglottitis and he took the following action:

- Reassured the young caller that he would be round immediately
- Gave instructions that the child should be nursed on his side
- Dialled the emergency ambulance number and made an urgent request for an ambulance to meet him at the house
- Selected several wide-bore needles to be inserted through the crico-thyroid membrane should that prove necessary

On arrival, the doctor observed the child to be febrile. There was neck extension, marked inspiratory stridor, copious drooling from the mouth, and central cyanosis.

No attempt was made to examine the throat. Oxygen was given and the child was immediately transferred to the waiting ambulance. The doctor accompanied the child in the ambulance for the 8-mile journey to hospital, prepared to provide an emergency airway with wide-bore needles if necessary. During the journey the hospital was alerted and a request made for a senior anaesthetist to be standing by.

On arrival, the child was transferred urgently to theatre where he had an endotracheal tube inserted under general anaesthetic. Direct laryngoscopy revealed a friable cherry-red and swollen epiglottis. He was transferred to the intensive care unit where was nursed for 8 days and received intravenous antibiotics. An initial trial of extubation failed as he was still having severe stridor and he was extubated finally after 6 days. Blood cultures isolated *H. influenzae* type b which was consistent with the diagnosis.

Follow-up by the general practitioner

The hospital was telephoned early the following morning for a report on the child's progress. An early morning visit was carried out to the family home to meet the mother, father, daughter aged 12, and younger daughter aged 3 years. As there was a child, apart from the index case, under the age of 4 years in the household rifampicin[69] (20 mg per kg per day in a single dose) was prescribed for all members of the household for 4 days. The parents were informed that they should closely observe the 3-year-old child, over the next few days. Follow-up visits were carried out over the next week and no secondary cases occurred.

At the time this event occurred (1990) the Hib vaccine was not available. Now the GP would ensure that the 3-year-old sibling was fully immunized.

Acute laryngotracheitis (croup)

'Croup' is an old term for acute laryngotracheitis. Although it is not anatomically strictly an upper respiratory tract infection, clinically, it is logical to consider it along with epiglottitis as another important infective cause of obstructed breathing especially in young children. It is, in fact, an acute laryngitis with stridor, occurring in up to 6% of children. There is a male/female ratio of 1.5:1.0 and an age span ranging from 2 months to 9 years, with the highest incidence around the age of 2 years. It is a virus infection, usually involving parainfluenza type I, although respiratory syncytial virus (RSV), measles, or influenza A or B may be responsible. The peak incidence is in winter. In older children mycoplasma has occasionally been implicated.

Clinical features

After two or three days of an upper respiratory illness, the child will develop a harsh, barking cough, and stridor, almost always much worse at night. Fever may be present. Physical examination usually shows a child with minimal to severe distress, the latter with dyspnoea, stridor, flaring of the ala nasi and intercostal recession. The lungs are usually clear on auscultation but transmitted upper airways sounds and some wheeze may be heard. The white blood count may be raised. Most children with croup can be managed at home, although deaths can occur and careful management is necessary.

The condition should not be confused with the much more life-threatening and dramatic epiglottitis.[23] (See Table 6.4) Other serious conditions must be included in the differential diagnosis:[24]

- Peritonsillar abscess (quinsy)
- Bacterial tracheitis
- Subglottic stenosis
- Laryngeal diphtheria
- Paraquat poisoning

Treatment

Management of a patient with croup is demanding for the GP, particularly, as many of these children are seen at night. Clinical confirmation of the diagnosis is important (this is not a condition that can be managed by telephone advice) and the parents will need constant reassurance. The child should be nursed in a warm humid environment and be closely observed for increased respiratory problems. Most GPs advise that the parents place the child in a steamy room while they wait for the doctor to arrive. Boiling the electric kettle with the lid off in the child's bedroom is effective, taking

Table 6.4 *Clinical distinctions between epiglottitis and acute laryngotracheitis (croup)*

	Epiglottitis	**Acute laryngotracheitis (croup)**
Age	1–5 years	3/12–3 years, peak at 2 years
Sex	Boys>girls	Boys>girls
Prodrome	Absent	Coryza
Sore throat	Uncommon	Characteristic
Hoarseness	No	Yes
Dysphagia	Common	Uncommon
Characteristic cough (seal's bark)	No	Yes
Drooling	Characteristic	Rare
Neck extension	Yes	No
Fever	Yes	Yes
Systemic toxicity	Marked	Mild
Inspiratory stridor	Yes	Yes
Cyanosis	With impending obstruction	Uncommon
Chest signs	Not prominent	Pneumonia may be present

Table 6.5 *Indications for hospitalization in acute laryngotracheitis (croup)*

- Heart rate >140 per minute
- Respiratory rate >60 per minute
- Cyanosis
- Confusion
- Severe intercostal recession
- Age less than 3 years
- Significant stridor at rest

care to keep it well away from the sick and other children of the household; warm drinks and liquid paracetamol are also beneficial and it is a common experience for the GP to arrive at the bedside to find that the child has almost recovered from his/her distress. Viruses are the causative agent in most cases of croup and if after careful examination of the ears and chest other diagnoses can confidently be excluded, there is no indication for the use of antibiotics. The most important aspect of management is to remain available, to use telephone follow-up, and to re-visit promptly if there is any deterioration.

Hospital admission may be necessary (Table 6.5) but this depends on many factors such as the severity of the attack, the age of the patient (particularly if very young), the ability of parents to cope, and living in remote area, particularly in adverse weather conditions. In hospital, humidified air with or without oxygen, is often provided by a mist tent. Benefit results from moistening of secretions making expectoration easier, soothing inflamed laryngeal mucosa, and reducing discomfort and hence coughing. In the USA, nebulized adrenaline has been demonstrated to be effective in reducing the croup score[25] in randomized controlled trials and is now a standard treatment for children admitted for croup.[26,27] UK hospital practice is also changing and the use of a form of nebulized adrenaline is now known to be as effective in reducing upper airway obstruction and is recommended for children admitted for moderate to severe croup.[28] It is not recommended for use outside the hospital environment in the UK.

Systemic steroids, usually dexamethasone, are also important in the management of croup in hospital and have been shown to reduce the croup score and the need for intubation. A single intramuscular injection of dexamethasone has been shown in a randomized placebo controlled trial to reduce the severity of the illness in the out-patient setting in the USA[28] and many American doctors now treat non-hospitalized children with croup with adrenaline, dexamethasone, and water mist.[29]

Recently, two randomized controlled trials of inhaled budesonide have been reported which demonstrate an improvement in the croup score in children with mild to moderate croup seen in hospital.[30,31] Further UK studies to evaluate the use of the drug outside hospital are needed but while these are awaited it is now reasonable for the GP to give a single dose of budesonide 2 mg by nebulizer to improve symptoms in children well enough to be managed at home.[32]

In approximately 1 in 500 children, a very severe form of croup develops with a secondary bacterial involvement. In this situation there is usually a very abrupt onset with a hoarse cough and the child becomes toxic in appearance and extremely dyspnoeic. Oedema of the larynx is accompanied by an exudate (pseudomembrane) and mucopurulent secretions extend into the smaller airways and alveoli. The infecting organism is likely to be *Staph. aureus* but other bacteria have been implicated, such as *Strep. pyogenes*. These children can become very ill requiring immediate intensive treatment in hospital.

Whooping cough (pertussis)

This is a prolonged URTI caused by the Gram-negative coccobacillus *Bordetella pertussis*. It is spread by droplet and is highly infectious. In the absence of adequate coverage by immunization there were epidemics in the UK every four years with 60% of cases occurring in the 0–4 year age group. Immunization coverage in Italy in the early 1990s was still only 40% and they reported that 1:14 cases of pertussis required hospital care and 1:850 died.[33] A British study of the natural history of the disease found that it is often relatively mild, that adults get whooping cough from their children and that the infection is commonest in 3-year-olds.[34] Adverse publicity in the UK has lead to some groups remaining susceptible and there is now a rising incidence, particularly among adolescents and adults.

Clinical features

The incubation period is 7–10 days which may be followed by a prodromal coryzal illness. This is followed by the characteristic coughing spasms interrupted by a noisy rapid inspiration (the whoop) which may end in vomiting. Infants may become apnoeic between spasms and the symptoms are both frightening and exhausting for child and parents alike. The illness may last for two months and in the later stages the cough is usually worse at night. Complications in small children include pneumonia and encephalopathy.

Pertussis in adults is a milder or subclinical disease but infections in this group may pose a threat to susceptible infants.

Treatment

Erythromycin should be given in confirmed cases to eliminate naso-pharyngeal carriage and reduce the chance of secondary transmission.

Patients who receive erythromycin within 7 days of the onset of the cough are significantly less likely to have a prolonged cough than those who do not receive it. The course should be given for 2 weeks; the antibiotic is not effective against prolonged cough if started later although there is some evidence that even later courses reduce the complication of pneumonia.

Otitis externa, otitis media, and mastoiditis

Epidemiology and impact on general practice

Patients present very commonly to the GP with earache and/or discharge from the ear. The mean weekly incidence is between 80 and 150 per 100 000 with about 45% of infections occurring in children under 4 years. Seasonal variations closely follow the pattern of the common cold with winter peaks and summer troughs.[4] The Third National Morbidity Survey (RCGP 1981) reported the overall episode rate of 'acute suppurative otitis media' as 27.6 per 1000. In the US, otitis media has been shown to be the most frequently recorded diagnosis of illness made by paediatricians. By the age of one year 62% of children will have had an episode of acute otitis media and 17% three or more episodes.[35] The long-term effects of such illness will be carried by a significant number into adult life. Although the incidence of acute otitis media falls after early childhood it causes significant illness in older age groups. The long-term consequences, including impaired hearing and chronic suppurative otitis media are well known to GPs. Children who have suffered recurrent episodes of acute otitis

Table 6.6 *Predisposing factors in diffuse otitis externa*

Local factors
- Trauma (e.g. scratching with dirty fingernail, unskilled syringing)
- Irritant and allergenic agents including topical antibiotics
- Active chronic suppurative otitis media
- Fungal
- Moisture: swimming, humid climates

General factors
- Generalized skin disease
- Seborrhoeic dermatitis
- Eczema
- Psoriasis

---

media perform less well than non-affected children in their future language and speech development.

Otitis externa

Aetiology

The microbiology of otitis externa is different in the acute or chronic form. The external ear canal is lined by keratinizing stratified squamous epithelium which acts as a barrier to infection which may be compromised by trauma or generalized skin disease. *Staphylococcus aureus* is the causative agent when pustule formation or folliculitis is involved whereas erysipelas of the external auditory meatus is due to group A streptococcus. The organisms associated with acute diffuse otitis externa (swimmer's ear) reflect the humid moist environment in which this condition is found. Hence, a variety of Gram-negative organisms, not infrequently *Pseudomonas aeruginosa*, are implicated.

Clinical features

Otitis externa may present either as an acute or chronic problem. The acute form, commonly associated with a pustule of the hair follicles in the external auditory meatus, causes intense pain worse on moving the pinna, and perhaps local lymphadenopathy. Rarely, erysipelas of the area presents with more severe pain and swollen glands. Swimmer's ear, a more diffuse acute infection of the ear canal characteristically occurs in humid warm conditions. The meatus becomes extremely itchy and then painful and red. Many factors have been identified as predisposing to diffuse external otitis (Table 6.6).

The two chronic forms of the disease, chronic otitis externa and malignant otitis externa, differ in their aetiology and long-term outcome. While the first condition may occur in the clinical context of chronic suppurative otitis media it usually results from inadequate treatment of an acute episode and is characterized by persistent oedema and thickening of the skin with healing by fibrosis. Malignant otitis externa is a rare but potentially life-threatening disease which presents with severe pain in and around the ear, including the mastoid, and with drainage of pus from the meatus. The infection can spread into the base of the skull and the brain. Since this condition usually occurs against a background of diabetes, immunosuppression, or general debilitation, it may be the presenting symptom of the underlying condition.

In the chronic forms of otitis externa, Gram-negative organisms may again be found, and it is important to exclude any underlying chronic suppurative otitis media (CSOM). In the malignant form of otitis externa *Ps. aeruginosa* is the major organism of concern. Infection with fungi such as *Aspergillus* (especially *niger*) and *Candida albicans* can also be troublesome in chronic forms of the disease. The agent involved in any particular case of otitis externa can be often be grown from swabs of the external meatus, but care must be taken to distinguish between pathogens, skin commensals, and bacterial overgrowth, particularly if antibiotics have been given.

Treatment

Acute otitis externa associated with *Staph. aureus* or with group A streptococcus requires specific treatment with the appropriate agent, either flucloxacillin or penicillin. In the acute diffuse form of the disease, attention must be directed towards appropriate aural care. The meatus should be carefully cleaned (solutions of alcohol and acetic acid may be of benefit), kept dry, and the patient should be discouraged from introducing implements (including fingers) into the canal. Topical broad spectrum antibiotic solutions, often combined with steroids to help reduce inflammation, may be of benefit. Ototoxic agents such as the aminoglycosides must not be used in the presence of a perforated tympanic membrane. Systemic antibiotics should not be required unless the soft tissues are heavily infected.

Antibiotics have little place in the management of chronic otitis externa where aural toilet and keeping the ear dry are of major importance. However, malignant otitis externa is a serious condition and requires urgent aggressive treatment, particularly as infection may spread to the meninges and the brain with potentially fatal consequences. These patients require urgent referral to an ENT surgeon as definitive treatment consists of adequate debridement of infected tissues and antipseudomonal antibiotics for up to 6 weeks. A combination of an aminoglycoside (i.e. gentamicin) and a ureidopenicillin (i.e. piperacillin) has been standard therapy, but recent reports have pointed to the efficacy of the 4-quinolone, ciprofloxacin, in this condition.

Table 6.7 *Bacteria causing acute otitis media*

Pathogen	Children with the pathogen (mean %)
Streptococcus pneumoniae	33
Haemophilus influenzae	21
Streptococcus pyogenes	8
Moraxella catarrhalis	3
Staphylococcus aureus	2

Otitis media

Aetiology

The bacterial agents associated with acute otitis media are well documented. Approximately one-quarter of paediatric cases have a viral aetiology (particularly respiratory syncytial virus) and another 50% are due to infection with either *Strep. pneumoniae* or *H. influenzae*. Children under the age 5 years are more likely to harbour *H. influenzae*: in older children *Strep. pneumoniae* is the usual pathogen. Whilst most of the *H. influenzae* are non-typable, of the 10% which are type b, nearly 25% of children infected with these strains have an associated septicaemia or meningitis. More recently, *Moraxella catarrhalis* has been demonstrated to be an important pathogen.[38] Less common organisms which may cause acute otitis media include group A streptococcus and *Staph. aureus*, whilst *Chlamydia trachomatis* may cause acute otitis media in infants under 6 months of age. *Mycoplasma pneumoniae* has been associated with bullae on the tympanic membrane, but it is very rare to culture successfully the organism from inner ear fluid. (See Table 6.7.)

Clinical features

Acute otitis media is a potentially serious condition in which the patient, usually a child, presents with a fever, acute pain, and some loss of hearing. The condition is defined by the presence of fluid in the middle ear in addition to signs of acute illness. There may be a history of a preceding URTI, including a sore throat. If the tympanic membrane perforates a discharge may be present; at this point the pain usually subsides. Discharge usually makes it impossible to visualize the tympanic membrane although the pus tends to move or pulsate when the patient coughs in contrast to the purulent discharge of otitis externa.

In very young children, signs are often less specific, with vomiting, lethargy, irritability, and, less frequently, diarrhoea. Whilst the tympanic membrane is usually red in otitis media this is itself is not sufficient to make the diagnosis, since the presence of middle ear fluid is an absolute requirement. Erythema of the membrane alone may reflect inflammation of the whole of the upper respiratory tract without fluid actually being present in the middle ear. For practical purposes, however, the diagnosis is a clinical one since using tympanometry as an objective measure of middle ear fluid is a specialized technique which must be interpreted within the wider clinical context.[36] The use of a pneumatic otoscope which demonstrates movement of the tympanic membrane is helpful. The distinction, however, between an acute otitis media of viral aetiology and that of bacterial aetiology on clinical grounds cannot be reliably made. Equally, the severity of inflammation of the tympanic membrane is not a reliable predictor of the clinical course of acute otitis media.[37]

Chronic otitis media results from recurrent attacks of acute otitis media or when fluid remains in the middle ear for extended period of times, usually following an acute attack.

Mastoiditis

In its acute form, mastoiditis is almost invariably associated with acute otitis media and hence the early signs are those of the underlying illness (i.e. fever, pain, hearing loss, and pus discharging from the tympanic membrane if it has perforated). At a later stage the mastoid area becomes tender and red and some swelling may be observed. Classically, the pinna of the ear is pushed down and out. Whilst early antibiotic intervention in most cases of bacterial acute otitis media has considerably reduced the incidence of significant mastoid infection (now about 1 per 1000 cases) should a full-blown mastoiditis become established it can produce a significant morbidity and mortality.

Diagnosis and investigations

In acute otitis media, the likely bacterial agents involved are well known so that unless the eardrum has already perforated and pus is available the diagnosis is on the basis of clinical findings. Rarely, the patient is so toxic and ill that referral for blood cultures and/or aspiration of the middle ear contents is required, but usually a trial of antibacterial agents is embarked on first.

In *mastoiditis*, it is usually possible to obtain a sample of the middle ear discharge although care should be taken not to contaminate it with organisms from the external meatus. X-rays of the mastoid region may show opacity of the air spaces.

Treatment

The medical treatment of acute otitis media requires adequate analgesia (paracetamol) and antibiotics which cover the major bacterial spectrum of infection. Whilst many clinicians use amoxycillin as first-line therapy, the increasing isolation of beta-lactamase-producing organisms requires that this view be reassessed. Studies have demonstrated that up to 20% of *H.*

influenzae may produce beta-lactamase. Furthermore, the increase in prevalence of *M. catarrhalis* as a cause of otitis media[39] suggests that agents such as co-amoxiclav should be considered first in this condition. In patients with a good history of penicillin allergy, a cephalosporin (up to 10% cross-reactivity with penicillin allergy has been reported) or macrolide antibiotic (especially if it is thought prudent to avoid cephalosporins) may be a useful alternative.

Management of acute otitis media: the role of antibiotics

There are different approaches to the management of earache due to otitis media. The use of antibiotics has been questioned and this has implications for decisions to visit children who present at night.[40–42] Some doctors prefer to advise analgesia with follow-up next morning for children who are otherwise well whilst others visit in order to prescribe antibiotics. If the situation is managed by telephone advice it is essential to be available and willing to see the child quickly should the situation deteriorate. The Netherlands College of General Practitioners has developed a national standard which does not recommend the immediate use of antibiotics for the condition.[1] They recommend that they should be reserved in children over 2 years for when the patient has a fever or the earache has lasted for more than three days. However, some American and British studies support the clinical impression that antibiotics shorten the duration of symptoms.[43,44] In an overall review of these and other, studies Burke[45] supports a less restrictive policy towards antibiotic prescribing particularly as there is no conclusive evidence that their use leads to a persistent middle ear effusion. Placebo has never been shown to be better than antibiotics in any of the randomized controlled trials that have been conducted confirming that antibiotics are not actually harmful. There is general agreement on the need for larger well-designed studies; until they are reported most GPs will want to consider their immediate use for the following high risk groups:

- Children under 2 years old
- The presence of fever
- Patients with bulging tympanic membranes
- Pain duration >48 hours
- Recurrent attacks

The use of decongestants is widely recommended but there is little or no scientific basis for prescribing them.

All children with acute otitis media should be reviewed 6 weeks after an episode to examine the tympanic membrane and check the hearing. This consultation provides an opportunity to review the management of the whole episode with the parent and to plan for the future. It can be conducted as part of child health surveillance or the family sent a separate appointment to attend. The follow-up of these children makes a good subject for practice clinical audit.

Myringotomy

Recent studies of the role of myringotomy with or without appropriate antibiotic therapy raises the question of the place of drainage of the middle ear fluid in the management of acute otitis media. In a random-ized, prospective trial in infants with otitis media comparing myringotomy alone, co-amoxiclav alone or co-amoxiclav with myringotomy, the use of co-amoxiclav alone was more effective than myringotomy alone in clearing the infection, and the addition of myringotomy to co-amoxiclav therapy did not increase the rate of recovery.[39]

Management of chronic otitis media

There is probably little place for the use of antibiotics in chronic otitis media although there have been a few studies which suggest that prophylaxis with once a day amoxycillin may help to reduce the symptoms but not the effusion associated with it. Prophylaxis with 23-valent pneumococcal vac-cine, which contains all of the common pneumococcal serotypes associated with otitis media has been shown to be of benefit in reducing infections in children over the age of 2 years in the USA.

Most GPs have adult patients with chronic perforations of the tympanic membrane. Large central perforations are characteristic of tubotympanic chronic suppurative otitis media and may be repaired when the otorrhoea is resolved. It is worth referring these patients for an ENT opinion; patients with marginal perforations associated with attico-antral disease should be referred urgently because associated cholesteatomata may be difficult to see and may cause bone erosion.

Chronic otitis media with effusion (glue ear): Surgical treatment

Surgery is sometimes useful in this condition and referral of the patient for insertion of grommets (tympanostomy tubes) may be required to deal with the persistent presence of the middle ear effusion. Glue ear is the commonest reason for elective surgery in children; one child in 200 in England is treated each year. There are, however, doubts about the need for such frequent intervention and the GP should be aware of them.[46] The natural history of understood; 20–30% of children under 6 years develop the condition at some time and 90% of these middle ear infusions resolve within 3 months.[36]

Many questions about the efficacy of grommets in preventing the disabilities which may result from hearing impairment remain unanswered. The side-effects of the procedure include tympanosclerosis, increased incidence of chronic perforation, and possibly cholesteatoma. Antibiotics have been suggested as an alternative to grommets and a meta-analysis of 27 published, randomized, controlled studies suggests that the short-term use of antibiotics may have a limited but beneficial role in clearing the effusion.[47] Adenoidectomy has been shown to have definite benefits on the course of persistent middle ear effusion.[46] The GP must be aware of the services offered by the local audiology department in monitoring children with impaired hearing. An *Effective Health Care* bulletin[48] recommends observation and testing of children with bilateral hearing impairment of more than 25 decibels. Each practice should develop a policy for monitoring and referral of children with glue ear based on discussion of the questions raised above with the local ENT and audiology services. These issues should also be fully discussed with parents before referral is initiated.

Sinusitis

Epidemiology and impact on general practice

Only a small proportion of patients who have URTIs go on to develop acute sinusitis. Since the air passages in the sinuses are not fully developed until after puberty the infection is seen more commonly in adults than in children. Whilst some clinicians believe that acute sinusitis is more prevalent in people who smoke cigarettes, there are no studies to document and the observation is, at the moment, only anecdotal.

Aetiology

The facial sinuses should be sterile but a variety of bacterial and viral agents have been isolated from direct aspiration. Multiple studies of community-acquired acute maxillary sinusitis have demonstrated the predominance of *Strep. pneumoniae* and non-encapsulated *H. influenzae*.[49] These organisms, alone or in combination, account for nearly 60% of isolates. *Staphylococcus aureus*, group A streptococcus, *M. catarrhalis*, and viridans streptococci comprise most of the rest, with anaerobes being isolated in adult cases associated with dental disease. Viruses were isolated from 25% of cases and have led some workers to postulate that many cases of acute sinusitis are on a background of preceding viral infection. In chronic sinusitis the bacterial flora is much less predictable, with a range of Gram-negative and Gram-positive organisms and anaerobes being recovered. This condition is not, however, primarily an infective one but reflects damage done to the ciliated lining of the sinus and its inability to clear organisms effectively. Hence, chronic disease is influenced by repeated episodes of mucosal oedema and hypersecretion in response to infection or allergy.

Clinical features

Acute sinusitis presents in the context of a recent URTI or cold, or rarely, from the spread of a dental infection. Patients with infection of the paranasal sinuses complain of pain and facial tenderness accompanied by a nasal discharge and/or a post-nasal discharge. Headache may be a prominent feature, worse in the morning and on bending forward and sometimes the patient complains that his voice sounds 'nasal'. The patient may also complain of an unpleasant taste in his mouth and of bad breath. Occasionally, there is a fever, especially with marked involvement of the maxillary sinus, and a cough.

On examination, patients with acute sinusitis may have tenderness over the affected sinus and a purulent nasal discharge. There may be some facial swelling, especially around the eyes if the ethmoid sinus is involved. Very rarely, the infection extends into the orbit or into the brain leading to signs of meningitis or focal neurological signs due to a brain abscess.

Diagnosis and investigations

A recent history of a cold, URTI, or dental problems may help to direct the diagnosis towards acute sinusitis. Clinical examination often reveals reduction of the nasal airway with crust formation on a hyperaemic mucosa. A pale mucosa with polyp formation suggests an allergic component. Deviation of the nasal septum may be obvious and is a predisposing factor. Tenderness over the sinuses is also of value. It can, however, be difficult to distinguish clinically between a cold which is taking some time to resolve and acute sinusitis.[50] Some clinicians still use transillumination of the sinuses to help in the diagnosis since opacity of the sinuses suggests that the air passages may be filled with fluid. X-rays in patients over the age of one year may occasionally be helpful in visualizing fluid levels, or complete opacity although other appearances on plain radiograph are unreliable for diagnosis. The Royal College of Radiologists do not recommend that sinus X-ray be ordered in general practice because of its unreliability in diagnosis and the large radiation exposure.[51] Since the infecting organisms of acute sinusitis are predictable, as in acute otitis media, it is unnecessary to directly sample the sinus in individual, non-complicated cases. There is however a role for computerized tomographic scanning and magnetic resonance imaging assessment in the identification of underlying anatomical abnormalities which may be the basis for severe or recurrent infections.[52]

Treatment

General practitioners have to rely on clinical judgement alone to manage the majority of cases. The diagnosis has been shown to be unreliable and the doctor may be criticized for overprescribing antibiotics. A study of the predictive value of symptoms and signs in diagnosing maxillary sinusitis using ultrasonography as the gold standard, confirmed the GP's diagnosis in only 50% of cases.[53] The general condition of the patient, severity of the symptoms, and presence of clinical signs will determine the decision to treat with careful monitoring of the course of the illness allowing for subsequent adjustment of therapy. Nasal decongestants, such as phenylephrine, are of benefit as supportive treatment, analgesia is required and many patients find steam inhalations beneficial. If antibiotics are used they are directed against the major bacterial pathogens and, as for acute otitis media, the prevalence of beta-lactamase-producing organisms should be taken into account. Whilst amoxycillin has been a mainstay of therapy, agents such as co-amoxiclav or cefaclor may now be first-line treatment. The treatment should be continued for 14 days. Certainly, if a patient fails to respond adequately to therapy, which does not extend to beta-lactamase-producing organisms, then a change of antibiotic to such agents may be prudent.

Further investigation or referral is indicated if there are several attacks each year affecting more than one anatomical site or associated with exacerbation of asthma. Endoscopic sinus surgery has been noted to have success rates approaching 90% in chronic sinusitis,[54,55] and these patients should be referred early for assessment as these new techniques can make a huge difference to their quality of life.

Infections of the mouth, head, and neck

Epidemiology and impact on general practice

Infections of the head and neck may present to the dentist rather than the GP. The complications of such infections may, however, be seen as acute presentations in general practice. In any event, all GPs see patients with toothache, often at night with no dentist available to give immediate care. Joint meetings to decide guidelines for management can profitably be arranged. Complications can occur either by direct extension from a septic focus or by haematogenous spread and include such uncommon events as thrombophlebitis of the jugular vein, carotid artery erosion with haemorrhage, and septic cavernous sinus thrombosis. Finally, infections may present as maxillary sinusitis due to the proximity of the molars to its antrum or even as osteomyelitis of the mandible, including that associated with actinomycosis.

Infections of the oral cavity and soft tissues of the head and neck can be divided into those that have a dental origin and those that do not.

Dental infections

If pain is associated with dental caries then the all too well-known symptoms of toothache, often extremely acute, and sensitization of the tooth result. If an abscess is present there may be swelling and marked tenderness of the gum. In infections of the sublingual, submaxillary, or submandibular fascial spaces Ludwig's angina may occur. This is a clinical diagnosis which presents as bilateral infection, involves both the submandibular and sublingual spaces, begins in the floor of the mouth and rapidly spreads as an indurated cellulitis. The patient will be systemically toxic with a brawny, non-pitting swelling of the submandibular region, with oedema of the neck that may compromise the airway. Infection is often associated with a dental source of infection. If other spaces of the head and neck become infected, localized swelling and symptoms related to pressure on related anatomical areas will be present.

Infections of a non-dental origin

A variety of systemic diseases can present with oral manifestations of which measles, chickenpox, mumps, and sexually transmitted diseases are examples. The patient will present with the prodrome and perhaps the relevant rash.

Herpetic stomatitis may present early with complaints of tingling and sensitization. The patient is usually correct in his own diagnosis of the condition. A much more dangerous form of stomatitis, so-called gangrenous severe malnutrition, especially in children. Aphthous ulcers and stomatitis probably do not have an infectious origin.

The other major anatomical area presenting with sepsis in this region are the salivary glands. Both acute and chronic forms are recognized, the former presenting with swelling of the pre- and post-auricular areas, high fever, extreme pain and tenderness over the affected area, and the potential for complications including respiratory obstruction and osteomyelitis. The condition occurs most commonly in elderly and dehydrated patients. In the chronic form of the disease the infection of the gland tends to be low grade, with superimposed acute exacerbations of infection and ultimate destruction of salivary tissue.

Aetiology

A large variety of aerobic and anaerobic organisms are associated with infections related to the oral cavity. Infections of dental origin reflect the wide range of flora present in the mouth. They are usually polymicrobial and comprise representatives from the indigenous oral flora in which anaerobes outnumber facultative aerobic bacteria by 8:1. The indigenous flora of the mouth varies with a number of different factors including age, nutrition, dentition, oral hygiene, hospitalization, recent antibiotic therapy, and smoking habits.

Diagnosis and investigations

When pus can be aspirated from localized collections it should be cultured for both aerobic and anaerobic organisms. If systemic signs are present or the patient is toxic, blood cultures should also be examined.

Treatment

The requirement for surgical drainage of a localized collection of pus must be properly and adequately assessed since, as with any collection, this is the mainstay of treatment. Antibiotic therapy is adjuvant and is of benefit in controlling the spread of infection into local areas and perhaps into the blood. Many infections of the soft tissues of the head and neck, especially those of a dental origin, have been traditionally treated with penicillin, often in high doses. Certainly, dental infections are usually responsive to this agent, but the recognition of the importance of beta-lactamase-producing organisms, especially anaerobes in the *Bacteroides* group have raised concerns over this practice. If surgical drainage has been performed but the clinical response to penicillin in good doses (1200 mg, 4–6 hourly) is inadequate or if the patient is severely debilitated or immunocompromised, then metronidazole with the addition of an anti-Gram-negative agent, such as gentamicin, might be required. In non-dental infections involving *Staph. aureus*, flucloxacillin should be used.

Infections of the eye

The eye is a particularly vulnerable part of the body. Its delicate conjunctival covering, its close access to the brain, and its involvement in a number of systemic illnesses demands that we consider infectious conditions of the eye seriously and systematically. In presenting the infections of the eye we have therefore chosen to organize the section anatomically rather than by prevalence starting with the external structures.

The presentation of the infectious red eye to the GP can run the spectrum of benign self-limiting viral infection to sight or life-threatening sepsis which demands urgent attention. Infections of the eye are as follows:

- Periocular infections
- Conjunctivitis
- Keratitis
- Endophthalmitis

All GPs should be able to carry out a basic examination of the eye, including simple tests of visual acuity, and be competent in the use of the ophthalmoscope.

Epidemiology and impact on general practice[56]

During the period of a year a GP will conduct about 50 consultations for eye problems for every 1000 patients on the list: of these the majority will be for infectious conjunctivitis. The condition leads to about 14 episodes of new or new recurrent eye disease per 1000 of the practice population in a year, with most cases seen in children under the age of 4 years. In contrast blepharitis (2 episodes/1000), chalazion (2 episodes/1000), and anterior uveitis (0.6 episodes/1000) are less common. Other infections present occasionally, although trauma which may be complicated by infection is responsible for 20% of consultations for eye problems.

Many patients with eye infections present with a painful red eye but it is important for the GP to remember that the differential diagnosis also contains non-infectious causes such as iritis/uveitits and glaucoma (see Table 6.11).

Periocular infections

These infections include those related to the eyelids, the lacrimal glands,

Table 6.8 *Glossary of periorbital infections involving the lids and lacrimal apparatus*

Eyelids	
Blepharitis	Chronic inflammation of lid margins
Hordeolum	Known as a stye. Infection of the glands of the eyelid
	Internal: infection of meibomian gland
	External: infection of glands in lash follicles and skin of lid
Chalazion	Sterile inflammation of meibomian gland
Lacrimal glands	
Caniculitis	Low grade anaerobic infection of canals from lacrimal gland
Dacrocystitis	Inflammation of lacrimal sac
	Acute: acute pain with blockage of the ends of the lacrimal duct
	Chronic: obstruction of the sac with secondary infection
Dacroadenitis	Inflammation of lacrimal gland

the orbit, and the paranasal and cavernous sinuses. The vocabulary of the infections is really the most complicated problem and hence a glossary of infections of these areas, especially those involving the lids and lacrimal apparatus, is shown in Table 6.8.

Abscesses of the eyelid.   Styes (or external hordeolum) are extremely common and are infrequently presented to the doctor unless they are particularly painful or recurrent. They result from an acute infection of the eyelash follicle which usually points and discharges.

An acute chalazion results when there is infection of a meibomian gland and is more alarming because it is internal and may become chronic following a granulomatous reaction that is consequent on plugging and infection of one of the deeper glands of the eyelid.Infections of the eye

Treatment

These infections are usually managed in the first instance with warm compresses, analgesics, and topical antibiotics, remembering that fusidic acid is useful for staphylococcal infections. Mothers of small children must be reminded that the infection is spread by touching the lesion. Ointment may be easier to use than drops and time should be taken with inexperienced parents to explain how to administer the medication. Patients with a chalazion may ultimately require curettage.

Blepharitis.   This is a bilateral inflammation of the lid margins accompanied by scaling and crusts. *Staphylococcus aureus* is usually implicated. Lash follicles are destroyed and in severe cases the margins may become ulcerated. There is often accompanying seborrhoea of the scalp and overall the patient looks and feels miserable. All age groups are affected and effective treatment is usually with a combination of a medicated shampoo for the scalp and antibiotic ointment for the eyelids. Some patients with chronic blepharitis have dry eyes and the discomfort is eased by the instillation of tear film supplements such as hypromellose drops, 0.5%.

Orbital cellulitis. This is an extremely serious, acute infection of the orbital contents. The vast majority of infections, especially in children, follow spread from local structures, often after sinusitis. Whilst it is rare for orbital cellulitis to be the result of haematogenous spread in adults, in children it can occur following septicaemia with certain organisms. Trauma to the area, sometimes in association with an orbital fracture may also result in orbital cellulitis. Presenting features include fever, orbital oedema, nasal discharge, pain, headache, and local tenderness. As the infection progresses there may be proptosis of the eye with conjunctival injection and increasing loss of vision. Loss of vision indicates spread to the posterior orbit and is a medical emergency. Systemically, the patient may be very toxic and unwell, with a fever and elevated white cell count. Chandler *et al.*[57] classified the course of the infection into five stages, beginning with a preseptal cellulitis in which the orbit itself is not yet infected but there is orbital oedema due to local infection of the sinuses, followed by progressive infection which ends with life-threatening cavernous sinus thrombosis. Whilst cavernous sinus thrombosis is a rare complication of orbital cellulitis itself, cellulitis is almost invariably present if thrombosis of the sinus has occurred. Signs of cavernous sinus thrombosis include early neurological involvement, often with ophthalmoplegia, proptosis, decreased level of consciousness, and meningitis.

The agents responsible for orbital cellulitis reflect the local flora of the head and neck. *Staphylococcus aureus* is the most frequently isolated organism, but *Strep. pneumoniae* and beta-haemolytic group A streptococcus are also commonly implicated. In children below the age of 5 years, *H. influenzae* is important and may cause orbital cellulitis as a result of systemic infection elsewhere via haematogenous spread. Cultures from the site often contain a variety of organisms, especially anaerobes, reflecting the mixed flora of the area. Opportunistic infections with fungi, especially *Mucor* and *Aspergillus*, are well described in immunocompromised patients. *Aspergillus* species can also cause chronic infection in normal hosts, but takes the form of slow, progressive disease in which granulomatous formation is marked.

Diagnosis and investigations

Culture of discharge from the eye in which eyelid or lacrimal infections are suspected may reveal the causative organism but in practice most simple eyelid infections are managed empirically. Blockage of the lacrimal ducts needs to be assessed, possibly with cannulation and radiology. Bacteriological investigation of discharge or drainage from the sinuses are important in order to guide treatment. Blood cultures are essential to investigate cases of orbital cellulitis since it may be difficult to obtain positive cultures from the eye itself.

Treatment

Infections of the eyelids and lacrimal apparatus often respond to treatment with topical antibiotics. Whilst both blepharitis and hordeolum may respond to local measures, dacrocystitis and dacroadenitis usually require systemic therapy, with agents such as flucloxacillin or penicillin, if group A streptococci are implicated.

Systemic antibiotics are essential for the treatment of orbital cellulitis and patients in whom this condition is suspected should be referred at once. Surgical drainage of congested sinuses may be required if more conservative means such as nasal decongestants fail. Blind therapy should be directed against *Staph. aureus* initially with flucloxacillin, whilst in children under the age of 5 years, *H. influenzae* must be appropriately covered with an agent such as cefotaxime, especially if there is concern about the possibility of beta-lactamase production resulting in ampicillin resistance. Therapy should be specifically directed once culture and sensitivity results are known. If the infection does not settle, the possibility of an orbital abscess must be considered so that drainage can be performed. Cavernous sinus thrombosis clearly requires urgent treatment with high doses of intravenous antibiotics and some clinicians advocate the use of steroids and others of anti-coagulants in this condition. Fungal infection with *Mucor* or *Aspergillus* requires surgical drainage and debridement. Systemic amphotericin B may have some adjuvant benefit.

Conjunctivitis

Clinical features

Conjunctivitis is the commonest cause of a painful red eye in general practice. The diagnosis is made on the history, type of discharge, and appearance of the underside of the lid. The patient usually presents to the GP complaining of red and discharging eyes. The eyes may feel sore rather than painful and there is no complaint about vision. On examination, there is bilateral hyperaemia of the conjunctiva and a mucopurulent discharge. A membrane may be visible over the conjunctiva. There may be signs of an associated URTI, including fever and a sore throat, especially with a viral aetiology.

Although it is not always possible to differentiate between viral and bacterial causes of conjunctivitis, the discharge tends to more watery than purulent with viral conjunctivitis and itching with follicle formation, seen best by everting the upper lid, may be prominent features. Follicles have been compared to small grains of rice and are formed from collections of lymphocytes.

Aetiological agents

Bacteria. A great diversity of bacterial agents have been implicated in the aetiology of infectious conjunctivitis, mostly reflecting the wide range of

Table 6.9 *Causes of conjunctivitis*

Bacteria	Viruses
*Streptococcus pneumoniae**	Adenoviruses
Viridans streptococci	Herpes simplex
*Staphylococcus aureus**	Measles
Corynebacterium diphtheriae	Influenza
*Haemophilus influenzae**	Picornaviruses
*Neisseria gonorrhoea**	Varicella zoster
*Moraxella catarrhalis**	
*Chlamydia trachomatis**	

* These organisms are associated with ophthalmia neonatorum.

organisms associated with head and mouth flora. The most important of these are shown in Table 6.9. In adults, *Strep. pneumoniae* is the most common agent but *Staph. aureus* is also important. *Streptococcus pneumoniae* has also been implicated in outbreaks of conjunctivitis.[58] As might be predicted, in addition to these agents, *H. influenzae* has a significant role to play in children. Many other bacteria, both Gram-negative and Gram-positive and anaerobic as well as aerobic organisms have been cited in the literature as causal agents of conjunctivitis. Three bacterial conditions deserve special mention, the first two for their association with sexually transmitted diseases and hence with ophthalmia neonatorum and the last, conjunctivitis due to *C. diphtheriae*, which although very rare, is a potentially life-threatening condition with important public health implications.

Ophthalmia neonatorum

This is a catch-all phrase for conjunctivitis which occurs in the neonatal period. Historically, the use of silver nitrate drops as prophylaxis against gonorrhoea was the commonest cause of a mild, self-limiting chemical conjunctivitis in the neonatal period, but this practice has been discontinued in the UK. Whilst there are non-infectious causes of the condition, two important agents, *Chlamydia trachomatis* and *N. gonorrhoeae*, cause infection in the neonate after acquisition from an infected maternal genital tract. *Chlamydia trachomatis* causes an inclusion conjunctivitis in neonates and should not be confused with trachoma, a blinding disease associated with poor living conditions, which is also caused by *Chlamydia* but involves different serotypes from those associated with neonatal infection. Chlamydial conjunctivitis is increasingly common and more than 30% of infants born to infected mothers can be expected to acquire it at birth.[59] It presents usually 1–3 weeks after birth as a moderate to severe mucopurulent conjunctivitis and there is often marked swelling and erythema of the eyelids. The infection is bilateral in about 50% of cases but it is usually more severe in one eye. Untreated, the infection is relatively benign but rarely it is associated with a neonatal chlamydial pneumonia.

Gonococcal ophthalmia neonatorum is probably less common than chlamydial neonatal disease, reflecting the higher incidence of maternal chlamydial infection, but its true incidence is unknown. It presents with copious discharge, earlier than chlamydial conjunctivitis, and usually within 48 hours of birth. It has potentially serious consequences to sight, including corneal ulceration with possible subsequent perforation. Other bacteria which cause ophthalmia neonatorum but which are not recognized as sexually transmitted organisms are also shown in Table 6.9. *Moraxella catarrhalis* is important in that it can sometimes be confused with *N. gonorrhoeae*. Since this has important implications for the parents of the child it is essential that the microbiology of the isolate is properly documented and reported.

Viruses. Viral conjunctivitis accounts for some 15–20% of cases of conjunctivitis. With a few exceptions they cause self-limiting illness of brief duration, but they tend to be highly infectious. Adenoviruses are most frequently implicated in outbreaks of the disease and have been isolated from 8% of patients with acute conjunctivitis in an opthalmic casualty department.[60] Depending on the serotype, adenoviruses can cause slightly different illnesses. Thus, for example, a syndrome sometimes called pharyngo-conjunctival fever is most frequently caused by serotypes 3 and 7 whilst epidemic kerato-conjunctivitis (EKC) is associated most commonly with serotype 8. Both illnesses have an associated sore throat, fever, follicular conjunctivitis, and preauricular lymphadenopathy. In EKC there may also be an associated keratitis.

Adenovirus kerato-conjunctivitis has an average incubation period of 7 days and frequently affects young adults. Transmission occurs from the respiratory tract to the eye by coughing and sneezing and from eye to eye from contaminated fingers or fomites. More than half of patients begin with unilateral disease which becomes bilateral within 3–7 days. While the infection usually resolves within 6 weeks, about 10% of patients develop a chronic papillary conjunctivitis which produces a foreign body sensation, redness, swelling of the eyelids, discharge, and watering, and which may continue for many months. Papillae are formed by tufts of blood vessels giving the under-surface of the lid a roughened appearance.

Other common causes of viral conjunctivitis are listed in Table 6.9. More rarely, molluscum contagiosum, human papillomavirus, rubella virus, and mumps virus can involve the eye with a conjunctivitis.

Diagnosis and investigations

Most cases of conjunctivitis are managed and diagnosed empirically since the illness is usually benign and self-limiting. Conjunctival scrapings or swabs for bacterial and viral culture may be of benefit in recalcitrant cases. All cases of ophthalmia neonatorum should be investigated with bacterial, viral (especially for herpes simplex), and chlamydial cultures. A Gram film of the

Table 6.10 *Advice for patients with acute conjunctivitis*

- Do not touch the eye(s) with fingers, use tissues or handkerchiefs, and wash hands afterwards.
- Use tissues or handkerchiefs during coughing and sneezing because sneezing into another person's eye spreads the infection
- Use separate towels
- Sleep in a separate bed and avoid kissing or close contact
- Avoid swimming or sharing baths with others
- Stay away from work or school while symptomatic

discharge may demonstrate the characteristic Gram-negative diplococci of *N. gonorrhoeae* and give an early indication of the diagnosis. If a sexually transmitted aetiological agent is identified then care and tact will be essential to ensure appropriate investigation and follow-up of the parents.

Treatment

Most cases of mild conjunctivitis are self-limiting and do not necessarily require treatment. Chloramphenicol applied to the eye initially every 2–4 hours as drops or as ointment covers many of the non-STD (sexually transmitted) bacterial agents involved with the exception of some Gram-negative organisms for which topical neomycin or gentamicin might be required. Some authors have questioned the use of chloramphenical because of the rare but devastating complication of bone marrow aplasia. Framycetin or fusidic acid are safe and effective alternatives.[67] Because of the highly infectious nature of adenovirus conjunctivitis and the difficulties in precise diagnosis in general practice all patients with conjunctivitis should be given the advice shown in Table 6.10. In addition, great care must be taken when examining these patients to wash hands before and after examination and to use unidose eye drops for diagnosis and treatment.

Current recommendations for gonococcal ophthalmia neonatorum requires urgent treatment with intravenous benzyl penicillin, but reports of the use of ceftriaxone, especially for the treatment of penicillinase-producing *N. gonorrhoeae*, as single-dose therapy are encouraging.[62] Babies suspected of having this infection should be referred urgently.

Systemic erythromycin therapy for 3 weeks, sometimes with the addition of topical (but *not* systemic) tetracycline, is required for the treatment of neonatal chlamydial infection.

> *Case history*
>
> A 28-year-old married woman had a profuse discharge and an unhealthy looking cervix at her postnatal examination. A swab for Chlamydia was positive. She denied intercourse since the birth of the baby; the child was completely well. The couple declined referral to the STD clinic and her

Table 6.11 *Causes of a painful red eye*

- Conjunctivitis
  - bacterial
  - viral
  - allergic
- Blepharitis
- Episcleritis
- Corneal ulcers
  - viral
  - bacterial
  - protozoan
- Corneal foreign bodies
- Acute angle closure glaucoma
- Uveitis
  - acute iritis
- Orbital cellulitis

---

husband subsequently attended the practice. He confided that he had had intercourse with another partner during his wife's pregnancy. Eventually, with the help of the GP, he was able to discuss the relationship with his wife and to suggest to his other partner that she attend the STD clinic. Both adults received treatment for *Chlamydia* infection. The GP decided to treat the infant with erythromycin syrup (40 mg/kg of body weight daily in four divided doses for 2 weeks) to prevent the rare complication of chlamydial pneumonitis. There was, however, never any evidence that the child had contracted the infection.

Keratitis

Corneal inflammation, or keratitis, is a much more worrying condition than conjunctivitis since it can rapidly and aggressively threaten vision. Keratitis usually implies that the integrity of the cornea has been impaired often by trauma, including the trauma related to abnormal lid function, dry eyes, or contact lenses. Corneal ulceration may be an associated finding. If the patient has a systemic illness which impairs the immune function, such as diabetes mellitus then, given the appropriate setting, the potential for keratitis increases. Keratitis should be considered a medical emergency since it potentially threatens sight. See Table 6.11 for the causes of a painful red eye.

Clinical features

A comparison of the clinical features of conjunctivitis and keratitis is shown in Table 6.12. Unlike conjunctivitis, pain, sometimes extremely severe, is the major presenting symptom of keratitis and it is common for the patient to experience some loss of vision. There is usually intense photophobia. Unless there is an associated conjunctivitis the eye does not necessarily appear red

Table 6.12 *Clinical features of conjunctivitis and keratitis*

	Conjunctivitis	**Keratitis**
Pain	Absent or 'sore'	Present: may be agonizing
Discharge	Often copious	Scanty if at all
Visual changes	None	Impaired vision
Conjunctival inflammation	Present	May be absent
Photophobia	Absent	Present
Corneal appearance	Normal	Loss of transparency
Corneal ulcers	Absent	May be present

nor is there much by way of discharge, but there is a loss of corneal transparency which may be difficult to detect unless a cobalt light (Wood's light) is used to visualize the cornea, following instillation of fluorescein. The crucial consequence of corneal inflammation is ulcer formation on the cornea which may subsequently result in corneal perforation or scarring. In late, severe, untreated infection the aqueous and vitreous humours may become involved resulting in endophthalmitis.

Aetiological agents

Bacteria. More than 60 infectious agents have been documented as causes of keratitis including bacteria, viruses, parasites, and fungi. All of the organisms which have been implicated in conjunctivitis are also involved in this infection but, in addition, *Ps. aeruginosa* is, along with *Staph. aureus* and *Strep. pneumoniae*, among the most important aetiological bacterial agent. These three organisms cause more than 80% of bacterial keratitis. *Pseudomonas aeruginosa* produces an exotoxin which can break down the corneal stroma resulting in rapid perforation. In general practice this organism, along with other Gram-negative bacilli, presents a particular hazard to contact lens users. Contaminated eye make-up is also a potential community source of infection.

Conjunctivitis and keratitis in contact lens wearers

About 1.65 million people in the UK wear contact lenses and it is quite common for wearers to consult the GP with eye infections. They may contract simple conjunctivitis which is unrelated to the lens. The lenses should be left out for a week while treatment is completed and the lenses and case thoroughly sterilized, and a review made of lens hygiene. They are, however, more likely to have unusual pathogens such as Gram-negative organisms and an aminoglycoside may be a better first choice in these patients rather than chloramphenicol.

Occasionally, a microbial keratitis may develop, often due to *Ps. aeruginosa* and usually resulting from poor lens hygiene. Progression to an extensive grey ulcer with a hypopyon can occur within a few days. This is a sight-threatening emergency and any suspicion of this condition should prompt immediate referral. Patients should take their lenses and case with them as the causative organism may be cultured from them.

Finally, the amoeba, *Acanthamoeba*, has been associated with keratitis in contact lens wearers who fail to use appropriate cleaning solutions.[63] This free-living protozoan is found in soil, pond water, and mains water supplies. Keratitis due to this organism has increasingly been reported amongst soft contact lens wearers. The infection starts by contamination of contact lens cases by household or mains water supply, and if bacteria are also present then the amoebas can multiply rapidly with the bacteria as a food source. The resulting keratitis can have a devastating effect on vision and it is essential that soft contact lens wearers do not use tap water to rinse lens cases. These should be washed daily in boiled cooled water and kept dry when not in use. Overnight or extended wear should be avoided as it leads to corneal oedema which predisposes to the infection. The major risk factors for *Acanthamoeba* keratitis in a case control study of patients seen at Moorfield hospital between 1989 and 1992 were failure to disinfect daily wear soft contact lenses and use of chlorine-release lens disinfection systems.[64]

Viruses. Herpetic keratitis is the most common and the most important viral keratitis and is almost always caused by herpes simplex virus-1 (HSV-1). The prevalence is not known but studies of patients with acute conjunctivitis seen in London eye casualty departments found about 9% to have the infection.[60]

Epidemiology and clinical features of HSV eye infections. The disease is variable in its presentation with the primary infection presenting as an acute, moderate to severe follicular kerato-conjunctivitis commonly associated with small blisters or ulcers on the eyelid. About 80% of patients have the infection in one eye and present with redness, watering, discharge, itching, and lid swelling. Most patients have a severe papillary response, seen best on everting the upper eyelid, with follicles seen mainly on the lower palpebral conjunctiva.[65]

Approximately 20% of neonates infected with herpes simplex virus have ocular involvement, 7% of which will be a keratitis. Characteristic dendritic ulcers may be present and a small number will have a perforated cornea.

In adults, there is a high recurrence rate of up to 40% following an initial attack of HSV keratitis. Although many cases heal without treatment after 2 weeks, with the duration and severity of attacks decreasing with time, a small number of patients develop stromal scarring with subsequent visual loss. In a study of 108 patients conducted in London with follow-up for up to 15 years, 35 individuals developed recurrent infection but only 3 had a dendritic ulcer.[60] Dendritic ulcers are characteristic branching corneal ulcers which show on fluorescein staining and are one of the lesions that should be looked for during the examination of a red eye. The infection is accelerated by the use of steroid medications in the eye and *it is negligent* to use them in a red eye if herpes simplex virus infection has not been excluded.

A few patients go on to develop repeated attacks of corneal ulceration with scarring of the stroma and vascularization of the cornea. Subsequently, there may be involvement of the deeper layers leading to herpetic disciform keratitis with pain and visual impairment.

With the introduction of a specific, effective, antiviral agent, acyclovir, it is now common practice to treat HSV infection, since treatment reduces visual morbidity and the likelihood of recurrences. These patients should be supervised by an opthalmologist with urgent referral to establish the diagnosis in the first attack. Treatment for recurrences is with topical acylovir five times daily and should be started at once by the GP with early review in the eye department.

Ophthalmic herpes zoster. Herpes zoster (shingles) which is not as sensitive to acyclovir may present with involvement of the ophthalmic division of the trigeminal nerve; it is estimated that about 7% of all cases of zoster affect the eye. If these patients are managed in general practice they should be seen daily. If the rash extends to the tip of the nose (indicating involvement of the naso-ciliary branch of the trigeminal nerve) then early treatment with acyclovir (800 mg, 5 times/day) has been shown to reduce ocular complications which can vary from mild to devastating eye disease. If despite this the patient develops a red eye then urgent referral to an ophthalmologist is wise.

Diagnosis and investigations

Although many patients with conjunctivitis may be treated expectantly, this is not true with a clinical diagnosis of keratitis since the potential threat to vision is a real one. Corneal scrapings from the ulcer for urgent Gram-stain and culture should be performed for both aerobic and anaerobic bacterial culture and for viral culture. These patients should be referred to eye casualty at once or, if this is impossible, their management pending urgent referral must be discussed with the ophthalmologist over the telephone.

Treatment

Infective keratitis and corneal ulceration with their potential for corneal perforation constitute a medical emergency which requires admission to hospital in most cases. Both topical antibiotics, administered in a variety of ways (topically as a high concentration solution, subconjunctivally or by continual lavage) and intravenous antibiotics can be used, often in combination. The choice of antibiotic may be indicated by the Gram-film. An aminoglycoside and a third-generation cephalosporin such as cefotaxime or ceftazidime can provide broad spectrum empirical therapy until results of cultures are known. Supportive measures include, in some cases, steroid therapy although its place, especially in cases of herpes zoster keratitis, is still controversial. The antiviral agent, acyclovir, now has an essential therapeutic place in the treatment of ocular herpes.

The GP should follow-up the patient to plan the management of recurrent disease should it appear and to encourage the patient to continue review with the eye department. Some patients with herpetic disciform keratitis may need months of treatment with a combination of acyclovir and steroids which must be reduced gradually to prevent recurrence. The GP should arrange to see these patients from time to time rather than just issuing repeat prescriptions at the request of the ophthalmologist. Contact lens wearers should be reminded about hygiene and to follow instructions about wear *to the letter*, as many people take risks even after serious eye infections.

Specific therapy for more exotic parasitic or fungal infections require expert advice.

Endophthalmitis

This is an inflammatory condition within the bony cavity of the orbit. Infectious endophthalmitis is the result either of trauma to the eye (surgical or non-surgical) or by haematogenous spread of an organism from a distant site. Postoperative endophthalmitis has been well reviewed.[66] Whilst it frequently presents while the patient is still in hospital, it may present in more indolent forms after discharge to the community and the trend to day surgery will inevitably lead to more presentations in general practice. The most common preceding surgical procedure is cataract extraction with intraocular lens implantation.[67]

Clinical features

Pain and reduced visual acuity are the major presenting clinical complaints of endophthalmitis. If there has been recent eye surgery the diagnosis should be urgently considered and the patient referred back to the surgeon at once. On examination, there is inflammation of the conjunctiva with lid and corneal oedema and a hypopyon may been seen. In the absence of a history of surgery or trauma, the patient is likely to be immunosuppressed or present with a systemic infection or soft tissue focus.

Aetiological agents

An enormous range of organisms have been implicated in infective endophthalmitis. Bacterial agents, viruses, fungi, and parasites have all been involved, with *Staph. aureus*, *Staph. epidermis*, and Gram-negative organisms, especially *Ps. aeruginosa*, being the major bacterial pathogens following operative procedures. A number of nosocomial outbreaks have also been reported related to contaminated fluids or equipment, often involving Gram-negative organisms. There is some relationship between the acuteness of the presentation and the organism in that *Staph. aureus* infections tend to present within a week of surgery, whilst infections with coagulase negative staphylococci present later (2–6 weeks post-surgery), and more indolently. Bacterial endophthalmitis which is not related to surgery or trauma is caused by haematogenous spread and is seen most commonly in ill, immunosuppressed patients. A focus is usually present resulting in endophthalmitis being associated with such systemic infections as endocarditis (and may present as Roth spots in the retina), meningitis, breast abscess, soft tissue, and intra-abdominal sepsis. In such cases, the organisms isolated from the eye usually reflect the underlying condition and infecting agent. Fungal endophthalmitis presents much more indolently than bacterial infection. Whilst it can occur after surgery or trauma, it is more commonly seen in the context of immunosuppression, antibiotic use, steroids, or intravenous drug abuse. *Candida albicans* is the most frequent agent implicated, but *Aspergillus* species, *Cryptococcus neoformans*, and *Mucor* are also important fungal causes. Amongst the viral agents, the herpesviruses can progress from causing a keratitis to endophthalmitis, usually an iridocyclitis.

Cytomegalovirus (CMV) is an important cause of congenital chorioretinitis and is now also of major concern in patients with AIDS. Both groups of patients may also be infected by *Toxoplasma gondii*, but *Toxocara* is the commonest parasitic cause of endophthalmitis and poses a serious threat to vision in young children.

Cytomegalovirus (CMV). Congenital infection with CMV is often marked by involvement of the eye, resulting in chorioretinitis in nearly one-third of affected infants. Other eye manifestations of infection include cataracts, iritis, and optic atrophy. In addition, there may be severe systemic infection, with jaundice, purpura, hepatosplenomegaly, pulmonary infiltrates, and intracerebral calcification. A small number of infants die *in utero* and survivors may be severely affected with microcephaly, mental retardation, and hearing loss. Although the virus may infect up to 1% of pregnant women, most infants are not affected. However, late manifestations occur in approximately 10% of infected cases and often involve neurological deficit, frequently with impairment of hearing. Careful follow-up of infected infants who are apparently well at birth is therefore necessary. In normal young adults CMV infection causes a mild hepatitis and 'mononucleosis' type illness which is self-limiting. CMV infection is currently much more frequently seen within the context of AIDS and other forms of acquired immunosuppression such as lymphoproliferative diseases and renal transplantation.

Cytomegalovirus chorioretinitis. Blurred vision often heralds the onset of the infection, with gradual loss of vision that is irreversible as the disease progresses. On fundoscopy the appearance of the chorioretinitis are distinctive, with widespread retinal haemorrhages, exudates, and oedema. Eventually, as healing occurs, atrophic lesions are seen. Regular ophthalmic examination in patients with AIDS is important since these eye signs are one of the earliest manifestations of systemic CMV infection. Early treatment with the antiviral agent, ganciclovir, is currently the best treatment available, but must be lifelong in order to prevent relapse. Some GPs have begun giving this on an out-patient basis as part of shared care to enable more community care of patients with this complication of AIDS.

Table 6.13 *Guidance to parents to prevent toxocariasis*

Did you know that your child is at risk from local cats and dogs?
Cats and dogs are important parts of many people's lives. They offer companionship, friendship and fun to children, families and elderly people. But they can also threaten the health of our children by carrying worms (called *Toxocara*) which can cause blindness.

There are 4 simple rules which can reduce this risk:

1. Always wash hands after handling soil or playing in a sandpit and before eating
2. Do not allow dogs or cats to foul children's play areas
3. Cover sandpits when not in use to avoid cats fouling them
4. Regularly de-worm kittens and puppies, cats and dogs

Toxocariasis. Infections with the nematodes, *Toxocara canis* or *Toxocara cati* are the commonest parasitic causes of endophthalmitis. They are also one of the causes of visceral larva migrans (VLM). Children become infected by ingesting soil contaminated with ova from dog and cat faeces, systemic involvement may include pulmonary infiltrates, hepatomegaly, and occasionally neurological symptoms. Eosinophilia is usually present. Eye manifestations are caused by migration of the larva to the eye and can result in a retinal granuloma or in chronic endophthalmitis, with loss of vision. Clinically it is important to distinguish it from a retinoblastoma with which it can be confused. Toxocariasis is responsible for about 10% of cases of uveitis in children; it tends to occur in slightly older children (their average age is about 8 years) than those who suffer from VLM and may be due to relatively mild infections with less immunological response. Hence, eye involvement in toxocariasis often unfortunately occurs in the absence of any other visceral features and without an eosinophilia. The child rarely notices any visual problem but loss of vision and disuse may produce a squint. At other times, it is only detected after routine acuity testing. Therapy may involve the use of an agent such as thiabendazole, especially in VLM, but the dead encysted larva which form part of the granulomatous eye lesion set up an inflammatory process in the eye which is best treated with systemic or intraocular steroids. However, prevention is the best treatment and should be encouraged by appropriate advice which is accessible and widespread.[68] A possible format for a leaflet or for the notice board is shown in Table 6.13.

Toxoplasmosis. Domestic cats and small rodents play an important part in the life cycle of toxoplasma, a protozoan which can cause retinochoroiditis. Most cases are believed to result from congenital infection acquired *in utero* and long-term follow-up of infected children show that most develop eye disease before the age of 20 years. The subject is covered in detail in Chapter

2, where it forms the basis for a case study for the primary care team in the ethical and practical issues involved in prevention of infection.

Diagnosis and investigations

Since sight may be severely and permanently compromised by endophthalmitis urgent diagnosis is essential. Although conjunctival material is most accessible, the organisms cultured from this site often do not reflect the situation within the eye. It is therefore critical to obtain samples from the site of infection (i.e. from within the orbit the of the eye). The recommended site for culture is the vitreous humour, since culture of the aqueous humour alone has been negative in 35–57% of series. Hence, hospital referral is mandatory for these patients.

Treatment

Definitive therapy for bacterial endophthalmitis has not yet been determined, with treatment issues revolving around the requirement for invasive surgery (vitrectomy or not) and the best route for delivering antibiotics. There is, however, consensus on the urgency to establish the correct diagnosis and the absolute requirement for timely intervention in order to obtain the best outcome.

References

1. De Melker R A, Kuyvenhoven M M. Management of upper respiratory tract infection in Dutch general practice. *Brit J Gen Pract* (1991) **4**: 504–7

2. Wald F. Sinusitis in children. *N Engl J Med* 1992 **326**: 319–23

3. Nicholson K *et al.* Respiratory viruses and excacerbations of asthma in adults. *BMJ* (1993) **307**: 982–6

4. Fleming D, Norbury C, Crombie D. Annual and seasonal variation in the incidence of common diseases. *Occasional Paper* 53. London: Royal College of General Practitioners. (1992)

5. Johnston S, Pattemore P, Sanderson G *et al.* Community study of role of viral infections in exacerbations of asthma in 9–11 year old children. *BMJ* (1995) **310**: 1225–9

6. Little P, Williamson I.Are antibiotics appropriate for sore throats? Costs outweigh the benefits. *BMJ* (1994) **309**: 1010–12

7. Shvartzman P. Are antibiotics appropriate for sore throats? Careful prescribing is beneficial. *BMJ* (1994) **309**: 1010–12

8. Demers D *et al.* Group A streptococcal disease. *Curr Op Infect Dis* (1993) **6**: 565–9

9. Shulman S. Complications of streptococcal pharyngitis. *Ped Infect Dis J* (1994) **13**: S70–4

10. Hjortdahl P, Melbye H. Does near-to-patient testing contribute to the diagnosis of streptococcal pharyngitis in adults. *Scand J Prim Health Care* (1994) **12**: 70–6

11. Pichichero M. Group A streptococcal tonsillopharyngitis: cost-effective diagnosis and treatment. *Annals Emer Med* (1995) **25**: 390–403

12. Pichichero M *et al*. Comparative reliability of clinical, culture and antigen detection methods for the diagnosis of Group A *beta-hemolytic* streptococcal tonsillopharyngitis. *Ped Ann* (1992) **21**: 798–805

13. Heiter B, Bourbeau P. Comparison of two rapid streptococcal antigen detection assays with culture for diagnosis of streptococcal pharyngitis. *J Clin Microbiol* (1995) **33**: 1408–10

14. Shvartzman P, Rosentzwaig A, Doignov F. Treatment of streptococcal pharyngitis with amoxycillin once a day. *BMJ* (1993) **306**: 1170–2

15. Tompkins D. Shannon A. Clinical value of microbiological investigations in general practice. *Brit J Gen Pract* (1993) **43**: 155–8

16. Dajani A, Taubert K, Ferrieri *et al*. Treatment of acute streptococcal pharyngitis and prevention of rheumatic fever: a statement for health professionals. Committee on rheumatic fever, endocarditis, and Kawasaki disease of the Council on cardiovascular disease in the young, the American Heart Association. *Ped* (1995) **96,4**: 758–64

17. Gordis L. The virtual disappearance of rheumatic fever in the United States: lessons on the rise and fall of disease. *Circulation* (1985) **72**: 1155–62

18. Vyse T *et al*. Hammersmith staff rounds. Rheumatic fever: changes in its incidence and presentation. *BMJ* (1991) **302**: 518–20.

19. Carr N, Wales S, Young D. Reported management of patients with sore throat in Australian general practice. *Brit J Gen Pract* (1994) **44**: 515–18

20. de Lange de Klerk *et al*. Effect of homeopathic medicines on daily burden of symptoms in children with recurrent upper respiratory tract infections. *BMJ* (1994) **309**: 1329–32

21. Strauss S. Epstein–Barr virus infections: Biology, pathogenesis, and management. *Ann Intern Med* (1993) **118**: 45–57

22. Wiselka M. Influenza: diagnosis, management, and prophylaxis. *BMJ* (1994) **308**: 1341–5

23. Cressman W, Myer C. Diagnosis and management of croup and epiglottitis. *Ped Clinics N Am* (1994) **41(2)**: 265–76

24. Bank D, Krug S. New approaches to upper airway disease. *Em Med Clinics N Am* (1995) **13**: 473–87

25. Jacobs S, Shortland G, Warner J *et al* Validation of a croup score and its use in triaging children with croup. *Anaesthesia* (1994) **49**: 903–6

26. Skolnik N. Croup. *J Fam Pract* (1993) **37**: 165–70

27. Cruz M, Stewart G, Rosenberg N. Use of dexamethasone in the outpatient management of acute laryngotracheitis. *Pediatrics* (1995) **96**: 220–3

28. Waisman Y, Klein B, Boenning D *et al*. Prospective randomised double-blind

study comparing L-epinephrine and racemic epinephrine aerosols in the treatment of laryngotracheitis (croup). *Pediatrics* (1992) **89**: 302–6

29. Connors K, Gavula D, Terndrup T. The use of corticosteroids in croup: a survey. *Ped Em Care* (1994) **10**: 197–9

30. Klassen T, Feldman M, Watters L *et al.* Nebulised budesonide for children with mild-to-moderate croup. *N Eng J Med* (1994) **331**: 285–9

31. Husby S, Agertoft L, Mortensen S. *et al.* Treatment of croup with nebulised steroid (budesonide): a double blind, placebo controlled study. *Arch Dis Child* (1993) **68**: 352–5

32. Inhaled budesonide and adrenaline for croup. *Drugs Therap Bull* (1996) **34**: 23–4

33. Pichichero M. Pertussis and pertussis vaccines *Curr Op Infect Dis* (1993) **6**: 558–64

34. Jenkinson D. Natural history of 500 consecutive cases of whooping cough: a general practice population study. *BMJ* (1995) **310**: 299–302

35. Teele D W. *et al.* Epidemiology of acute otitis media during the first seven years of life in children in greater Boston: a prospective cohort study. *J Infect Dis* (1989) **160**: 83–94

36. Maw R. Using tympanometry to detect glue ear in general practice: overreliance will lead to overtreatment. *BMJ* (1992) **304**: 67–8

37. Appelman C *et al.* Severity of inflammation of tympanic membrane as predictor of clinical course of recurrent acute otitis media. *BMJ* (1993) **306**: 895

38. Bluestone C, Stephenson J, Martin L. Ten-year review of otitis media pathogens. *Infect Dis* (1992) **11**: S7–11

39. Engelhard D *et al.* Randomised study of myringotomy, amoxycillin/clavulanate, or both for acute otitis media in infants. *Lancet* (1989) **32**: 141–3

40. Bain J. Justification for antibiotic use in general practice *BMJ* (1990) **300**: 1006–7

41. Froom J, Culpepper L, Grog P *et al.* Diagnosis and antibiotic treatment of acute otitis media: report from international primary care network. *BMJ* (1990) **300**: 582–6

42. van Buchem F, Peeters M, van't Hof M. Acute otitis media: Myringotomy, antibiotics or neither? *Lancet* (1981) **2**: 883–8

43. Kaleida P H *et al.* Amoxycillin or myringotomy or both for acute otitis media: results of a randomised clinical trial. *Ped* (1991) **87**: 466–74

44. Burke P *et al.* Acute red ear in children: controlled trial of non-antibiotic treatment in general practice. *BMJ* (1991) **303**: 558–62

45. Burke P. Otitis media: antibiotics or not? *Practitioner* (1992) **236**: 432–9

46. De Melker R. Treating persistent glue ear in children. *BMJ* (1993) **306**: 5

47. Williams R, Chalmers T, Stange K *et al.* Use of antibiotics in preventing recurrent acute otitis media and in treating otitis media with effusion. *JAMA* (1993) **270**: 1344–51

48. The treatment of persistent glue ear in children. *Effective Health Care* (1992) no **4**

49. Evans K. Diagnosis and management of sinusitis. *BMJ* (1994) **309**: 1415–22

50. van Buchem L, Peeters M, Beaumont J. Acute maxillary sinusitis in general practice: the relation between clinical picture and objective findings *Euro J Gen Pract* (1995) **1**: 155–60

51. Royal College of Radiologists. *Making the best use of a department of clinical radiology. Guidelines for doctors.* 2nd ed. London: *Royal College of Radiologists.* 1993

52. April M, Zinreich S, Baroody F *et al.* Coronal CT scan abnormalities in children with chronic sinusitis. *Laryngoscope* (1993) **103**: 985–90

53. van Dui JN *et al.* Use of symptoms and signs to diagnose maxillary sinusitis in general practice: comparison with ultrasonography. *BMJ* (1992) **305**: 684–7

54. Lanza D, Kennedy D. Current concepts in the surgical management of chronic and recurrent acute sinusitis *J Allergy Clin Immunol* (1992) **90**: 505–10

55. Lazar R, Younis R, Long T. Functional endonasal sinus surgery in adults and children. *Laryngoscope* (1993) **103**: 1–5

56. Sheldrick J, Vernon S, Wilson A. Demand incidence and episode rates of opthalmic disease in a defined urban population. *BMJ* (1992) **305**: 933–6

57. Chandler J, Langenrunner D, Stevens E. The pathogenesis of orbital complications in acute sinusitis. *Laryngoscope* (1970) **1980**: 1414–28

58. Shayegani M, Parsons L, Gibbons W *et al.* Characterisation of non-typable *Streptococcus Pneumoniae*-like organisms isolated from outbreaks of conjunctivitis. *J Clin Microbiol* (1982) **16**: 8

59. Darougar S, Monnickendam M, Woodland R. Management and prevention of occular viral and chlamydial infections. *CRC: Crit Rev Microbiol* (1989) **16**: 369–418

60. Wishart P, James C, Wishart M *et al.* Prevalence of acute conjunctivitis caused by Chlamydia, adenovirus and herpes simplex virus in an opthalmic casualty department. *Brit J Ophthalmol* (1984) **68**: 653

61. Doona M, Walsh J. The use of chloramphenicol as topical eye medication: time to cry halt? *BMJ* (1995) **310**: 1217–8

62. Laga M, Naamara W, Brunham R *et al.* Single dose therapy of gonococcal opthalmia neonatorum with ceftriaxone. *N Engl J Med* (1986) **315**: 1382

63. Sheal D. (Editorial) Acanthamoeba keratitis: A problem for contact lens users that is here to stay. *BMJ* (1994) **308**: 1116–17

64. Radford C *et al.* Risk factors for acanthamoeba keratitis in contact lens users: a case-control study *BMJ* (1995) **310**: 1567–70

65. Darougar S, Wishart M, Viswalingam N. Epidemiological and clinical features of primary herpes simplex virus occular infection. *Brit J Ophthalmol* (1985) **69**: 2

66. Elston R, Chattopadhyay B. Postoperative endophthalmitis. *J Hosp Infection* (1991) **17**: 243–53

67. Pflugfelder S, Flynn H. Infectious endophthalmitis *Infect Dis Clin N Am* (1992) **6**: 859–73

68. Kerr-Muir M. *Toxocara canis* and human health *BMJ* (1994) **309**: 5–6

69. Cartwright K, Begg N, Hull D. Chemoprophylaxis for *Haemophilus influenzae* type b. (Editorial) *BMJ* (1991) **302**: 546–7

CHAPTER SEVEN

Infections of the lower respiratory tract

This chapter deals with common and important lower respiratory tract infections (LRTIs) which principally manifest beyond the trachea and discusses their epidemiology, aetiology, clinical features, investigation, and management. Although GPs play a major part in dealing with these problems, one of their most important roles is to encourage patients to stop smoking thereby substantially reducing the impact of these infections on individuals and families.

Many GPs link their anti-smoking advice to the patient's presenting complaints and believe that this is the most effective way of intervening. Some doctors are less enthusiastic about discussing smoking with every smoker that they see even though there is evidence that a comprehensive approach will have a small beneficial effect.[1] In an important early study Russell[2] reported that 5% of smokers gave up completely for one year after minimal opportunistic intervention by the GP. It has now been established that it is effective to advise smokers to stop on each occasion that they consult and that additional measures such as leaflets and follow-up appointments to discuss smoking will have some effect. Advice to stop smoking should take into account the following factors:[3]

1. Heavy smokers may need to cut down and work towards a date for stopping completely. Nicotine chewing gum may be helpful.

2. People with low self-esteem and low expectation of success need encouragement and follow-up.

3. If finance is the only motive for stopping introduce others such as the health risks and the risks of passive smoking, particularly for small children.

4. Encourage them to get other family members to stop at the same time. Plan daily routine to avoid the company of smokers if possible. Tell friends and colleagues of their plan to stop.

5. Plan coping strategies for 'high-risk' situations such as parties or after eating.

Acute lower respiratory tract infections

Many of the LRTIs which are managed in general practice are relatively mild and self-limiting, are not investigated, and are managed symptomatically.

They frequently follow a sore throat or coryza and are described as 'acute bronchitis' or a 'cold on the chest' both by patients and in the medical records. The diagnosis is usually formalized only if the constitutional symptoms including fever, and the lower respiratory symptoms including wheeze, chest pain, breathlessness, and retrosternal soreness, reach a certain threshold. While many of these infections are viral, some studies indicate that the range of pathogens is similar to that which causes community-acquired pneumonia.[4] The decision to prescribe antibiotics in these circumstances is a difficult one and subject to all the factors discussed in Chapter 5.[5] If an antibiotic is given amoxycillin is usually the first choice and was at least as effective as clarithromycin, in a study of 442 adults in a general practice setting. Of these patients (none of whom were investigated), 45% were confined to bed for about 3 days, 76% were unable to perform their normal duties for 1–10 days, and 67% were off work for a median number of 5 days.[6] This study was performed at a time of low *Mycoplasma pneumoniae* activity and it might be that a macrolide would confer advantages during a peak of the four-yearly epidemic cycle. It is open to question (and the authors of this book agree) whether antibiotics made any difference at all to a proportion of these patients; they were given on the usual basis of clinical judgement and negotiation which needs a much better base in research than presently exists.

Chronic bronchitis

This is the commonest chest disorder seen in general practice with 20% of males and 5% of females over the age of 40 having symptoms which qualify for the diagnosis. It is a disease of smokers and ex-smokers. An alternative diagnosis such as asthma or bronchiectasis should be sought in lifelong non-smokers. While the disease is not primarily caused by infection recurrent bronchial infections are common. The risk factors for chronic bronchitis are shown in Table 7.1.

Table 7.1 *Risk factors for chronic bronchitis*

- Males
- Cigarette smoking
- Passive smoking
- Occupational hazards such as coal-mining
- Socioeconomic groups IV and V
- Urban living
- Atmospheric pollution
- Increasing age
- Family history of bronchitis
- History of recurrent bronchitis in childhood

In chronic bronchitis, a chronic airflow limitation is defined as existing in any person who regularly expectorates sputum for at least three months of the year and has done so for two years. It is a functional disorder, characterized by excess secretion of sticky mucus caused by hypertrophy of the mucuos glands and an increase in size and number of goblet cells.

Diagnosis and investigations

This is made from the history, clinical examination, and by use of a peak flow meter or vitalograph which will demonstrate irreversible airways obstruction. The condition must be distinguished from other chronic chest diseases such as bronchiectasis, pneumoconiosis, carcinoma of lung, late onset asthma, tuberculosis, and left-sided heart failure.

A chest X-ray may be necessary to exclude other chest diseases, or carcinoma of lung and serial lung function tests are an essential aid to long-term management. Sputum culture is of little value except to exclude tuberculosis.

Treatment

The general management of chronic bronchitis involves the considered use of many therapeutic agents:

- Physiotherapy
- Beta-2 stimulators
- Theophylline and derivatives
- Anticholinergic drugs
- Corticosteroids (inhaled and oral)
- Oxygen and oxygen concentrator (discuss with local pharmacist)
- Influenza vaccination
- Diuretics (if cor pulmonale)

The defence mechanisms of the lower respiratory tract are very efficient in healthy individuals and despite the upper respiratory tract being colonized by inhaled bacteria the lower respiratory tract usually remains sterile. Cigarette smoking and viral infections cause damage to the cilia of the epithelium in both upper and lower respiratory tracts, this interrupts co-ordinated ciliated movement which helps to repel bacteria and prevent their multiplication in static mucus.

The organisms responsible for exacerbations of chronic bronchitis are shown in Table 7.2, and *Streptococcus pneumoniae*, *Haemophilus influenzae*, and *Moraxella catarrhalis* are the commonest pathogens. Increasing numbers of *H. influenzae* produce β-lactamase and are resistant to ampicillin. At least 10–20% of *H. influenzae* isolates and 40–80% of *M. catarrhalis* strains are now resistant to this antibiotic. To overcome this problem one may use a β-lactamase inhibitor such as clavulanic acid. An alternative strategy

Table 7.2 *Organisms responsible for exacerbations of chronic bronchitis*

- *Haemophilus influenzae*
- *Streptococcus pneumoniae*
- *Staphylococcus aureus*
- *Moraxella catarrhalis*
- *Pseudomonas aeruginosa*
- *Klebsiella pneumoniae*
- *Escherichia coli*

is to prescribe a quinolone such as ciprofloxacin which is unaffected by β-lactamase but its activity against *Strep. pneumoniae* is limited. In patients with bronchiectasis or severe chronic obstructive airways disease high antibiotic doses may be necessary. In the UK, 3–4% of *Strep. pneumoniae* are penicillin-resistant but the figure may be much higher in other countries.[7] The GP must take note of this when treating infections acquired overseas. Penicillin resistance among *Strep. pneumoniae* is 13% in Pakistan, around 12% in Australia, and as high as 36% in Spain. Erythromycin has some *in vitro* activity against *H. influenzae*, but it is doubtful whether adequate penetration of the chest occurs *in vivo* for it to be of value. It has no activity against *M. catarrhalis*. Clarithromycin may now be a reasonable alternative for treatment when infection with *M. catarrhalis*, *H. influenzae*, *Strep. pneumoniae*, or *Staph. aureus* are likely.

The antibiotic treatment of acute exacerbations of chronic bronchitis is by no means straightforward. Some situations may respond well to first-line treatment such as ampicillin, amoxycillin, or trimethoprim but the more expensive quinolones, co-amoxiclav and new macrolides have an important place in management. It is important that the patient realizes that antibiotics are only part of the approach to managing the condition and that avoidance of smoking, both active and passive, is the first imperative.

Bronchiolitis

Parainfluenza and respiratory syncytial virus (RSV)

Parainfluenza and RSV are single-stranded RNA viruses that replicate in the cytoplasm of the epithelial cells which line the respiratory tract. Both viruses cause most severe illness in children under the age of 5 year Parainfluenza is frequently found in the autumn and causes laryngotracheobronchitis (croup). Respiratory syncytial virus is most often found in the winter months in epidemics involving children under 2 years. The illness can be particularly severe in these children leading to bronchiolitis and pneumonia requiring hospital admission. Bronchiolitis presents with fever, sometimes coryza and cough. Respiratory distress is characterized by intercostal indrawing and subcostal recession on inspiration. Auscultation of the chest reveals rhonchi, inspiratory wheeze, and fine crepitations with the signs worsening over 2–5 days. The illness usually resolves within a week and death is rare in healthy babies. Antibiotics are unhelpful, but admission to hospital should be considered early, with close monitoring of the situation while the child remains at home.

Respiratory syncytial virus may also cause bronchitis in adults and in the very elderly or immunocompromised in whom infection may be very severe. When infections do occur in other adults they are most commonly found in those in contact with young children (e.g. staff from nursery schools, play groups, and hospital units).

Respiratory syncytial virus is often implicated in exacerbations of asthma in children and recurrent 'wheezy bronchitis' has been reported following bronchiolitis caused by RSV.[8] The infection varies considerably in severity and up to 10% of hospitalized patients require artificial ventilation. In the hospital setting, ribavirin administered by aerosol may be used in treatment for patients who are known to have RSV infection. Parainfluenza virus in children, particularly the very young, also requires close observation. If any sign of respiratory distress develops urgent admission must be arranged as intubation may occasionally be required. It is always worrying to the GP to know that these infections are prevalent in the practice area. Confidence and quality care are ensured by availability, sympathetic well-trained reception staff, meticulous attention to follow-up arrangements, including use of the telephone, and the realization that parents really do have an instinct about serious illness in their children. A vaccine against RSV is being developed and will be a welcome addition to the childhood immunization programme.

Pneumonia

The term 'pneumonia' implies an acute inflammation of the parenchyma of the lung. The diagnosis involves confirmation of the physical signs or radiological evidence of consolidation.

Classification

There are several ways to classify pneumonia:

- Primary or secondary
- Radiological
- By organism
- Bacterial: typical or atypical

Primary pneumonia occurring in otherwise healthy patients, previously free of any lung disease, is distinguished from *secondary* pneumonia where an underlying cause is present. Causes include bronchogenic carcinoma, bronchiectasis or an underlying cause outside the chest, such as neurological disease or gastrointestinal problems producing aspiration. Secondary pneumonia may also result from reduced host antimicrobial defence mechanisms in patients who are immunocompromised or have a chronic debilitating disease, such as leukaemia.

As far as the GP is concerned the conventional classification of pneumonia into lobar, lobular, and bronchopneumonia is unhelpful in determining aetiology and therapy. Radiologically, it is usual to distinguish between lobar pneumonia and bronchopneumonia but in the general practice setting the distinction is not always clear-cut.

Classification by the infecting organism also poses problems as the GP is unlikely to have this information when treatment is commenced.

In this chapter we propose a practical classification:

- Community-acquired pneumonia
- Hospital-acquired (nosocomial) pneumonia
- Recurrent pneumonia
- Pneumonia in the immunocompromised patient
- Aspiration pneumonia
- Geographical pneumonia

Community-acquired pneumonias are primary pneumonias (Table 7.3) acquired in the community and are often managed at home or in a community hospital. *Hospital-acquired (nosocomial) pneumonias* are defined as a pulmonary infection that develops two days or more after hospital admission. *Recurrent pneumonia* implies three or more separate attacks of pneumonia in one patient. *Pneumonia in the immunocompromised patient* is an increasing problem involving patients with HIV/AIDS, and those on immunosuppressive therapy. *Aspiration pneumonia* is usually associated with altered consciousness or dysphagia. *Geographical pneumonia* implies unusual bacterial, viral, fungal, and protozoal infections that should be considered in persons living in, or returning from, countries abroad.

Epidemiology

Despite antibiotic treatment, pneumonia remains a major cause of morbidity and mortality; mortality being more common at the extremes of age and in secondary pneumonia. Death rates from pneumonia declined considerably in the 1950s when penicillin and sulphonamides were first used in treatment. While there is a continued slow decline in those under 40 years of age, certified deaths from pneumonia in the elderly continue to rise and pneumonia still causes more deaths than any other infectious disease in the UK.

In a well-designed Finnish study of all cases of pneumonia occurring during a one-year period in a rural population of 46 979, the incidence rate was 36/1000 in children aged 0–4 years and was higher than in any other age group. It was 16/1000 in children aged 5–14 years; only three children aged 0–14 had an underlying condition. The authors propose that

Table 7.3 *Cause of community-acquired pneumonia*

Bacterial pneumonia
Streptococcus pneumoniae
Staphylococcus aureus
Haemophilus influenzae

Atypical pneumonia
Mycoplasma pneumoniae
Legionnaires' disease (*Legionella pneumophila*)
Chlamydia pneumoniae
Chlamydia psittaci (psittacosis/ornithosis)
Coxiella burnetti (Q fever)

Tuberculosis
Mycobacterium tuberculosis

Viruses
Influenza types A and B
Parainfluenza types I, II, III
Respiratory syncytial virus (RSV)
Adenoviruses types I–V, and VII
Enteroviruses (coxsackie and echoviruses)
Cytomegalovirus
Varicella zoster virus
Herpes simplex
Measles virus

Protozoal, fungal, and helminthic
Pneumocystis carinii (particularly in the immunocompromised)
Cryptococcus (particularly in the immunocompromised)
Histoplasma

---

the study is relevant to rural populations in industrialized countries.[9] In another Finnish study of 195 children hospitalized with community-acquired pneumonia which determined the aetiology using a wide range of diagnostic tools, pneumococci and respiratory syncytial virus were the most commonly responsible microorganisms.

Non-capsulated forms of *H. influenzae* were involved in 9% of the infections, *M. catarrhalis* in 2%. Other causative agents included *M. pneumoniae*, *Chlamydia* species and parainfluenza virus. About 37% of the infections were viral, 32% were mixed viral/bacterial and 30% were bacterial alone.[10]

In a British multicentre study of 453 adults admitted to hospital with community acquired pneumonia, there was a total mortality of 6%,[11] while in another study of 73 patients over 65 years of age admitted to a single hospital the mortality reached 33% even though death from pneumonia as a terminal event in severe chronic illness was excluded.[12]

Pneumonia is most common in men, the young, and the elderly, in debilitated individuals and those living in overcrowded or congested community situations. Deaths from pneumonia peak in the winter months when the most common infections are influenza, staphylococcal and pneumococcal pneumonia. Some atypical pneumonias, such as *Legionella* pneumonia are more often found in summer and autumn.[13]

Community-acquired pneumonia

A study of community-acquired pneumonia in adults in British hospitals in 1982–3 suggested that pneumococcal infections were still the most common cause of community-acquired pneumonias. In this study, 453 adults in 25 hospitals entered a prospective study of community-acquired pneumonia and a microbiological diagnosis was established in 67% of patients. *Strep. pneumoniae* (34%), *M. pneumoniae* (18%), and influenza A virus (7%) were the commonest microorganisms. The authors recommended that antibiotics should be given as early as possible and always chosen to cover *Strep. pneumoniae* and in addition, *M. pneumoniae* during outbreaks and *Staph. aureus* during influenza epidemics.

Pneumococcal pneumonia affects about 1 in 1000 adults each year with a mortality of 10–20%. Atypical pneumonias, particularly, *M. pneumoniae,* account for 15–20% of cases, viruses are implicated in 10–20% of cases and are frequently complicated by secondary bacterial infection. Pneumonia due to *M. pneumoniae* occurs in epidemics every 3 to 4 years which last for 18 months to 2 years.[14] Infection rates are greatest in school-age children and young adults, and during epidemics the organism causes 30–60% of pneumonias in individuals between the ages of five and twenty years. Infection is spread by infected respiratory secretions, particularly in families and remote populations with close contact. Military recruits and college students are particularly susceptible.

Hospital-acquired (Nosocomial) pneumonia

A pulmonary infection that develops two or more days after hospital admission for some other reason is defined as a nosocomial pneumonia. Studies from the USA show that Gram-negative bacillary infection accounts for almost 50% of all nosocomial pneumonias and Gram-positive bacteria make up only 10–20% of the organisms found. Anaerobic infection is likely and mixed infections may occur, particularly when aspiration has occurred. Sputum specimens are frequently contaminated in the oropharynx, rendering culture an unreliable means of diagnosis. The possibility possibility of *Legionella* infection should always be borne in mind in these circumstances.

The GP is sometimes presented with nosocomial pulmonary infection in a recently discharged hospital patient and must make treatment decisions on a 'best guess' basis unless relevant microbiology is available from the hospital. As the care of patients is increasingly shifted into the primary care setting with

Table 7.4 *Pathogens implicated in hospital-acquired pneumonia*

- Gram-negative bacteria
  - *Pseudomonas* spp. (50% or more)
  - *Klebsiella* spp.
  - *Escherichia coli*
  - *Proteus* spp.
  - *Serratia* spp.
- *Staphylococcus aureus*
- *Streptococcus pneumoniae*
- Other streptococci
- Anaerobes
- *Legionella* spp.
- Fungi

very early discharge from hospital to care in community beds or at home, this situation is likely to become even commoner. At the very least, the GP should discuss the case with the local microbiologist to discover the local patterns of nosocomial infection and to ensure that the choice of antibiotic is appropriate (see Table 7.4).

Clinical features, diagnosis, and treatment

While the signs of a classical lobar pneumonia are learned by every medical student the general practice presentation of pneumonia takes many forms. Some of the points which should be included in the history are shown in Table 7.5, this type of information is valuable in assessing the likely organisms and as a pointer to further investigation and referral.

The onset of a serious bacterial pneumonia is often abrupt and unambiguous with characteristic symptoms, including cough, pleuritic chest pain, and fever. There is usually a sustained elevation of temperature. In the initial stages the cough is non-productive but subsequently there may be a characteristic production of muco-purulent yellow or green sputum which may also be bloodstained. Dyspnoea may be present. In many cases an upper respiratory tract infection (URTI) precedes the onset of pneumonia. In the elderly and the very young, the presentation of bacterial pneumonia may be very different. Elderly patients can present at a fairly early stage with confusion and very few, if any, chest symptoms. Neonates may present with tachypnoea, tachycardia, disinterest in bottle or breast, or lethargy.

In adults with a classical lobar pneumonia, usually caused by the pneumococcus,[15] rigors are common and the physical examination reveals pyrexia, tachypnoea and tachycardia, and the white blood count is usually elevated. At an advanced stage, confusion, cyanosis, and laboured breathing may be apparent. Fine but distinct crepitations may be heard before the signs of

Table 7.5 *Some questions to consider in the patient with pneumonia*

Is this a secondary pneumonia?
Consider the patient's underlying general physical condition and history of chronic illness

Is there any underlying respiratory disease?
e.g. influenza (post-influenzal staphylococcal pneumonia), measles, chicken pox

What are the social circumstances?
e.g. hostel accommodation with poor nutrition. Consider *Mycobacterium tuberculosis*

Recent stay in a hospital or hotel?
Consider *Legionella pneumophila*

Contact with farm animals or birds?
Consider Q fever, psittacosis

Returning traveller?
Consider *Salmonella typhi*

Risk factors for HIV?
Consider *Pneumocystis carinii, Mycobacterium tuberculosis, Cytomegalovirus* (CMV), *Candida, Aspergillus fumigatus*

---

lobar consolidation are present, a pleural rub is common. In lower lobe pneumonia, pain may be referred to the abdomen, opening up a broad differential diagnosis.

Many patients with community-acquired bacterial pneumonia are not young and healthy and they present with a different pattern of infection. These patients include the elderly, nursing home patients, diabetics, people with alcohol dependence, and those with chronic obstructive airways disease. In these people the infection may be due to organisms such as *Staph. aureus, H. influenzae, Klebsiella pneumoniae,* and *Enterobacter aerogenes. Streptococcus pneumoniae* or *H. influenzae* pneumonia are likely pathogens in patients with chronic leukaemia, sickle-cell disease, and those with a history of splenectomy.

Atypical pneumonia

The term 'atypical pneumonia' refers to a group of pneumonias, including *M. pneumoniae, Coxiella burnetti* (causing Q fever), and *Chlamydia psittaci* causing psittacosis. Also sometimes included under this heading are the Legionellaceae family, some viral pneumonias, and a new chlamydial strain, *Chlamydia pneumoniae.*

Atypical pneumonias usually occur in younger people. Children over

Table 7.6 *Features which help to distinguish bacterial from atypical pneumonia*

	Bacterial	**Atypical**
History	Rapid onset with high fever + rigors	Insidious over 5–7 days
Radiology	Intra-alveolar	Mainly interstitial
Sputum	Purulent, occasionally bloodstained	Generally mucoid
Age	Any age	Predominantly younger adults
Pleuritic pain	Common	Uncommon
Examination	Signs consolidation often present	Consolidation
Serology	Negative	Rise in titre
White blood cell current (WBC)	Raised, usually >15 000 × 109/l polymorphs	Normal or slightly raised differential WBC normal

the age of 5 years and young adults are at greatest risk. The contrasting clinical features of atypical and bacterial pneumonias are shown in Table 7.6.

Mycoplasma pneumoniae

Mycoplasmas are the smallest of the free-living organisms, are widespread in nature and are well recognized as common pathogens. They are different from true bacteria in having no cell wall and also from viruses. Unlike viruses, they are capable of cell-free growth in artificial media and are susceptible to certain antibiotics. At least 12 *Mycoplasma* species have been isolated from humans, but only 3 species are generally accepted as human pathogens; *M. pneumoniae* being principally a respiratory pathogen. In recovering from respiratory infection with *M. pneumoniae*, the host responds by the production of specific local and systemic antibodies to the organism. Immunity to infection is not complete and cases of second infection do occur. Re-infection accounts for most patients aged over 45 years and may be associated with severe symptoms.

In the UK, a joint British Thoracic Society/Public Health Laboratory Service study of community-acquired pneumonia in adults in 1982–3 showed that *M. pneumoniae* was responsible for 18% of cases and was the most commonly identified organism after *Strep. pneumoniae*.

In general practice, *M. pneumoniae* infection is infrequently diagnosed and it may be that many mild infections are missed. The clinical picture of the disease is typically of an influenza-like illness, with fever, headaches, lassitude, and cough. *Mycoplasma pneumoniae* infections may in addition manifest as, or be associated with, pharyngitis, otitis media, sinusitis, bronchitis, and bronchiolitis. The incubation period ranges from 9 to 21 days, the onset is insidious with prodromal symptoms of malaise, fever, and upper respiratory tract symptoms. A non-productive cough is usually present. Moderate pyrexia may be present but rigors are unusual. Physical signs are often minimal or absent except for a few rales. Occasionally, extra respiratory disease results. A causal relationship may exist between *M. pneumoniae* infection and erythema multiforme, aseptic meningitis, meningo-encephalitis, pancreatitis, myocarditis, and pericarditis.

Treatment

The clinical course of *M. pneumoniae* infection is usually mild and can be managed at home. Hospitalization may be necessary in the immunocompromised, where an additional underlying disease is present and in re-infection in patients over 45 years when illness may be severe.

Mycoplasma pneumoniae usually responds to erythromycin, 0.5 g, 6- to 8-hourly, and the newer macrolide, clarithromycin, is very active against this organism. Tetracycline is a suitable second-line treatment but not for children under 8 years of age and pregnant women. Usually, 2–3 weeks of erythromycin is recommended to prevent relapse. Mycoplasmas are resistant to all penicillins, cephalosporins, and trimethoprim.

Legionnaires' Disease (*Legionella pneumophila*)

The Pennsylvanian American Legion held its 58th convention at the Bellevue Stratford Hotel, Philadelphia from 21 July to 24 July 1976. On 27 July a delegate died from pneumonia and within a very few days 28 more had died, and more than 180 were affected with pneumonia.

Following intensive laboratory investigation a bacillary organism was isolated. *Legionella pneumophila* is a short Gram-negative flagellated bacillus. The Legionellaceae comprises at least 22 species of legionella and 10 serotypes of *L. pneumophila*. They are found widely in man's environment. Hot water tanks, cooling towers, and shower heads act as a foci of infection. Outbreaks occur both abroad and in the UK. Most outbreaks occur during the summer. It may survive in tap water at room temperature for more than a year and is often found in hot water and heating systems where sediment and warmth encourage growth. Cooling fans in air conditioning units may nebulize infected droplets over a wide area. Legionnaires' disease appears in three different forms—as explosive epidemics, as endemic infections, or as sporadic cases. Endemic infections have usually been associated with new hotels, hospitals, or buildings. Small outbreaks have occurred in many hospitals in the UK. Such a nosocomial infection is particularly dangerous as it affects already ill or debilitated patients and those at high risk. The clinical features of legionnaires' disease in the community ranges from subclinical through mild to fulminating pneumonia. It is three times more common in men than women, is rare in children, and the usual age range is 20–75 years, with the highest incidence in the 40–70-year-olds. Immunosuppressed patients, alcoholics, diabetics, and smokers are at special risk.

A characteristic clinical presentation is sometimes seen: the patient has a high fever, non-productive cough, headache, confusion, and gastrointestinal symptoms. Rigors may occur with a temperature of less than 39°C. There is accompanying malaise and myalgia. Severe headache, delirium, and confusion may, on occasion, dominate the clinical picture and tend to mask the true diagnosis of pneumonia. The chest signs are often sparse and not commensurate with the apparent severity of the illness. A few crackles may be heard and local consolidation may be present. It is not uncommon for a pleural effusion to develop.

Treatment

If the diagnosis of legionnaires' disease is suspected, then hospital management is usually indicated. If, for logistic reasons this is not possible, then treatment should be commenced with erythromycin 500–1000 mg, 6-hourly. The legionellae are susceptible *in vitro* to a number of antimicrobial agents, including erythromycin, clarithromycin, rifampicin, chloramphenicol. Penicillins, cephalosporins, and aminoglycosides are ineffective therapy for *L. pneumophila* pneumonia.

In hospital, treatment is most usually commenced with erythromycin 1 g, 6 hourly intravenously, and oral erythromycin is substituted when clinical improvement occurs. Therapy is usually continued for three weeks following clinical response. In the hospital setting, patients who do not appear to be responding well to treatment with erythromycin may, in addition, be given rifampicin 600 mg every 12 hours. Some authorities recommend a combination of erythromycin and rifampicin in any immunocompromised host who develops *L. pneumophila* pneumonia. There is some evidence that other antimicrobials, such as tetracyclines and co-trimoxazole, may be effective but are not recommended as first-line treatments.

The macrolide, clarithromycin, is a potent intraphagocytic antibiotic and may in the future be shown to be clinically superior to erythromycin in the treatment of *L. pneumophila* pneumonia.

Chlamydia pneumoniae

Chlamydia pneumoniae, is a new species of *Chlamydia*, which was identified in 1986, and is a common cause of pneumonia and other acute respiratory tract infections. Approximately 10% of community-acquired pneumonias have been associated with *C. pneumoniae* infection which is now recognized as among the four or five most commonly identified causes of all pneumonias.[16] Infection with *C. pneumoniae* is both endemic and epidemic.

Chlamydia pneumoniae antibody has been found in 25–45% of adults from different areas of the world. It is uncommon in individuals under the age of 8 years and its prevalence increases sharply in older children and young adults, reaching a plateau by the age of age 30.

Man is thought to be the natural host for *C. pneumoniae*. In epidemics of pneumonia in Finland associated with *C. pneumoniae* antibody, no avian source for the pneumonia has been identified. The emergence of *C. pneumoniae* as a previously unsuspected pathogen reflects the difficulty in cultivating the organism and the changing pattern of respiratory infections.

Clinical features

Current data suggests that 70% of *C. pneumoniae* infections may be either asymptomatic or only mildly symptomatic. In teenagers experiencing their first infection the illness may be biphasic, initially presenting with pharyngitis followed, after 1–3 weeks, by bronchitis and pneumonia. Asymptomatic infections are common in adults but the infection may be serious in the elderly. If pneumonia occurs in this group it is often complicated and severe. Patients with chronic disease, such as chronic obstructive pulmonary disease and cardiac failure, are at particular risk.

Investigations

Clinical laboratory findings in C. *pneumoniae* infections are unremarkable. The white cell count is often normal and the ESR elevated. Chest X-ray in C. *pneumoniae* pneumonia characteristically shows single lesions that are subsegmental and may be in any part of the lung. Consolidation is uncommon. Patients with bilateral lesions are more likely to develop pleurisy.

Laboratory diagnosis is based on the isolation of the organism and serological finding. Isolation is difficult. Two serological tests are used in diagnosis:

1. Complement fixation test measuring antibodies against all *Chlamydia*.

2. *Chlamydia pneumoniae* specific antigen.

Treatment

Both clinical experience and laboratory studies have shown that tetracycline and erythromycin are effective against C. *pneumoniae* organisms. Intensive and prolonged therapy may be required. Current recommendations are erythromycin or tetracycline (but not in children) 2 g per day for 10–14 days or 1 g per day for 21 days. The clinician should not be surprised if the patient requires additional antibiotic therapy.

Newer macrolides may, in future, have a considerable place in treatment. Clarithromycin exhibits excellent *in vitro* activity against C. *pneumoniae*.

Chlamydia psittaci (psittacosis/ornithosis)

Psittacosis is a zoonotic infectious illness of wild and domestic birds that is caused by C. *psittaci*. It is an intracellular parasite with world-wide distribution and was first identified in parrots, although almost any species of bird and, indeed, some mammals can serve as hosts. Transmission to man occurs either indirectly through inhalation of infected excreta or directly through contact with an infected bird. Psittacosis is an occupational hazard to pet-shop owners and outbreaks may occasionally occur among workers in poultry-processing plants. Asymptomatic adult birds carry the infection. Psittacosis is not food-borne, but person to person spread has been recorded but is thought to be rare.

The incubation of the illness is usually from 7 to 15 days. Clinical manifestation may be either of a mild respiratory illness or severe disease with multiorgan involvement in which pneumonia usually is the most prominent manifestation. Severe headache is common and there may be associated anorexia, arthralgia, sore throat, and malaise.[17] A cough may be present. When fever occurs a relative bradycardia may be present. The cough is usually dry and hacking but may be productive at a later stage. Severely affected patients may become cyanotic, profoundly dyspnoeic, and encephalitis can occur as a complication. On examination, fine inspiratory crackles may be heard. Hepatosplenomegaly may be found and occasionally macules resembling rose spots are seen. In very severe cases jaundice may occur. Chest x-ray often reveals extensive pulmonary involvement and much greater than that anticipated from physical examination.

Diagnosis and investigations

While a history of contact with birds may be found, this is not always the case. The white blood count ranges from modest leucopenia to a slight leucocytosis. Confirmation of the diagnosis is normally obtained by serological methods when a fourfold rise and complement fixing antibodies in acute and convalescent sera is found. A single elevated titre (<1:64) in a patient with a compatible history and clinical findings provides fairly good presumptive evidence of the diagnosis.

Immunity to psittacosis is transient and repeated cases among bird fanciers, etc. is well documented.

Treatment

This is with tetracycline 2–3 g per day. As relapses are common, therapy should be continued for 21 days. Second-line treatment is with erythromycin.

Home or hospital management of pneumonia?

Often, the great dilemma for the GP is the decision whether to treat at home, move to a GP community hospital bed or admit to an acute medical hospital unit. Some poor prognostic features for patients with community-acquired pneumonia are shown in Table 7.7.

Investigation of a patient with pneumonia in general practice

The investigations that might be reasonable to carry out for general practice management of patients with pneumonia are shown in Table 7.8; some of the

Table 7.7 *Features indicating a poor prognosis for patients with community-acquired pneumonia*

History
- Pre-existing debilitating disease
- Extremes of age

Social circumstance
- Poverty
- Lack of relatives or committed neighbour
- Isolated location (particularly during winter months)

Examination
- Confusion
- Marked tachypnoea
- Hypotension
- Cyanosis

Investigation
- Low white blood cell count
- Raised blood urea
- Multilobe involvement

Table 7.8 *Investigation of pneumonia*

Sputum for:
Gram-stain
Culture

Blood for:
Full blood count
Blood urea and creatinine
Liver function tests
Serological detection of antibodies
Blood cultures

Chest X-ray

tests are infrequently used (e.g. blood cultures) but as GP community beds become more common, they will be used more frequently in practice.

Chest X-ray

There is little difference in the method of presentation and subsequent clinical findings between the various forms of bacterial pneumonia. A chest X-ray may help to identify and quantify the severity of the infection, but may not be possible during acute illness at home. Domiciliary chest X-rays tend to be of poor quality and are rarely of value. If an X-ray is carried out in a hospital department a more satisfactory picture is obtained. Most commonly, a localized bronchopneumonia pattern is seen which is non-specific and unhelpful. However, dense lobar or multi-lobar consolidation, or large pleural effusions support the diagnosis of a bacterial pneumonia. Upper lobe consolidation with a downward bowing of the fissure, suggests *Klebsiella* pneumonia. Multiple bilateral cavities suggest infection due to *Staph. aureus* and if the illness is post-influenzal, the diagnosis is likely. Cavitation may also suggest Gram-negative infection, *Strep. pneumoniae* or an anaerobic infection. A diffuse patchy picture progressing to numerous small abscesses that coalesce to form one or several abscesses is suggestive of *Pseudomonas* infection. In *Mycoplasma* pneumonia, X-rays often show more extensive disease than is suggested by clinical examination. The X-ray in legionnaires' disease may show diffuse patchy shadows. In more than a quarter of cases, a small pleural effusion is seen. The radiographic picture resolves only slowly and may take up to six months before returning to normal.

In Nottingham, a prospective one-year study was carried out of community-acquired pneumonia, defined as an acute lower respiratory tract infection, for which antibiotics were prescribed.[12] In 236 of 251 episodes of pneumonia investigated, acute radiographic changes were present in 93 (39%). A pathogen was identified in 129 (55%) episodes, and hospital admission was required in 52 (22%) episodes.

Laboratory investigations

Immediate Gram-stain of the sputum may suggest a diagnosis of pneumococcal pneumonia but this procedure is unlikely in the general practice setting. Cultures of sputum may be of benefit but should not be allowed to delay onset of treatment. An elevated cold agglutinin titre may be found in some 50% of cases of *Mycoplasma* pneumonia by the second week of illness but may also be present in other types of pneumonia. Isolation of the organism from sputum is not always possible and takes from one to three weeks. An initial antibody titre of 1:128 suggests the diagnosis, but for confirmation, acute and convalescent sera titres must be obtained and demonstrate a fourfold rise. The blood picture can be helpful in distinguishing between legionnaires' disease and pyogenic pneumonia in that the white cell count may be only slightly raised and is certainly usually less than 15 000/mm³. Lymphopenia may be present. In severe illness other features may include abnormal liver function tests, hypoalbuminaemia, raised blood urea, haematuria, and proteinuria. Confirmation of the diagnosis may be carried out using an indirect fluorescent antibody test to detect specific serum antibodies. Acute and convalescent sera are examined. The antibody rise may be delayed for up to three or more weeks, so unfortunately the serological diagnosis may be retrospective. However, a presumptive diagnosis can be made if a single titre of at least

Table 7.9 *First-line treatments for community-aquired pneumonia*

- Parenteral benzylpenicillin (1.2–2.4 g daily IM in divided doses) on the basis that *Streptococcus pneumoniae* is most common cause

- Erythromycin (2 g daily by mouth). First choice if there is a history of penicillin allergy or suspicion of increasingly common *Mycoplasma pneumoniae* infection. Also effective against infection with *Moraxella catarrhalis*

- The macrolide clarithromycin 250 mg *twice daily* for 7 days. May be increased to 500 mg twice daily for up to 14 days in severe infections. Spectrum of activity includes:
  - *Streptococcus pneumoniae*
  - *Staphylococcus aureus* (methicillin-susceptible strains)
  - *Moraxella catarrhalis*
  - *Legionella pneumophila*
  - *Haemophilus influenzae*
  - *Mycoplasma pneumoniae*
  - *Chlamydia pneumoniae* and *C. trachomatis*

- Flucloxacillin (500 mg 6-hourly by mouth) if staphylococcal pneumonia suspected, because of concurrent influenza epidemic.

- Co-amoxiclav. Suitable treatment for infection with *H. influenzae* and *M.* catarrhalis

---

1:256 is obtained. If the diagnosis is suspected admission should be always be discussed.

Home treatment of community-acquired bacterial pneumonia

Having weighed up all the clues produced from a knowledge of epidemiology, history, presentation, and clinical examination, and having decided to treat the patient in the community, the GP has to resort to 'best guess' treatment while investigations are arranged. 'Best guesses' are improved substantially by a discussion of the case with the medical microbiologist! First-line treatments are shown in Table 7.9.

If a severe infection is treated at home antibiotic treatment should be given parenterally during the first 24 hours, changing to oral, as clinical improvement occurs, although some authors report that an oral regime is effective for most patients.[18] There must be close supervision of patients with pneumonia, particularly those patients with poor prognostic features. Home helps, relatives and neighbours, and the primary health care team all have a role to play in the supervision and management, particularly of the elderly.

Domiciliary physiotherapy has a vital role in aiding recovery and preventing costly hospital admission. Avoidance of dehydration is important and if the practice team is unable to maintain clinical supervision or the patient does not have adequate domestic support the patient should be admitted to hospital.

Return to work

No firm guidelines can be given concerning return to work following an episode of pneumonia but the GP should consider the following factors:

- Age of patient
- Type and severity of illness
- Concomitant conditions
- Nature of work
- Motivation

Generally, pneumonia leaves a patient exhausted and depressed, and full recovery may take up to three months. They should be encouraged to spend an adequate time convalescing. Patients who smoke should be strongly encouraged to stop, and follow-up arranged to give them support.

Complications

If the patient with pneumonia fails to improve this may suggest a wrong diagnosis, inappropriate treatment, the interplay of certain host factors, or the presence of complications. The exacerbation of underlying chronic disease such as heart failure or asthma also delays recovery. Examples of these include:

1. *Wrong diagnosis.* The responsible organism may be unusual or unexpected, resistant to the chosen antibiotic, or there may be unidentified pre-existing lung disease.
2. *Inappropriate treatment.* The choice of antibiotic or the route of administration may not be ideal.
3. *Host factors.* These include poor compliance, allergy to the chosen antibiotic, severe debility, pre-existing disease, or a previously undiagnosed immunocompromised patient.
4. *Complications.* These include lung abscess, empyema, metastatic endocarditis or septic arthritis, and deep vein thrombosis.

Recurrent pneumonia

Patients who suffer three or more separate attacks of pneumonia are said to have recurrent pneumonia. Recurrent pneumonia in one area of the lung suggests a local or bronchiole abnormality. When it is present in different sites a more generalized disease is likely.

Causes of recurrent pneumonia

Local causes include bronchial obstruction due to tumour or foreign body and local disease such as localized bronchiectasis, and pulmonary sequestration. Generalized pulmonary disease associated with recurrent pneumonia includes chronic bronchitis, bronchiectasis, sinusitis with post-nasal drip, cystic fibrosis, and immobile cilia syndrome. Non-respiratory causes include recurrent aspiration (oesophageal problems, alcoholics, epileptics), and immunodeficiency states.

Pneumonia in the immunocompromised patient

This is a difficult and, sadly, ever-increasing problem. The increasing use of immunosuppressive therapy in transplantation and oncology, together with the dramatic increase in the prevalence of AIDS has highlighted this particular area of respiratory (as well as other) opportunistic infections. The approach to the management of such infections is threefold:

1. Primary prophylaxis.
2. Treatment of active infection.
3. Prevention of recurrences (secondary prophylaxis).

With the increase in the prevalence of AIDS, GPs will be faced with the difficulty of diagnosing many of the bacterial, protozoal, fungal, and other viral conditions associated with its immunosuppression. Significant pulmonary disease occurs in almost all patients with AIDS. Investigators have found that the development of opportunistic infections is related to the level of CD4 + T cells in the blood. Healthy individuals have about 1000 such cells in every cubic millimetre of blood. In HIV-infected individuals, the number declines by an average of about 40–80 every year. As the helper-T-cell count falls, so does the risk of opportunistic infection. When the count falls to between 400 and 200/mm³ first infections commonly appear. While some of these may be relatively benign in the form of candida, shingles, etc., other more serious opportunistic infections soon develop. It has been shown that *Pneumocystis carinii* is most likely to occur if the CD plus T-cell count drops below 200. Without preventative therapy some 20% of patients with a count of less than 200 will have a first bout of *P. carinii* pneumonia within a year. The pulmonary manifestations of HIV infection are shown in Table 7.10. In AIDS, infection with *P. carinii*, cytomegalovirus, mycobacteria, *Legionella*, and *Cryptococcus* are the most common. There is little doubt that primary and secondary prevention of *P. carinii* in the AIDS patient can prolong life. Decisions regarding treatment are most usually taken in conjunction with a hospital-based specialized unit or genitourinary physician.

Table 7.10 *Pulmonary manifestations of HIV infection*

Opportunistic infections diagnostic of AIDS
Pneumocystis carinii pneumonia
Broncho-pulmonary candidiasis
Pulmonary cryptococcosis
Pulmonary toxoplasmosis
Disseminated histoplasmosis
Disseminated *Mycobacterium avium* complex
Cytomegalovirus pneumonia

HIV-related pulmonary disorders
Tuberculosis
Nocardiosis

Pneumocystis carinii

Clinical features

About 80–85% of patients with AIDS develop *P. carinii* infection at some stage of their illness. Transmission is by droplet infection and the patient may, in the first instance, present with excessive dyspnoea on mild exertion. There may be an accompanying non-productive cough, fever, or tachypnoea. Chest signs may be minimal and consist of inspiratory crackles. The classical X-ray picture of *P. carinii* is a diffuse bilateral perihilar pulmonary infiltrate. A normal chest X-ray is found in some 5% of patients with symptomatic *P. carinii* infection. Infection can only be diagnosed with confidence by staining the organism within lung tissue or secretions. In the immunocompromised patient, the organisms invade the alveoli where an inflammatory response occurs. The alveoli become filled with fluid impeding the uptake of oxygen.

Prevention

The introduction of preventative therapy should be considered at an early stage after due consideration of clinical findings, CD4 count, and assessment by the GP and a specialist. Prevention is by either:

1. *Inhaled pentamidine*, which is thought to prevent microbial replication by inhibiting the synthesis of DNA.

2. *Oral co-trimoxazole* which may produce severe nausea, skin rashes, and, on occasion, Stevens–Johnson syndrome.

The treatment of active infection should be carried out in consultation with a specialized unit and, in the first instance, as a hospital in-patient.

Cytomegalovirus (CMV)

Cytomegalovirus may cause bronchopneumonia or interstitial pneumonia. Normally, there are associated systemic features, such as lymphadenopathy and hepatosplenomegaly. It is rare to have CMV pulmonary infection as a primary infection in a healthy adult, the infection being much more likely in immunosuppressed patients. In such situations the infection may be associated with other organisms, such as *P. carinii* or *M. tuberculosis*. The treatment of CMV pneumonia in the immunosuppressed patient is usually with ganciclovir but which should be administered as an in-patient under specialist advice.

Pulmonary tuberculosis

Epidemiology

Tuberculosis (TB) notifications in England and Wales increased by 1.5% in 1988 and 5.3% in 1989 reversing the decline which has been seen since the beginning of the century. While there is a slight reduction in the figures for 1990, the actual figures in 1990 were still greater than those in 1988. In 1989, 5432 cases of TB were reported from the Communicable Disease Surveillance Centre and there were 443 deaths.[19, 20] Similarly in the USA, TB notifications plateaued in 1986 but have since risen, reversing a 40-year trend. In 1993, the World Health Organization designated the world-wide increase that has occurred a global emergency. Cases of TB had become so rare in the UK population that the relevance of a national BCG vaccination programme in schools has been questioned by some authorities. The dangers of losing interest in case finding and prevention programmes in developed countries in the face of increasing poverty and deprivation have been well reviewed.[21] The lack of an overall strategy for tackling the disease in the UK has been raised with attention drawn to the widespread variations in BCG programmes and policies for the screening of immigrants.[22] The infection is a present threat to the most vulnerable members of society and GP should remember that fact.

On a world-wide scale, TB still represents a very major public health problem being a disease linked with poverty, malnutrition, and overcrowding. In developing countries it is estimated that over 5000 people per day die from tuberculosis.

In 1986, there was thought to be a prevalence rate of approximately 5 cases per 100 000 in the white population in the UK and 126 cases per 100 000 in UK South Asian ethnic groups. The infection was found particularly in those who had recently come to live in the UK from the Indian subcontinent. In the UK, indigenous population TB is most common in men over 55 and it commonly manifests as a respiratory disease. In contrast, among South Asians the disease is often seen in younger people, many under the age of 35, and up to 50%

present with non-respiratory infection. Children of South Asian parents born in the UK have ten times the incidence of tuberculosis seen in white children but less than half that of South Asian children born abroad. Tuberculosis may be contracted while visiting relatives in the Indian subcontinent but present on return to the UK. The maximum incidence of TB in South Asian immigrants is within five years of arrival, and it is estimated that some 10% develop the disease during that period.

Finally, there is a significant overlap in clinical disease between TB and HIV with new and reactivation of old foci of infection occurring as a result of immunosupression. It is important not to overstate the contribution of this factor to the overall picture; at present, HIV is thought to account for only 4.2% of all incident cases.[23]

In some areas of the country, a GP may expect to see two or more cases of TB a year and it is important to be alert to the wide variety of ways in which it presents.

Case study

One of the authors saw four new presentations of TB in one year in an inner city practice. None of the patients were from minority ethnic groups: a man of 67, a heavy drinker, had pulmonary TB; another woman of 58 presented with glands in the left supra-clavicular fossa which at first seemed to be malignant; and a woman of 62 presented with a mysterious rash over her shins which turned out to be TB! She had had a nephrectomy 30 years previously 'for an infection'. There was also a death from tuberculous meningitis in a baby of 3 months living in a squat with a mother addicted to heroin.

Aetiology

Tuberculosis is caused by infection with *M. tuberculosis*. This is a very virulent organism and is most commonly transmitted through air and droplet infection from coughing and sneezing. The small droplets are able to reach the alveoli and are not prevented from doing so by simple masks. An immunological response to the presence of the bacillary protein develops some 3 to 6 weeks following contact and results in a positive tuberculin test. Spread to regional nodes occurs (paratracheal and hilar) leading to the formation of a Ghon's focus. The bacilli may travel via the bloodstream to distant sites, perhaps to be reactivated later, particularly if an immunocompromised state should develop. In most healthy individuals, cellular immunity prevents spread and the infection is contained.

Clinical features

The cardinal presenting symptom of respiratory tuberculosis is cough which persists and worsens. It may be wrongly attributed to smoking, thus delaying the diagnosis. Any persistent cough in an at-risk person must be investigated by chest X-ray. Further suspicion will be aroused if there is unexplained chronic ill health and fatigue, or weight loss. Haemoptysis may occur. Respiratory TB may present with chest infection, pneumonia, or pleurisy, the diagnosis being suspected when there is a failure to respond to conventional antibiotic treatment.

Late diagnosis contributes to mortality from TB and the GP must, therefore, develop a high index of suspicion, particularly in those at potential risk. On chest X-ray, TB usually manifests as upper zone shadowing sometimes with cavitation. While the picture may be classical, it may resemble other diseases and confirmation of the diagnosis by bacteriological examination of the sputum is important. Mediastinal lymphadenopathy with radiographically normal lungs occurs in some 15–20% of Asian patients with respiratory TB. The differential diagnosis includes sarcoidosis, carcinoma, and lymphoma. Some patients present with pleural pain, breathlessness, and fever; a pleural effusion may be present. While miliary tuberculosis was formerly a disease of the young, it is more often seen in the elderly and may present as general debility and anorexia rather than with chest symptoms. Transmission of infection with *M. tuberculosis* is from human to human and involves aerosols of microdroplets of upper respiratory tract secretions. Even when conditions favour transmission (household contacts with months to years of exposure) only approximately 50–65% of the exposed children (5–9 years of age) and around 20% of contacts of all ages become infected. In contrast, transmission rates for measles are in the order of 81%. Certain factors do, however, increase the infectivity of a patient, including extensive cavitation in tuberculosis of the lung, laryngeal involvement, acid-fast bacilli in sputum smear, overcrowding, and unprotected cough in confined surroundings.

Case history

A healthy Turkish man of 35 who had been living in the UK for 10 years returned to visit his family for three months in 1995. Two weeks after he returned to the UK he visited the GP with an acute respiratory illness complaining of cough, wheeze, fatigue, and generalized aching. There were no localized signs in the chest. He was treated with co-amoxiclav and salbutamol and asked to return if he did not improve. Over the next month he made a partial recovery: on examination there were coarse crepitations and occasional wheezes over both lungs. The GP entertained the working diagnosis of *Mycoplasma* pneumonia and prescribed erythromycin which made the patient sick. As he did not recover, a chest X-ray was ordered. The GP was telephoned urgently by the hospital radiologist since the radiological findings were diagnostic of TB. Sputum culture subsequently confirmed the diagnosis.

The patient refused to accept the diagnosis, as he was ashamed, and insisted on a second opinion sought privately even though the family had little money. None of the family in England were affected and he refused to inform his family in Turkey. He made a complete recovery on anti-TB medication.

Points for discussion with the GP registrar

Several issues arise from this case history, which might form the basis for discussion: the clinical management and the timing of the chest X-ray: developing relationships and protocols with hospital diagnostic departments:

under what circumstances can the diagnosis of *M. pneumoniae* infection be purely a clinical one; requests for non-NHS second opinions by people who cannot afford them; and the stigma of tuberculosis.

Primary tuberculosis. Infection of a patient with *M. tuberculosis* usually, in the first instance, produces a subclinical syndrome manifest only by the development of skin test reactivity to tuberculin purified protein derivative (PPD, Mantoux test). Occasionally mild chest symptoms may be present.

Progressive primary tuberculosis. This occurs as a result of failure to develop a cellular immune response sufficient to limit the primary infection. This is most usually seen in a child or in an immunosuppressed or elderly adult.

Reactivation tuberculosis. This is an example of disease occurring in a previously sensitized host. Factors that influence the reactivation of latent foci are those associated with attenuation of T-cell responses and include tumours such as Hodgkin's disease, AIDS, steroid therapy, viral infections, malnutrition, old age, and possibly stress.

Treatment

This is a specialized area and should always be on the advice of a consultant chest physician. Many patients are now treated as out-patients and the GP usually shares the responsibility for prescribing and follow-up with the chest physician. The combination and duration of drug treatment will depend on factors such as the severity and site of the disease and the ethnic origin of the patient. It is usual for the treatment of pulmonary tuberculosis to last for approximately 6 months and modern regimes are very effective with cure rates of 97–100%. The principles of chemotherapy are to avoid resistance by treating the patient long term with at least two drugs to which the organism is most likely to be sensitive. Triple therapy, which includes isoniazid, is used initially (first 2 months) while sensitivity results are awaited.

The key drugs in modern short course therapy are rifampicin, isoniazid, and pyrazinamide. Ethambutol may also be used in initial treatment. Treatment begins for 2 months with at least three of these drugs and subsequently isoniazid and rifampicin are usually given for a further 4 months. The side-effects and drug interactions of anti-tuberculous drugs are listed in Table 7.11. Pyridoxine is usually administered with this protocol to prevent the peripheral neuropathy associated with isoniazid use. Patients who drink heavily and who are being treated for TB should have their liver function tests monitored especially closely while on treatment. If jaundice develops all drugs must be stopped until it settles and the condition reassessed. Anticoagulant therapy must be very carefully monitored

The GP must be aware of the needs of minority ethnic groups when managing tuberculosis. Rifampicin is contained in a cellulose capsule which may produce a moral dilemma for Muslims or Jews. To an Asian, Chinese,

Table 7.11 *Side-effects and drug interactions of anti-tuberculous drugs*

Drug	Side-effect
Isoniazid	Hepatitis
	Peripheral neuropathy
	Rash
Rifampicin	Rash
	Hepatitis
	Malaise
	Anorexia
	Rarely acute renal failure or thrombocytopenic purpura particularly if therapy is irregular or intermittent. Urine is strongly coloured
Pyrazinamide	Nausea
	Anorexia
	Rash
	Occasional hepatitis
Ethambutol	Optic neuritis

Drug interactions

Isoniazid:
may potentiate anti-epileptic effects of phenytoin, ethosuximide, and carbamazepine

Rifampicin:
induces liver enzymes giving reduced efficacy of: warfarin, phenytoin, oestrogen-containing oral contraceptives, corticosteroids

or African patient, TB may be regarded as a curse, spell, or punishment. The stigma and fear of TB is still in the minds of many older people in the UK especially if they endured extreme poverty as children. Further reading on this topic[24] and discussion with local community workers can help to increase the sensitivity and hence the effectiveness of the primary health care team in this area.

Complications

These include pleural effusion, empyema, pneumothorax, pyopneumothorax, laryngeal disease, cor pulmonale from extensive disease, adult respiratory distress syndrome, and enteritis.

Prevention

Contact tracing is an important way of identifying new cases of tuberculosis. In two recent surveys 10–14% of all new cases were discovered in this way. All patients with TB must by law be notified to the Consultant in

Communicable Disease Control or in Scotland to the Chief Administrative Medical Officer.

Other approaches to the prevention of TB are discussed in detail in Chapter 2.

Bronchiectasis

Bronchiectasis is defined as damage to and destruction of the central conducting airways of segmental or subsegmental size resulting in abnormal widening of one or more branches of the bronchial tree. Changes are usually found at lung bases.

Aetiology

Bronchiectasis may be transient as found in pneumonia (pseudobronchiectasis) but is usually permanent and may follow severe pneumonia, inhalation of a foreign body, or pertussis infection in childhood. The condition may also follow extensive infections with *M. tuberculosis* or fungal infections. Once damaged, the airways become dilated facilitating further bacterial insults. Retraction of the surrounding lung tissue due to inflammation and scarring increases the effect of dilatation and chronic disease may result (Table 7.12).

Clinical features

The hallmark of bronchiectasis is chronic cough and the expectoration of purulent sputum. Occasionally, haemoptysis due to damage to a small capillary may occur. Fever and exertional dyspnoea are manifestations of established advanced disease. Finger clubbing is commonly seen.

Table 7.12 *Causes of bronchiectasis*

- Measles
- Pertussis
- Tuberculosis
- Obstruction by foreign body or tumour
- Pneumonia
- Congenital abnormalities:
  - cystic fibrosis
  - immunodeficiency diseases
  - Kartagener's syndrome (situs inversus, sinusitis, and bronchiectasis)

Investigations

Many of these patients will see chest physicians but there is no reason why the GP should not monitor their progress, thereby avoiding unnecessary visits to the hospital out-patient department. The blood picture in an acute infection shows a neutrophil leucocytosis. Hypochromic anaemia may be present. The sputum is often copious, and a mixed flora is grown on culture. The chest X-ray may reveal air fluid levels or at least thickened bronchi. A CT scan and bronchography will give more detailed picture of damage. Fibreoptic bronchoscopy is indicated in the presence of haemoptysis. Spirometry and arterial blood gases are useful in assessing the degree of airflow obstruction and the degree of hypoxemia in severe cases. ECG is of value in assessing right ventricular hypertrophy and cor pulmonale.

Treatment

This is based on antibiotic therapy and active physiotherapy. Smoking must be abandoned and all possible support and help given to that end. Mucocilliary clearance is impaired and active physiotherapy is vital to prevent further damage and subsequent chronic respiratory illness. Postural drainage and breathing exercises must be professionally taught and religiously carried out. Where bronchospasm is a feature an inhaled B-receptor agonist may prove necessary. Numerous different organisms may be associated with infection and the antibiotic choice for acute exacerbations may include: ampicillin, amoxycillin, erythromycin, clarithromycin, trimethroprim, and oxytetracycline. Very occasionally, long-term antibiotics are necessary.

Surgery is indicated when other forms of treatment have failed to control symptoms. The surgical resection of localized areas of bronchiectasis can be palliative or curative. Recurrent episodes of haemoptysis may, in consultation with a respiratory physician, be an indication for referral for surgical opinion.

Prevention

Bronchiectasis is prevented by:

- Avoidance of smoking
- Early cessation of smoking
- Prompt and effective treatment of childhood respiratory infections
- Pertussis immunization
- Adequate physiotherapy following severe pneumonia

Cystic fibrosis

Epidemiology

Cystic fibrosis (CF) is the most common lethal genetic disease of the white race. It affects 1 in 2000 whites, 1 in 17 000 blacks, and 1 in 90 000 Asians. It is transmitted as an autosomal recessive trait so that about 1 in 23 of the population carries the gene.

Aetiology

This is a genetic condition resulting from a gene mutation on the long arm of chromosome 7. An abnormal regulator protein leads to a disruption of chloride channel controls and chloride and water are not excreted while sodium and water are absorbed. The clinical consequence is thickened secretions on mucosal surfaces with an altered electrolyte composition.

Clinical features

Cystic fibrosis is a multisystem disease characterized by viscous secretions and dysfunction of multiple exocrine glands, resulting in pancreatic insufficiency, malabsorption, chronic pulmonary infection with emphysema, and high chloride concentration in sweat. Forty per cent of patients present with respiratory disease, 30% with malabsorption, failure to thrive, and intussusception, 20% at birth with meconium ileus, and 10% in other ways.

In the 1930s when the disease was first described, life-expectancy was about six months. The median survival in the 1940s was two years, and now in the 1990s it is over 30 years

Pulmonary disease

Over 90% of the deaths of CF patients are caused by lung disease. At birth and before the first infection the lungs are histologically normal. Pulmonary manifestations usually become apparent during the first few months of life. The common sequence of events is an initial viral infection followed by bacterial infection. An intense inflammatory response occurs, hypertrophy, and hyperplasia of mucus-secreting apparatus follows and ultimately there is destruction of bronchial wall and bronchiectasis. If progress is not arrested at an early stage in the cycle, localized suppurative bronchopneumonia with marked necrosis results. New blood vessels form an extensive vascular plexus in the bronchial walls and leads to bronchopulmonary shunting. Progress of the disease is related to interaction between the host and various organisms. A transient hypogammaglobulinaemia has been described and immune complexes related to *Ps. aeruginosa* are found. There have been inconsistent reports of improvement with corticosteroid therapy, but most clinicians believe that lung damage results primarily from inflammation. *Staph. aureus* predominates early in the course, but later *Ps. aeruginosa* of particular serotypes rarely seen in other patients are present. *Pseudomonas cepacia* and *H. influenzae* are also commonly found. *Klebsiella, Escherichia coli,* and anaerobes are less commonly isolated.

Cystic fibrosis should be suspected in any child with:

(1) persistent respiratory symptoms, particularly if associated with failure to thrive;

(2) severe or recurrent bronchiolitis;

(3) persistent wheeze not typical of asthma;

(4) persistent X-ray changes, particularly involving right upper lobe of lung;

(5) moist productive cough;

(6) clubbing, with any other suggestive features.

Investigations

These children will usually be investigated by specialists although it is reasonable to organize preliminary tests while awaiting referral.

• *Chest X-ray.* Bronchial wall thickening, hyperinflation and on occasion atelectasis will be in evidence. In adults in particular cystic bronchiectatic changes may be seen as 'tram tracks' and ring shadows.

• *Lung function tests.* FEV 1 and FVC are reduced and the residual volume is increased.

Carrier screening and prenatal diagnosis

As the disease is genetically determined the parents of an affected child require genetic counselling. Adults who have a family history of the disease will expect an opportunity to discuss the chances of having an affected child before they embark on pregnancy. The gene for cystic fibrosis was cloned in 1989 and as a result it is possible to detect carriers in the general population.[25,26] Screening could detect 72% of carrier couples with a 1 in 4 risk of having an affected child, and one of the proposed approaches to implementing such a programme is to carry it out during routine antenatal consultations in general practice. General practitioners are generally positive about being involved in screening although they express a need to know more about the epidemiology, genetics, and clinical features of the condition before becoming involved.[27]

Prenatal diagnosis is available, but before it is contemplated the parents must have adequate opportunity to consider the implications and their attitude to abortion. While the advice may well come from specialists there is an important role for the family doctor in providing a continuing forum for the couple to explore their feelings. Diagnostic techniques include ultrasound, amniocentesis (intestinal isoenzyme level), and chorionic villus sampling (recombinant DNA techniques).

Neonatal screening using radioimmunoassay testing on blood samples is being developed but is presently unreliable.

Treatment

The diagnosis of cystic fibrosis in a family is a crisis requiring close involvement and communication between the patient, relatives, hospital consultant,

Table 7.13 *Respiratory complications of cystic fibrosis*

- Pneumothorax
- Haemoptysis
- Pulmonary hypertension
- Cor pulmonale
- Lobar atelectasis
- Clubbing
- Sinusitis
- Nasal polyps
- Respiratory failure

physiotherapist, and members of the primary health care team. A great deal of reassurance and organization of the support network is vital. Everybody concerned must be involved in the construction and implementation of a management plan, which should include:

1. Normal immunization schedule including Hib. In addition, pneumococcal and influenza vaccination should be given.

2. Early and aggressive treatment of any chest infection. Some authorities advocate prophylactic antibiotics against staphylococci during the first two years of life.

3. Awareness by the GP of the likely organisms and the appropriate treatment for lung infections:
   Staph. aureus: flucloxacillin,
   H. influenzae: amoxycillin
   Ps. aeruginosa: ciprofloxacin (on specialist advice)

4. Advice should always be sought from local microbiologist

5. Possible use of antibiotics by aerosol.

6. Physiotherapy

7. Attention to physical development and fitness.

8. Consideration of alternate day systemic steroids in severe disease.

Indications for hospitalization

Many families affected by cystic fibrosis become experts on all aspects of the disease and develop a close relationship with the hospital team which cares for them. It is important that the general practice team does not lose contact and become mere providers of antibiotics. Building this relationship depends on taking time to understand the disease and its effects and maintaining close contact with the hospital team. These children suffer many complications (Table 7.13), and in order to prolong life and improve its quality the GP must be aware of the indications for admission to hospital which include:

- Poor response to oral antibiotic therapy resulting in the need for parenteral therapy
- Haemoptysis
- Failure to thrive
- New radiographic signs

References

1. Coleman T, Wilson A. Anti-smoking advice in general practice consultations: general practitioners' attitudes, reported practice and perceived problems. *Brit J Gen Pract* (1996) **46**: 87–91

2. Russell M, Wilson C, Taylor C. Effect of general practitioners' advice against smoking. *BMJ* (1979) **2**: 231–5

3. Lennox A. Determinants of outcome in smoking cessation. *Brit J Gen Pract* (1992) **42**: 247–52

4. Macfarlane J, Colville A, Guion *et al.* Prospective study of aetiology and outcome of adult lower respiratory tract infections in the community. *Lancet* (1993) **341**: 511–14

5. Gonzales R, Sande M. What will it take to stop physicians prescribing antibiotics in acute bronchitis. *Lancet* (1995) **345**: 665–6

6. Macfarlane J, Prewitt J, Gard P. Comparison of amoxycillin and clarithromycin as an initial treatment of community-acquired lower respiratory tract infections. *Brit J Gen Pract* (1996) **46**: 357–60

7. McDougal L K *et al.* Analysis of multiply antimicrobial resistant isolates of *streptococcus pneumoniae* from the United States. *Antimicrob Agents Chemother* (1992) **36**: 2176–84

8. Korppi M, Reijonen T, Pöysä L. A 2- to 3-year outcome after bronchiolitis. *Am J Dis Child* (1993) **147**: 628–31

9. Jokinen C *et al.* Incidence of community acquired pneumonia in the population of four municipalities in Eastern Finland. *Am J Epidemiol* (1993) **137**: 977–88

10. Korppi M *et al.* Aetiology of community-acquired pneumonia in children treated in hospital. *Europ J Ped* (1993) **152**: 24–30

11. Research Committee of the British Thoracic Society and the Public Health Laboratory Service. Community acquired pneumonia in adults in British Hospitals in (1982–1983): a survey of aetiology, mortality, prognostic factors and outcome. *Q J Med* (1987) **62**: 195–220

12. Woodhead M *et al.* Prospective study of the aetiology and outcome of pneumonia in the community. *Lancet* (1987) 21 March: 671–4

13. Hosher H, Jones G, Hawkey P. Management of community acquired lower respiratory tract infection. (Review article). *BMJ* (1994) **308**: 701–5

14. Mycoplasma pneumoniae. (Editorial). *Lancet* (1991) **337**: 651–2

15. Obaro S, Monteil M, Henderson D. The pneumococcal problem. *BMJ* (1996) **312**: 1521–5

16. Bourke S. Chlamydial respiratory infections *BMJ* (1993) **306**: 1219–20

17. Tattersfield A, Macfarlane J. A complicated case of community acquired pneumonia. *BMJ* (1996) **312**: 899–901

18. Chan R, Hemeryck L, O'Regan M *et al*. Oral versus intravenous antibiotics for community acquired lower respiratory tract infection in a general hospital: randomised controlled trial. *BMJ* (1995) **310**: 1360–2

19. Raviglione M *et al*. Secular trends of tuberculosis in Western Europe. *Bull WHO* (1993) **71**: 297–306

20. Watson J (Editorial). Tuberculosis in Britain today. Notifications are no longer falling. *BMJ* (1993) **306**: 221–2

21. Joseph S. Tuberculosis, Again. *Am J Public Health* (1993) **83**: 647–8

22. Evans M. Is tuberculosis taken seriously in the United Kingdom? *BMJ* (1995) **311**: 1483–5

23. Centers for disease control and prevention: Estimates of future global tuberculosis morbidity and mortality. *MMWR* (1993) **42**: 961–964

24. Sumartojo E. When tuberculosis treatment fails: a social behavioral account of patient adherence. *Am Rev Respir Dis* (1993) **147**: 1311–20

25. Watson E, Williamson R, Chapple J. Attitudes to carrier screening for cystic fibrosis: a survey of health care professionals, relatives of sufferers and other members of the public. *Brit J Gen Pract* (1991) **41**: 237–40

26. Harris H, Scotcher D, Hartley N. Pilot study of the acceptability of cystic fibrosis carrier testing during routine antenatal consultations in general practice. *Brit J Gen Pract* (1996) **46**: 225–7

27. Boulton M, Cummings C, Williamson R. The views of general practitioners on community carrier screening for cystic fibrosis. *Brit J Gen Pract* (1996) **46**: 299–301

CHAPTER EIGHT

Infections of the central nervous system

The three major groups of infections of the central nervous system: meningitis, encephalitis, and focal suppurative disease—all require urgent therapy if serious sequaelae are to be avoided. This therapy will almost always need to be undertaken in hospital and, hence, the principal requirement of the general practitioner is the ability to recognize the danger signals that should urge prompt referral. The importance of these infections stems from their catastrophic effect if they are mismanaged rather than their frequency, but as they all present in primary care they are described in some detail here.

The central nervous system (CNS) is covered by three layers of meninges. The innermost layer, which is tightly applied to the surface of the brain and spinal cord is the pia mater. Outside this, and more loosely applied to the surface, is the arachnoid; between the pia and the arachnoid is the cerebrospinal fluid (CSF). The outermost layer of the meninges is the dura mater which is adherent to the periosteum of the skull. The dura is invaginated at several points to form four septa containing the venous sinuses: (1) the falx cerebri superiorly between the two cerebral hemispheres; (2) the falx cerebelli; (3) the tentorium cerebelli; and (4) the diaphragma selli.

The CSF is largely secreted by the choroid plexuses within the cerebral ventricles and flows outwards through the foramina of Luschka and Magendie (in the roof of the fourth ventricle) into the subarachnoid space. It then circulates over and around the brain and spinal cord by bulk flow and is reabsorbed through the arachnoid villi in the superior sagittal sinus. The normal volume of CSF in the adult is 110–140 ml and there is turnover of the total volume at least three times each day.

Acute meningitis

Despite the advances in antimicrobial chemotherapy and increased under-standing of the pathophysiology of meningitis, the mortality has not changed much in the past 30 years.[1] Any improvement in outcome depends upon an earlier recognition of meningitis and the rapid differentiation of those cases with a bacterial aetiology since it is any delay in the institution of effective antimicrobial therapy that is associated with a high mortality.

Epidemiology

The epidemiology of meningitis is complex and depends greatly on the age of the individual. The overall incidence is uncertain as most viral cases are not reported and even for bacterial meningitis there is considerable under notification: in the UK, however, the annual incidence of bacterial meningitis is probably about 3–5/100 000 population in the absence of epidemics. The disease is commonest in young children and it has been estimated that at least 1/1000 children will develop meningitis by the age of 10 years. Boys are more likely to be affected than girls.

Aetiology

Few organisms consistently cause meningitis as a primary manifestation of disease (Table 8.1) and outside the neonatal period there are only three major pathogens: *Neisseria meningitidis, Haemophilus influenzae,* and *Streptococcus pneumoniae.* Even when neonatal meningitis, almost always caused by *Escherichia coli* or the group B streptococcus, is included, only five

Table 8.1 *The causes of meningitis*

Common pathogens
Meningococcus
Pneumococcus
Haemophilus influenzae
Enteroviruses
Mumps virus

Rarer causes
Mycobacterium tuberculosis
Listeria monocytogenes
Gram-negative bacilli
Staphylococci
Leptospira
Borrelia burgdorferi (Lyme disease)
Human immunodeficiency virus (HIV)
Other viruses
Amoebae
Cryptococcus neoformans

In the new-born
Group B streptococci
Escherichia coli
Listeria monocytogenes
Other Gram-negative bacilli
Staphylococcus aureus

bacterial pathogens need to be considered in the vast majority of instances. Until the 1980s, the meningococcus was the most common bacterial pathogen in the UK, but subsequently there were rising *H. influenzae* rates and this pathogen then overtook *N. meningitidis* in frequency. The introduction of Hib vaccine, however, reversed this trend dramatically. The majority of *H. influenzae* cases occurred in children under 3 years of age: beyond this age the organism became progressively less important as a meningeal pathogen. The incidence of meningitis falls to low levels in early adult life but in adults over the age of 45 years it again becomes more common, primarily due to an increasing incidence of *Strep. pneumoniae* infections. The rate in those over 60 years is about twice that of adults aged 30–59.

Pathogenesis

The bacteria that cause meningitis usually initially colonize the mucosa of the nasopharynx, then invade the bloodstream and cross the blood-brain barrier. Each of these steps requires virulence factors which are poorly understood. Similarly, the precise mechanisms that enable some viruses to cause meningitis and meningoencephalitis after delivery to the nervous system by the haematogenous route remain to be determined.

Although infection usually reaches the CNS via the bloodstream, it can occur as a result of direct implantation of organisms following head injury or surgery, or as a result of anatomical abnormalities such as dermal sinuses. Bacteria probably enter the CSF via the blood vessels in the choroid plexuses and then spread along the normal channels of CSF flow.

In the absence of infection the CSF is devoid of any cellular components and the immunoglobulin and complement levels are very low. It is thus an immunologically naive site and infection readily gains a hold and causes meningitis. Infection within the subarachnoid space involves the pia and arachnoid (known collectively as the leptomeninges) and may spread across the foramina of Luschka and Magendie into the ventricles.

As a result of the initial inflammatory response in meningitis, there is an increase in the antibody levels within the CSF and an influx of polymorphonuclear leucocytes (PMNs). The lack of other defence mechanism within the CSF renders these cells relatively inefficient at phagocytosis. The bacteria causing meningitis do not usually spread outside the subarachnoid space and the disturbances of brain function seen in purulent meningitis are primarily due to inflammatory responses. Various bacterial products released within the CNS activate a cascade of inflammatory mediators and these are then responsible for many of the pathological processes which cause damage to the brain. Gram-negative bacteria initiate the inflammatory cascade by release of endotoxin and Gram-positive bacteria such as pneumococci by release of other cell wall components, particularly teichoic acid. These bacterial products induce the release of tumour necrosis factor (TNF) and interleukins from macrophages and other mononuclear cells and there is now also ample evidence that some components of polymorphonuclear phagocytes themselves are cytotoxic for brain cells. The results of the inflammatory responses are impairment of the blood–brain barrier and the development of cerebral oedema and raised intracranial pressure. Exactly how these adverse effects are induced by the inflammatory products is unclear but the levels of various cytokines, particularly TNF and interleukin-1, within the CSF are correlated with a poor outcome in purulent meningitis.

The cerebral oedema produces major changes upon the cerebral circulation resulting in cerebral ischaemia and further cerebral oedema. The cranial nerves, particularly the facial and auditory nerves, may also be affected as they traverse the subarachnoid space in meningitis. Cranial nerve function is particularly likely to be affected in chronic forms of meningitis such as that caused by *Mycobacterium tuberculosis* and fungi.

Meningitis may produce either communicating or obstructive hydrocephalus. Communicating hydrocephalus results when exudate within the subarachnoid space clogs up reabsorption of CSF across the arachnoid villi. Although there is ventricular dilatation, the raised pressure is distributed throughout the subarachnoid space and the ventricular system. In obstructive hydrocephalus, however, the inflammation blocks the ventricular system at one of its narrow points and leads to dilatation of the ventricular system. In this form of hydrocephalus, lumbar puncture can precipitate brain herniation and be lethal.

Clinical features

Meningitis may be acute or chronic and acute meningitis may be aseptic (usually but not always due to viruses) or purulent (generally bacterial). The clinical features of all forms of meningitis are, however, very similar and the critical distinction between bacterial and viral causes can rarely be made by the GP, whose primary role must remain the referral of suspicious cases for further investigation in hospital. Meningitis of whatever aetiology is usually eventually associated with the features of meningism (headache, photophobia, and spasm of the spinal muscles producing neck rigidity and a positive Kernig's sign), and fever. In bacterial meningitis there may also be cerebral oedema and raised intracranial pressure leading to alterations in consciousness and seizures.

The diagnosis of meningism is made by taking the weight of the patient's head by putting both hands under the occiput while the patient is lying down and passively flexing the patient's head forward to a right angle. Spasm of the spinal muscles, and sometimes pain, limits flexion of the neck, often towards the end of the test: any resistance makes the test positive. Kernig's sign is elicited by flexing the (supine) patient's hip to 90 degrees, and then attempting to extend the knee. In normal individuals the knee should be able to be extended to at least 45 degrees above the horizontal without hamstring spasm. Spinal spasm can also be detected in young children by the 'tripod' sign. Here, the child, when asked to sit up, does not lean forward but supports him- or herself with both arms held extended behind the trunk.

Such classical features of meningitis are easy to recognize but in many cases of bacterial meningitis the presentation is insidious and patients will seek medical attention before any such florid symptoms or signs develop.[2]

It can be extremely difficult to spot the subtle signs of meningitis in these patients but, even though any single GP is only likely to see a handful of cases of bacterial meningitis in a lifetime, he/she must maintain a constant level of awareness and get into the habit of considering the possibility of meningitis in any patient with one of the cardinal 'meningeal' symptoms—vomiting, headache, stiff neck, lethargy, or confusion—occurring on the background of an upper respiratory tract infection.

In neonates, the elderly, and immunocompromised patients the signs are often even more subtle (often only fever and irritability or poor feeding in the presence of marginal changes in cerebral function). Meningism is very difficult to detect in children under 18 months of age. If the infant still has a fontanelle then it can be helpful to assess whether this is full, since a full fontanelle is present in some infants with meningitis. If there is genuine doubt and the person is not very unwell, then it may be acceptable to arrange to see them again a few hours later in order to reconsider the possibility of meningitis. Even so, disaster may occasionally strike and given that the adage in hospital practice is: 'If you think of doing a lumbar puncture, do one,' then for the GP the adage should be: 'If you think meningitis is possible, refer to hospital.' In hospital, there are much better opportunities for close observation.

Once the presence of meningitis has been suspected the paramount need is the separation of bacterial meningitis from non-bacterial causes since any delay in effective therapy for the former is associated with a high mortality. Such a separation can only definitively be made by examination of the CSF but consideration of the speed of progression of the illness and the presence of certain clinical features may give important clues. A rapidly progressive meningitis is almost always due to pyogenic bacteria and warrants immediate referral. Of even more concern is the presence of a petechial or purpuric rash. This is almost pathognomonic of meningococcal meningitis, which is one of the true medical emergencies. Any delay in treatment can literally be fatal and the GP should be prepared to administer a parenteral antibiotic immediately to these cases: intravenous benzyl penicillin is traditional but almost any of the newer beta-lactam antibiotics or chloramphenicol would be equally suitable.

Case history

A young mother called the GP at the end of evening surgery. Her 2-year-old son had been listless over the past few days and irritable that afternoon. The doctor visited on the way home and confirmed the mother's findings. There were no localizing signs and no rash and he promised to call back at 10.30 pm. Two hours later he received a phone call to say the child was much worse and had developed a rash. He phoned the ambulance and arranged to meet at the house where he found a seriously ill child covered in a petechial rash. He gave immediate IM benzyl penicillin and accompanied the child to hospital in the ambulance. Fortunately, the outcome was a complete recovery.

Points for discussion with the GP registrar

- Tolerating uncertainty in the management of ill children
- The management of emergencies in the home and drugs for the doctor's bag
- Implications for the doctor—patient relationship if the child had died on the way to hospital

The ultimate decision regarding management of most cases of meningitis will be made after the patient has reached hospital. Most patients will not have any specific clinical findings and will have had symptoms for more than 24 hours. Any of the organisms listed in Table 8.1 may be responsible for the illness in this group and a decision regarding treatment depends the results of lumbar puncture (LP). The microscopical and biochemical examination of the CSF usually gives some indication of the type of organism responsible for the meningitis (Table 8.2). There is, however, a good deal of overlap between the findings in the different categories and a Gram-stain and subsequent culture of the CSF is mandatory in all cases. Other patients will have a very acute and rapidly progressive illness and this is almost always due to pyogenic bacteria. In these cases, providing an initial brief examination fails to reveal papilloedema or focal neurological signs, a LP and blood cultures will usually be obtained and empirical therapy directed at the likely pathogens (see below) started quickly before the CSF result is available. Papilloedema is unusual in meningitis and its presence or the presence of depressed consciousness or focal signs should prompt a search for an intracranial space-occupying

Table 8.2 *Cerebrospinal fluid changes in various forms of meningitis*

Normal	Pyogenic bacterial	Viral meningitis	TB meningitis
Appearance			
Clear	Turbid/purulent	Clear/opalescent	Clear/opalescent
Cells			
0–5/mm³	35–2000/mm³	35–500/mm³	35–1000/mm³
Predominant cell type			
Lymphocytes	Neutrophils	Lymphocytes	Lymphocytes
Glucose			
2.2–3.3 mmol/l[a]	Very low	Normal[b]	Low
Gram-stain organisms			
No	Usually	No	Yes; Ziehl–Neilson

[a] Approximately 60% of blood level.
[b] Occasionally low in mumps meningitis.

lesion; an urgent CT scan is needed in these patients before LP can be contemplated.

Treatment

It is not uncommon for parents of a child with meningitis to wish to discuss the hospital management with the GP as the overwhelming nature of the experience may inhibit them from so doing during the critical phase. An overview of the likely approach follows.

Once an lumbar puncture (LP) has been performed a decision can be made on the need to start therapy (or to change to more specific therapy for those who have already been given empirical antibiotics). If an organism is seen within the CSF the decision is usually quite straightforward, but if not the question is whether there is anything to suggest that the meningitis is caused by an organism other than a virus. Prior therapy with an antibiotic, perhaps administered for a non-specific febrile illness or for mild respiratory symptoms, may prevent organisms from being detected on the Gram's stain but the cellular response usually remains recognizably purulent and antibiotics will be prescribed. Considerable help is now available to the hospital clinician from the results of tests for bacterial antigens within the CSF. Sometimes, if the patient is not too ill, the doctor will defer antibiotic therapy, carefully observe the patient, and repeat the LP some hours later. Changes in the CSF to a more typical viral or bacterial picture may thus be detected and the patient managed accordingly.

The choice of antibiotics for bacterial infections depends on a number of criteria:

- Sensitivity of the likely pathogens
- The need for bactericidal therapy—the lack of an effective immune response within the CSF makes this imperative
- Adequate penetration of the antibiotic into the CSF. Almost always this will entail intravenous administration in order to achieve high blood, and hence CSF, levels.

The antibiotics suitable for proven infections are discussed below. Except for neonates and certain other special instances, the empirical therapy of presumed acute bacterial meningitis is now best given with a third-generation cephalosporin, which will be effective against meningococci, *H. influenzae* (which is still a possibility in children under the age of 5 or 6 years, despite Hib vaccine) and the increasing number of penicillin-resistant pneumococci. There is no evidence that giving more than one antibiotic in these circumstances is of additional benefit and it merely exposes the patient to an increased risk of side-effects. Antibiotic therapy for meningitis is usually somewhat arbitrarily given for 7–14 days, but for meningococcal infections this can probably be shortened to 5–7 days.

Given that much of the cerebral damage of meningitis is ultimately caused by cytokine activation by bacterial cell wall products, it is possible that antibiotics, by killing bacteria and releasing further cell wall products, could make the condition worse. This has led to a search for methods of treating bacterial meningitis that might limit the inflammatory response. One such approach is the use of corticosteroids. It has now been shown that the use of corticosteroids in bacterial meningitis may limit the complication of deafness in children with *H. influenzae* meningitis. This benefit has not yet been conclusively shown to extend to children with other forms of bacterial meningitis or to adults, but dexamethasone therapy is now often administered for the first 4 days of therapy in infants and young children with meningitis.

The gross mortality statistics are difficult to interpret since the prognosis of the various types of meningitis differs markedly. For meningococcal meningitis without the Waterhouse-Friderichsen syndrome of gross septicaemic shock, the mortality is less than 5%, whereas in neonatal meningitis and pneumococcal meningitis the mortality even in the best hands is still around 20%. In those who survive the most common complication is deafness, which follows about 5–10% of cases of meningitis, particularly that due to *H. influenzae*.

When a tragedy happens

It is the nature of medicine and life that wrong diagnoses are made and patients die. Tragedies occur for a wide variety of reasons, but few situations are more distressing than the death of a neonate or infant with a delayed diagnosis of septicaemia or meningitis. In such circumstances parental anger may well be directed at the GP as a component of the bereavement reaction. It is essential that the doctor appreciates and understands the reaction and must never respond in a similar mode. Calm, empathic communication is essential to achieve mutual understanding and sustain a trusting relationship. Numerous follow-up visits will be necessary to the parents. At such a time, it is essential that the GP who may reproach him/herself obtains the moral support, understanding, and caring of partners who should arrange protected time for the doctor to cope with his/her own feelings and those of the bereaved parents.

The chances of such a misfortune occurring are lessened by remembering the following points:

1. With any ill pyrexial child very careful attention should be given to the history as related by the parents and particularly the mother.

2. Careful clinical examination must be carried out and in the case of a neonate or infant there must be a high index of suspicion for diagnosis of septicaemia or meningitis.

3. Education of parents in the management of the pyrexial child is important and a practice leaflet outlining management is recommended.

4. Admission to hospital is necessary following a first febrile convulsion in a child under the age of 18 months.

5. Communication and dialogue between GP and parents is an essential part of management and follow-up.

Chronic meningitis

A number of infections can cause the clinical syndrome of chronic meningitis. The onset is more subacute or chronic with slowly increasing meningism, confusion, lethargy, and vomiting. These symptoms sometimes wax and wane with short-lived episodes of more severe neurological deterioration. The causes of this syndrome are the intracellular bacteria and other organisms and there are often clinical signs of associated systemic disease. The usual aetiologies of this syndrome in the UK are tuberculosis and cryptococcosis (in immunocompromised individuals), although imported cases of brucellosis, histoplasmosis or other fungal infections of the nervous system are seen very infrequently. Non-infectious forms of meningitis, such as sarcoidosis and neoplastic meningitis, need to be excluded. The diagnosis of these forms of meningitis is established in the hospital laboratory.

Bacterial meningitis

Meningococcal meningitis

Neisseria meningitidis (the meningococcus) is a Gram-negative bacterium that is carried asymptomatically in the nasopharynx of many individuals. There are several serogroups of meningococci, based upon the antigenic composition of the polysaccharide capsule, and the prevalence of each particular serogroup differs with time and geography for reasons that are not clear. Group A, for instance is the cause of regular large epidemics of meningitis in parts of sub-Saharal Africa and was once responsible for major outbreaks in the UK. Epidemics of meningitis caused by A and C strains have also occurred recently in South America, the Middle East and in Asia (Nepal and India, in particular). Recently, group B has become the chief strain in Europe. In addition, the predominant strains of group B meningococci also change with time. In the UK, the increase in meningococcal disease over the past decade has been associated with a group B, type 15 strain that seems to be peculiarly able to cause disease in teenagers and young adults as well as in children.[3] Other types are also still encountered.

The carriage rate for meningococci in the nasopharynx of the normal healthy population is about 10%. In most cases, this nasopharyngeal colonization leads to the development of antibodies that prevent mucosal invasion but occasionally, for poorly understood reasons, acquisition is followed by septicaemia and meningitis. Transmission of the organism from person to person is usually the result of direct contact such as kissing or prolonged close contact. This is predominantly a sporadic disease of children and young adults (60% of cases occur in children under the age of 5 years, with a second small peak in the late teens and early twenties) but small outbreaks of infection sometimes occur in susceptible populations. Most cases occur in the winter months.

There is usually an abrupt onset of symptoms with rapid progression to confusion or coma. The meningitis is part of a septicaemic process and the rash of meningococcaemia is an important diagnostic sign. The frequency of the rash depends on how hard it is sought. About half the cases will have a rash by the time a GP sees them[4] and two-thirds of patients have a rash upon admission to hospital. The rash may initially be macular and pink but later it becomes petechial or purpuric. A purpuric rash is a poor prognostic sign.

In about 10% of cases there is no meningitis and septicaemia dominates the clinical picture. The overwhelming majority of such patients will have a rash and in some the septicaemia is fulminant with widespread skin lesions, disseminated intravascular coagulation, and circulatory collapse. This is the Waterhouse–Friderichson syndrome which has a very poor prognosis. The diagnosis of meningococcal septicaemia and meningitis is made by finding purulent CSF containing Gram-negative diplococci, detecting specific meningococcal antigens within the CSF, or culturing the organism from blood cultures. Organisms can also sometimes be detected within the skin lesions.

The general practice management of a child with suspected meningococcal disease. In 1988, the chief medical officer wrote to all GPs urging them to consider giving parenteral penicillin to all suspected cases of meningococcal disease before admission to hospital. In 1992, a study of the administration of penicillin before admission to patients with meningococcal disease revealed that only 28% had received it.[5] Patients who had received the drug had a much better prognosis. Begg[6] has postulated that the reluctance to administer the drug stems from fear of anaphylaxis and worry that the hospital investigations will be compromised. He emphasizes that neither of these reasons are sufficient to weigh against a life-saving intervention (Table 8.3).

Treatment is with high dose intravenous benzyl penicillin, a third-generation cephalosporin or chloramphenicol, given in hospital for 5–7 days. The overall mortality is about 5–10% and neurological sequelae are relatively infrequent.[7]

Meningococcal septicaemia or meningitis are notifiable diseases and in order to institute effective control measures, cases need to be advised immediately. The risk of second cases within the household contacts of the index case is significantly greater than in the general population. In order to minimize this risk chemoprophylaxis is given to close contacts who might either be incubating the disease in their nasopharynx or who might act as source of transmission to other household members. The current recommendations are to give adult contacts either ciprofloxacin (500 mg single dose) or rifampicin (600 mg every 12 hours for 2 days). A two day course of rifampicin is offered to contacts aged between 3 months and 12 years. The doses are 10 mg/kg 12 hourly (aged 1 to 12 years) or 5 mg/kg 12

Table 8.3 *Meningococcal infection and the role of the general practitioner*

- Be aware of the local prevalence of the infection.
- Be alert to the possibility and remember the speed at which the infection develops. If you think of it, admit the patient. Arrange very careful and frequent follow-up for ill children with no localizing signs. Be particularly vigilant if you are handing over to a colleague
- Carry benzylpenicillin in your bag and ensure that it is in date
- Treat patients with suspected disease immediately with parenteral (preferably IV) benzyl penicillin. Only a documented history of anaphylaxis is relevant
- Administer 1200 mg benzylpenicillin to adults and children over 10 years, 500 mg for children 1–9 years, and 300 mg for children under 1 year
- Remember to inform the public health department and to liaise in respect of prophylaxis for contacts
- Stay in telephone contact with the hospital and the family and be prepared to provide support and explanation as the situation evolves
- Be prepared to support GP colleagues who are upset by the death of a young patient in their care

---

hourly (aged 3 months to 1 year). Contacts are all those living in the same house as the index case and to those who have been mouth-kissing contacts in the week preceding diagnosis. School contacts are not usually in need of prophylaxis unless more than one related case occurs at the school. Mass chemoprophylaxis is not indicated, even if there is obvious public demand: it is the public health doctor's job to co-ordinate its administration and to assuage public concern although this is ideally done in collaboration with local general practices (see Chapter 2).

Recipients of rifampicin should be warned not to take alcohol and that their urine will be coloured orange while taking the antibiotic. Family contacts should be warned to report feverish illnesses to their GP and those with headache and fever should be admitted to hospital and regarded as presumptive cases (even if they have been given prophylaxis).

Polysaccharide vaccines are available that provide effective short term (5 years) immunity against meningococci of groups A, C, Y, and W135, but it has not been possible to produce a vaccine against group B meningococci. Vaccines are poorly immunogenic in children under 2 years of age and even in adults antibodies take 10–14 days to develop; vaccination is not, therefore, effective in controlling infection in household contacts.

Vaccination may be offered to those travelling to countries experiencing a major epidemic of meningococcal disease and is compulsory for certain individuals (Haj pilgrims visiting Saudi Arabia for instance). Risk is greatest to travellers under 35, particularly young children.

Pneumococcal meningitis

Streptococcus pneumoniae (the pneumococcus) is a capsulated Gram-positive diplococcus that causes about 15% of cases of bacterial meningitis. Meningeal infection occurs at any age but is of particular importance in the first year of life and in the adult and elderly patient: between 50% and 60% of cases occur in those less than 1 year old, or greater than 50 years of age. It is more common in males and is particularly prevalent in the late autumn, winter, and early spring. Alcoholics and those splenectomized or with splenic dysfunction, including patients with sickle-cell disease, are at increased risk of pneumococcal disease. It is also by far the most common cause of meningitis following closed head trauma, and if there is a basal skull fracture and dural tear repeated attacks may occur. Other high-risk groups are those with hypogammaglobulinaemia, nephrotic syndrome, or malignancy. In half the cases, the *Strep. pneumoniae* is presumed to have originated from nasopharyngeal carriage but in others there is a focus of pneumococcal infection in the lungs, paranasal sinuses, or middle ear.

Pneumococcal meningitis presents like any other form of bacterial meningitis. In children, the illness is often preceded by an upper respiratory tract infection (URTI) followed by insidious development of irritability, lethargy, and signs of meningism. It is often the most severe of the common forms of meningitis with coma and seizures appearing early in the course. Convulsions are common and may be generalized or focal. Focal neurological signs, particularly cranial nerve palsies, are seen at presentation in more than a quarter of cases.

Strains of pneumococci that are relatively resistant to penicillin are now becoming sufficiently widespread for a third-generation cephalosporin (ceftriaxone or cefotaxime), rather than benzylpenicillin, to be the drug of choice for pneumococcal meningitis, at least until the organism isolated can be shown to be penicillin-sensitive. The mortality is higher and permanent sequelae are more frequent after pneumococcal meningitis than after other forms of bacterial meningitis. The mortality remains at about 25%. About 25% of survivors have some form of neurological sequelae (e.g. deafness, convulsions, developmental retardation), and in the very young or very old these problems are even more common.

It is not possible to determine whether the pneumococcal vaccine is effective in preventing pneumococcal meningitis. The vaccine does appear to protect against pneumococcal pneumonia and bacteraemia in different groups at particular risk of invasive pneumococcal disease, but protection against meningitis does appear to be less effective, possibly because of the number of pneumococcal serotypes that cause meningitis but that are not included within the 23 serotypes in the vaccine.

Haemophilus meningitis

Haemophilus influenzae is a small Gram-negative bacterium that may exist with or without a capsule. Meningitis (and indeed almost all forms of invasive infection) is caused primarily by capsulate strains of the organism that are classified by their capsular polysaccharide as type b and the disease has become very rare since the introduction of Hib immunization. The nasopharynx is the primary site for bacterial colonization and invasion by *H. influenzae*. Carriage of the organism is common at all ages but only about 5% of carriers harbour encapsulated strains and very few of these are type b.

Before Hib immunization meningitis due to *H. influenzae* was almost exclusively a disease of children between 4 months and 6 years of age. There was a slight predominance in boys and at any one time about 1% of children under 6 years were colonized with *H. influenzae* type b, generally in the nasopharynx.[8] It was the most common form of bacterial meningitis before the introduction of Hib immunization. Most cases are sporadic but secondary cases do occur in household contacts or children attending the same daycare facility as the index case.

The disease usually develops insidiously over several days in a child who has had symptoms suggestive of a URTI or ear infection. Pharyngitis and otitis media are associated with *H. influenzae* meningitis in 50% and 67% of cases, respectively. A high index of suspicion is required in order to make the diagnosis of meningitis and it can be extremely difficult to determine the exact time of onset of meningitis. Occasionally, the infection can have a fulminant course progressing to coma within a few hours. Convulsions are not uncommon in the early stages of *H. influenzae* meningitis and do not necessarily portend a poor outcome. Subdural effusions are also common in very young infants with meningitis and again do not indicate a poor outcome: most will resolve spontaneously.

A substantial number of *H. influenzae* strains are now resistant to ampicillin, and strains resistant to chloramphenicol are also becoming a problem in some areas of the world. The third-generation cephalosporins are effective against ampicillin-resistant and chloramphenicol-resistant *H. influenzae* and they are now considered the drugs of choice for this form of meningitis. Cefotaxime is probably the optimal therapy in the UK and should be continued for 7–10 days; once the organism has been shown to be sensitive the treatment can be changed to the cheaper ampicillin or chloramphenicol. The mortality is 5–10%. The rates of neurological sequelae vary depending upon the age of the child. Furthermore, although a significant percentage infected early in life have detectable learning or behavioural difficulties, these are often minimal and most children with *H. influenzae* meningitis have a good prognosis.

Recent studies have supported the routine administration of steroids in children with *H. influenzae* (and possibly other bacterial) meningitis: their use reduces the mortality and morbidity (particularly deafness) associated with this disease.

Household contacts under the age of 4 years are at increased risk of disease within a month of an index case and chemoprophylaxis is now recommended to eradicate nasopharyngeal carriage within the household.[9] Rifampicin prophylaxis [20 mg/kg body weight (10 mg/kg/day for infants less than 1 month old), up to a maximum dose of 600 mg, once daily for 4 days] should be given to all members of a household when there is a child at risk. There is still uncertainty as to whether all daycare contacts of an index case should also be given prophylaxis but this is probably a prudent policy if there are children under 2 years old attending the nursery or if more than one case has occurred.

Neonatal meningitis

Meningitis is more common in the first month of life than at any other time and continues to cause significant morbidity and mortality. In the UK, its incidence is about 1/2500 live births and is particularly seen in low birth weight infants (below 2.5 kg). The organisms that are chiefly responsible are group B streptococci (GBS) and *Escherichia coli*, particularly strains carrying the K1 capsular polysaccharide antigen. Other less common organisms include *Listeria monocytogenes, Pseudomonas aeruginosa*, and *Staphylococcus aureus*. The bacteria either arise from the mother's genital tract and colonize the infant during birth or are introduced as a result of invasive procedures. The classical features of meningitis are often absent in the new-born and the diagnosis of neonatal meningitis requires a high index of suspicion. Non-specific abnormalities such as poor feeding, respiratory distress, diarrhoea, vomiting, and irritability may predominate. Brief convulsions are common but are rarely *grand mal* in type and may not be recognized as such. Meningitis caused by GBS presents in two distinct ways, depending on its time of onset after birth.

1. *Early-onset (first week of life)*. The infant has a fulminant illness with a high mortality. Septicaemia and respiratory symptoms (often confused with respiratory distress syndrome) are prominent. This is particularly common in premature infants and is rarely seen by the general practitioner.

2. *Late-onset (after the first week of life)*. This is a more insidious illness occurring from 10 days to 8 weeks after delivery and may well present to the GP or health visitor. It is not associated with prematurity, meningitis is a prominent feature, and the prognosis is much better with a mortality of about 15%.

The treatment usually recommended for neonatal meningitis is a combination of ampicillin and gentamicin, which will cover both GBS and *E. coli*. Since there is controversy over the need for gentamicin to be given intraventricularly, however, many paediatricians now use one of the third-generation cephalosporins, such as ceftriaxone or cefotaxime, instead of this combination. Proven GBS infection can usually be treated with ampicillin or penicillin alone.

The prognosis of neonatal meningitis remains poor with mortality up to 50% in premature infants and neurological and psychological sequelae in one-third of the survivors.

Other types of purulent meningitis

Shunt-associated meningitis. Up to 25% of patients with ventriculo-atrial or ventriculo-peritoneal shunts for hydrocephalus develop meningitis. Half of these infections are due to *Staph. epidermidis* and many of the remainder are due to Gram-negative bacilli. Systemic and intraventricular therapy with antibiotics (vancomycin seems best for staphylococci) often fails to eradicate the infection and removal of the shunt may be necessary.

Meningitis due to Gram-negative enteric bacilli. This is an increasingly common form of meningitis in patients with head injuries, those who have had neurosurgery, and elderly diabetics or alcoholics. The signs of meningitis in these groups are often mistakenly attributed to the underlying condition. Therapy with the third-generation cephalosporins is a significant improvement over the aminoglycosides but the mortality still remains high.

Listeria meningitis. Although this form of meningitis can occur in normal adults it is chiefly a disease of neonates or pregnant, debilitated, or immunocompromised adults (especially recipients of renal transplants). The organism *L. monocytogenes* is a Gram-positive bacillus which can multiply at refrigerator temperatures. Many foodstuffs are contaminated and infection may be acquired from foods which are eaten raw or under-cooked or are eaten cold after pre-cooking. High-risk foods are soft cheeses, pâté, and cook–chill foods, unless thoroughly reheated before eating.

Tuberculous meningitis

Tuberculous meningitis may be a manifestation of miliary (disseminated) spread during primary tuberculosis in children or adolescents or due to rupture of a subependymal tubercle later in life. The clinical presentation is very variable. Usually it has a subacute or chronic progression with a period of general ill-health, low grade fever, and malaise which lasts for a week or two before meningeal symptoms appear. There is then increasingly severe headache, irritability, vomiting, and drowsiness followed by further depression of consciousness, seizures, and focal neurological signs, particularly cranial nerve palsies. Sometimes, however, tuberculous meningitis can present as an acute meningitis, clinically indistinguishable from acute pyogenic meningitis.

In a small minority of patients, choroidal tubercles can be seen in the fundi as round pale or pink lesions about the size of the optic disc but, in general, as for all forms of meningitis the diagnosis depends on the CSF examination. It is still prudent to regard any subacute meningitis with a low CSF sugar content as tuberculous meningitis until proved otherwise. Diagnosis can be confirmed by finding the organism on microscopy of the CSF (a large quantity of CSF, up to 10 ml, should be sent for examination if tuberculosis is suspected) but often treatment has to be given on suspicion when the other CSF results, particularly the glucose level, are suggestive. In children, the chest X-ray may show evidence of pulmonary tuberculosis but, in adults, the X-ray is generally normal.

Therapy of tuberculous meningitis must take into consideration the ability of drugs to cross the blood–brain barrier. The two drugs that attain the best CSF levels are pyrazinamide and isoniazid (up to 10 mg/kg body weight/day: at this dose pyridoxine should also be given to prevent isoniazid toxicity). These two drugs are usually given together with rifampicin and either streptomycin or ethambutol for the first 2–3 months of therapy. Treatment is then usually continued with isoniazid and rifampicin for a further 7–10 months. Modern drug regimens have made intrathecal streptomycin unnecessary.

The use of steroids remains controversial but they are usually recommended for patients with high CSF protein levels and impending spinal block, those with significantly elevated intracranial pressure, and those with focal or general neurological signs. Most patients will recover completely if therapy is started before consciousness is depressed but some develop hydrocephalus or spinal arachnoiditis. Close monitoring and CT scanning is necessary during the early stages of therapy.

Viral meningitis

This is a common problem and probably accounts for 80% or more of all cases of meningitis and about half of the cases referred for evaluation in hospital. The illness is usually mild and many cases undoubtedly go unrecognized. In others, the clinical picture is similar to that of early bacterial meningitis and hence the need to examine the CSF in all such cases. Most cases occur in children and young adults. Many different viruses have been implicated in meningitis but the majority of isolates are enteroviruses (Coxsackie, echoviruses, and polioviruses, see below), or mumps virus. Enterovirus infections are more common in the late summer and early autumn, sometimes in epidemics. Some cases are associated with other features of enteroviral infection, such as the rash of hand, foot, and mouth disease, the oral lesions of herpangina, or a variety of other rashes. Mumps virus infections tend to occur in the late winter and early spring. Recent or concomitant parotitis would favour mumps but in about 50% of cases the meningitis occurs in the absence of any salivary gland swelling.

Whatever the cause, the management of suspected viral meningitis is purely symptomatic and recovery is usually rapid and complete. It is, however, important for CSF to be examined and if the CSF shows an excessive number of lymphocytes and a raised protein but no organisms are seen on Gram-staining (aseptic meningitis) then, although the likeliest cause is a viral infection, the other causes of such a CSF picture, particularly tuberculous and fungal meningitis, require consideration.

Poliomyelitis

Globally, the three poliovirus serotypes are the most important enteroviruses. Vaccination has largely eliminated poliomyelitis world wide but rather paradoxically, the disease has become more common in some developing countries as living standards improve. This is because the improved sanitation delays infection beyond early infancy and the risk of paralytic disease is related to age. The condition only remains endemic in parts of Africa and Asia. Transmission is usually by the faecal-oral route but may be through the pharyngeal secretions of an infected person. Transmission by water is also believed to occur.

About 90% of all infections with polioviruses are asymptomatic. In the other 10%, after an incubation period of a week or two, there is a 2–3 day non-specific febrile illness with no neurological symptoms. Some of these individuals will have features of aseptic meningitis but only a very small minority (perhaps 0.1% of those infected) develop paralytic disease a few days later. These unfortunate patients develop muscle pains, often in the neck or back, which are relieved by movement. Frank weakness and asymmetric flaccid paralysis then gradually develop, with proximal muscles more affected than distal and legs more than arms. Sensory loss is very rare and should suggest another diagnosis (e.g. Guillain-Barré syndrome). The maximum degree of paralysis is evident within a week and is very variable.

There is no specific therapy for poliomyelitis. Management involves rest and splinting to prevent contractures during the acute phase, followed by mobilization and rehabilitation. Recovery may continue for several months but paralysis persisting beyond this time is permanent. The two types of polio vaccine and their use are described in Chapter 2.

Fungal meningitis

Cryptococcal meningitis

Meningitis due to the yeast *Cryptococcus neoformans* is by far the most important cause of fungal meningitis and is typically seen in patients whose immunity is depressed by steroids, diabetes, or lymphoproliferative disorders. In addition, about 10% of patients with AIDS develop cryptococcal meningitis. The infection is a chronic meningitis with scattered focal collections of fungal cells embedded in the gelatinous polysaccharide capsular material distributed within the brain sulci. The symptoms tend to be intermittent over several weeks and meningism is less common than headache, confusion, changes in behaviour, and depressed consciousness. Papilloedema and cranial nerve palsies are common. The organism may be visualized in the CSF using an India ink preparation or cryptococcal antigen may be detected using latex agglutination or ELISA. Patients with AIDS have little evidence of an inflammatory response within the CSF and yet the fluid is often full of cryptococci.

Treatment is with intravenous amphotericin B in normal dose (0.6–1 mg/kg body weight/day) or at a lower dose combined with oral flucytosine for 6–10 weeks. Fluconazole, an antifungal azole, is also effective and has less severe side-effects than amphotericin B. An added advantage is that, for AIDS patients who need to be continued on prophylaxis indefinitely in order to delay the reactivation of cryptococcal disease, fluconazole can be administered orally.

Encephalitis

Although meningitis and encephalitis are often considered separate entities there is usually a degree of overlap so that meningo-encephalitis probably more correctly reflects the extent of the pathological process. There are, however, some illnesses in which widespread inflammation of the brain parenchyma regularly occurs so that disturbances of consciousness, personality, though, and motor function predominate. Some of these (e.g. herpes simplex encephalitis, rabies, and toxoplasmosis), are caused by organisms that directly invade the brain tissue. This is a primary encephalitis and is characterized pathologically by dead or dying neurones surrounded by an inflammatory infiltrate. Other infectious agents can cause a clinical picture suggestive of encephalitis without actually invading CNS parenchyma. Some viral infections, for instance, are complicated by demyelinating diseases, either of central myelin to cause encephalitis, or peripheral myelin (giving rise to a Guillain-Barré syndrome, see below), probably as a result of sensitization to a component of myelin. In these conditions, the microscopic changes are those of perivascular demyelination and mononuclear cell infiltrate. A third group of illnesses are the non-inflammatory encephalopathies, where there is cerebral oedema and raised intracranial pressure but no inflammation and a lack of cells in the CSF. Whether by direct or indirect pathogenic mechanisms, these forms of encephalitis have considerable similarities in their presentations.

Finally, a primary invasive encephalitis can be chronic in its course, progressing over many months and sometimes commencing many years after the initial infection. These chronic infections are exemplified by subacute sclerosing panencephalitis (SSPE) and the slow virus infections.

Although there is an extensive list of viruses and other organisms that may cause encephalitis, in the UK there are a relative few that are seen with any frequency. The most common cause of direct viral invasion is herpes simplex virus with a lesser number of cases due to enteroviruses and mumps.[10] Chickenpox, glandular fever, and herpes zoster are occasionally followed by an encephalitis. Rabies and a number of virus infections transmitted by mosquitos, ticks, and other arthropods (arboviruses), although they cause a great deal of infection in other parts of the world, are only very rarely imported into this country (see Chapter 15). Encephalitis can occur with mycoplasmal infections but most other non-viral infections that can present with encephalitic features (e.g. tuberculosis or cryptococcosis), tend to present with significant meningeal components to the illness.

In post-infectious encephalitis there is often an abrupt onset 2–10 days after an exanthematous or respiratory infection: other forms of encephalitis may develop over a period of 2–3 days. Patients with encephalitis usually have signs and symptoms of meningeal inflammation but, in addition, have alterations of consciousness and prominent mental changes. Any of these symptoms presenting after a minor infection signals the need for immediate referral to hospital. Convulsions are common and focal signs reflecting damage to any part of the brain or spinal cord usually develop. Upgoing plantar reflexes and other signs of spasticity are particularly common but hemiparesis, cerebellar signs, or transverse myelitis may dominate the clinical picture. The presence of fever, seizures, and fluctuating clinical signs tend to distinguish an encephalitic illness from a metabolic or toxic encephalopathy.

Routine laboratory investigations do not help a great deal in establishing the aetiology of encephalitis and all patients require admission to hospital for brain scanning and CSF examination. The purpose of the investigations is principally to diagnose causes of encephalitis that require specific therapy in addition to full supportive measures. This essentially means herpes simplex encephalitis, since there are no effective antiviral drugs for other forms of viral infection. All forms of encephalitis tend to cause a predominance of lymphocytes within the CSF, although the number of cells can be very variable. The EEG will show a diffuse inflammatory process with bilateral slow wave activity and occasional spike discharges. Herpes simplex encephalitis tends to produce focal changes on CT scanning or EEG examinations but the only specific means of rapidly diagnosing herpes encephalitis used to be histological examination and immunological probing of brain tissue obtained at brain biopsy. Brain biopsy is, however, hardly ever performed in the UK, physicians preferring to treat empirically for herpes simplex with parenteral acyclovir in all cases of encephalitis and attempting to confirm the diagnosis by other means.

The specific diagnosis of the aetiology of encephalitis usually depends upon immunological techniques either to detect viral DNA (by the polymerase chain reaction, PCR) or antigens within the CSF or to determine specific antibody responses. Specific IgM can be sought and another method of obtaining evidence of CNS infection by a particular agent is to determine the ratio of antibody to the organism in the CSF and the serum: if this is higher than the ratio of a control globulin then it suggests local production of an antibody in response to infection within the CNS.

Patients with encephalitis can make dramatic recoveries even from deep and prolonged coma and hence full supportive measures should be implemented in all cases. The mortality varies with the aetiological agent from less than 1% to more than 50%. There is no evidence of any benefit from the use of corticosteroids in parainfectious encephalitis although they are widely used.

Specific pathogens

Herpes simplex encephalitis

In the UK, the commonest form of sporadic encephalitis is that due to herpes simplex virus (HSV) but even so it only occurs in 1–3 per million of the population per annum. Most GPs will thus never see a case. It occurs at all ages, in each sex, and is not seasonal. Even though most cases occur in persons with evidence of previous infection with herpes simplex virus, such infection is almost universal and a past history of herpes labialis or other cutaneous disease is of little help.

The disease has the typical clinical features of any encephalitis with an acute onset of fever, early deterioration in consciousness, frequent seizures, and rapid progression. Superimposed on this, however, are features that reflect the particular predilection of the virus for the temporal or frontal lobes. The necrosis and oedema that results often produces focal symptoms (anosmia, olfactory, or auditory hallucinations, etc.), and focal temporo-frontal abnormalities are commonly detectable on the EEG, isotope scan, or CT scan. The diagnosis is best confirmed prospectively by detection of viral DNA by PCR in the CSF but evidence of secretion of specific antibody in the CSF is available in retrospect.

As soon as the diagnosis of herpes encephalitis is suspected acyclovir (10 mg/kg body weight, 8-hourly) should be started. This is the drug of choice for HSV encephalitis and is clearly beneficial providing therapy is started before severe brain necrosis has occurred. Therapy should be given for 2 weeks. With such therapy more than 50% of patients can return to normal activity within 6 months. The percentage is much higher in younger patients and those who are not deeply unconscious on initiation of therapy. For the elderly patient in coma at presentation, acyclovir may well be life-saving but the long term outcome is bleak with almost all survivors left with major neurological sequaelae. Until proof of HSV infection is obtained, investigations aimed at other treatable causes of the symptoms should be continued.

Varicella zoster virus encephalitis

Encephalitis is a rare complication of herpes zoster, usually occurring in the elderly with cranial zoster or in immunocompromised individuals. The illness tends to appear a week or so after the appearance of the skin lesions but it is not clear whether it is due to direct viral invasion of the CNS or to a hypersensitivity reaction (see below). Untreated, the illness lasts for about two weeks and most patients recover with no sequaelae. Whether acyclovir improves the outcome has not been tested in a controlled fashion.

Post-infectious encephalitis

This rare form of encephalitis has been reported as a sequel to (among others) measles, chickenpox, mumps, glandular fever, influenza, other childhood exanthemata, and certain vaccines. It is characterized by patchy demyelination in the brain and spinal cord. It is believed to be due to a cell-mediated hypersensitivity reaction to part of the basic protein of CNS myelin, triggered in some way by the preceding infection. Characteristically, it occurs 2–12 days after the onset of infection (slightly longer after vaccination), and is extremely variable in severity. It is rarely seen in children under 2 years old. Recovery is the rule but the course is extremely unpredictable and the mortality is probably 25–30%. A similar percentage may be left with neurological or developmental sequaelae. There is no clear evidence to suggest any benefit from corticosteroid or other therapy.

Cerebellar ataxia

This is an encephalopathic illness that uncommonly follows chickenpox (and sometimes other viral infections) in childhood. It appears about one week after the onset of the rash and is manifest by truncal ataxia, vertigo, and vomiting. Speech is slurred and occasionally nystagmus is present. Often, the only abnormality in the CSF is a raised protein concentration; a few lymphocytes may also be present. There is usually a complete resolution of symptoms within 1–3 weeks. Antiviral therapy is not warranted.

Reye's syndrome

This is an acute encephalopathy that occurs in children between 2 and 16 years old and is associated with an acute fatty liver and cerebral oedema. It usually follows influenza, varicella, or other virus infections and its occurrence has been linked to ingestion of aspirin. There is often nausea and vomiting for 1–2 days before changes in conscious level and hepatic failure. Mortality depends on the degree of coma and hepatic insufficiency and may approach 40%. Intensive supportive measures aimed at reducing cerebral oedema are needed.

Chronic and progressive viral encephalitis

There are several chronic and progressive neurological conditions caused by viruses or prions (the agents of transmissible spongiform encephalopathies). The chronic viral infections are exemplified by subacute sclerosing panencephalitis (SSPE, due to measles virus) and progressive multifocal leukoencephalopathy (PML, due to papovavirus).

SSPE is a progressive inflammatory encephalitis involving grey and white matter that commences several years after clinical measles. It is extremely rare and appears to be caused by a defective form of the measles virus. The clinical features are a progressive decline in intellectual performance and abnormal behaviour, combined with seizures and myoclonic jerks. Characteristic features are seen on the EEG and the CSF contains high concentrations of antimeasles antibody. Death occurs after a few months and there is no effective therapy.

PML is a subacute demyelinating disease of the CNS that occurs in immunocompromised patients and which is caused by the JC virus, a member of the polyoma group of papovaviruses. It is due to reactivation of latent virus and occurs in those with defective cellular immunity, particularly patients with AIDS. The clinical manifestations are diverse and reflect the widespread foci of demyelination seen on MRI scanning. There is no effective therapy and death occurs within a few months of the appearance of the first neurological symptoms.

The spongiform encephalopathies are caused by a bizarre group of transmissible agents termed 'prions'. The term was chosen to designate a proteinaceous infectious particle which was resistant to formaldehyde, heating, and various other physical procedures that hydrolyse or modify nucleic acids. The diseases caused by these agents have in common a number of fundamental properties:

- their pathology is almost exclusively confined to the nervous system
- they produce a reactive astrocytosis in the CNS with a complete lack of inflammatory response;
- they have a very long incubation time
- their infectivity is associated with cerebral deposits of amyloid proteins with a molecular weight of 27–30 kDa.

Their pathogenesis is, however, extremely bewildering.

Creutzfeld–Jacob disease

Creutzfeld–Jacob disease (CJD) is a human form of these illnesses which is characterized by dementia, ataxia, and myoclonic jerks starting in late middle age and leading to death within a year or so. The overall incidence is about one case per million of the population. A presenile dementia with myoclonic jerks is almost always CJD. The diagnosis can be confirmed by EEG, which usually has a characteristic pattern of rhythmic, periodic bursts of high-amplitude biphasic or triphasic complexes.

The transmissibility of prion diseases in laboratory animals and in humans is clear; accidental transmission of CJD has followed corneal transplantation, injection of human growth hormone prepared from cadaveric pituitary glands, and contaminated surgical instruments. Most cases of CJD are, however, sporadic with no epidemiological evidence of transmission from other humans or from infected animals. Furthermore, 5–10% of cases of CJD occur in familial clusters and hence CJD seems the only known human disease which is both transmissible and genetic. Modern molecular biology has shed some light on this apparent contradiction. The 27–30 kDa 'prion' protein is present in equal amounts in normal and infected neurones. The function of the normal cellular protein is still unknown. It seems likely, however, that in prion disease the host is induced to synthesize a modification of the normal protein and thus it seems that this protein is not the principal part of an infectious agent but is a constituent of the cerebral amyloid produced in excess as a pathological response or due to a mutation.

There is no general agreement about the nature of the putative unconventional agents that are responsible for prion disorders. One hypothesis is that, after transmission from one host to another, the prion protein is able to self replicate rather as a crystal grows from a 'seed' but this theory (and others) still leaves many questions to be answered.

Bovine spongiform encephalopathy (BSE)

Much public disquiet has resulted from the recognition that similar prion-associated spongiform encephalopathies occur in sheep (scrapie) and cattle (bovine spongiform encephalopathy or BSE). Scrapie was in fact the first prion disorder to be described and the appearance of BSE in cattle has been blamed on the feeding of infected sheep offal to cows. If this were the case and BSE reflected trans-species infection with a common prion 'infective particle', then there is concern that humans could acquire CJD by ingestion of contaminated sheepmeat or beef. No cases of CJD from contaminated sheep meat have been described but recent evidence of a new variant form of CJD with distinctive pathological features, a rapid clinical course, and occurrence in a younger age group has raised the spectre of possible transmission of the BSE prion to humans.[11]

Cases of new variant CJD in cattle farmers have also raised concerns of other routes of transmission for those in close contact with infected animals and the inability of scientists to prove that BSE could not be transmitted to humans has lead to anxiety among the general population.[12] No scientific proof of such transmission has been obtained, but in 1987 the UK government took steps forbidding the feeding of offal to other food mammals and strict precautions were recommended in abattoirs to prevent contamination of meat with neural tissue. The description in 1996 of new variant CJD led some to believe that these measures were inadequate (although the long incubation period of the spongiform encephalopathies suggests that the prion might have been acquired before the control measures were implemented). This has led to British beef being banned from markets world-wide and the start of a cull of older animals.

Neurological infections in travellers

A large number of viruses, transmitted by mosquitoes or ticks may cause encephalitis in travellers.

Tick-borne encephalitis

This arboviral infection is transmitted to man by the bite of an infected tick. Hill walkers in Central and Eastern Europe and Scandinavia are most at risk as are campers and hikers. The greatest risk is in late spring and summer. Ticks are found in warm forest areas and where there is dense undergrowth. The illness begins after an incubation period of 1–2 weeks with an influenza-like illness lasting for a few days. After a lull of about 10 days the second phase follows in approximately 25% of individuals: this produces severe headache, fever, and encephalomyelitis, characteristically affecting the brainstem and cervical spinal cord. Death is rare. Vaccination is available and recommended for those at risk (see Chapter 15).

Japanese B encephalitis

This is is a mosquito-borne viral disease occurring in many areas throughout the Indian subcontinent, South East Asia, and the Far East. Risk is higher in rural areas where the mosquito breeds in rice fields and particularly where rice growing and pig farming coexist. Clinically apparent infections comprise only 0.2–4% of those infected, but among symptomatic individuals the disease can be severe and fatality rates of 20–50% have been reported. The disease occurs primarily among young children and the elderly. Symptoms usually begin 1–2 weeks after a bite from an infected mosquito. The illness may begin rather like influenza but then progresses with headache, neck stiffness, and coma.

The endemic areas of Asia include, during the monsoon season, the lowlands of Nepal, Bangladesh, northern India, Burma, northern Thailand, China, Taiwan, Korea, and eastern Russia; and throughout the entire year, Indonesia, Malaysia, Laos, Philippines, Sri Lanka, southern India, and Thailand, Democratic Kampuchea, and Vietnam.

An effective vaccine is available and stocks are held at some specialist centres (see Chapter 15). Travellers should also employ personal protection measures against being bitten by *Culex* mosquitoes.

Rabies

This is a severe viral encephalitis which to all intents and purposes is always fatal. Virtually all mammals can be infected but thanks to quarantine measures and vaccination of domestic pets it is absent from several countries, including the UK, Scandinavia, Australia, and Japan. Virtually all other parts of the world should be considered infected. Dogs account for about 90% of cases of human rabies in those parts of the world where dogs are not vaccinated but in areas where rabies vaccine has been widely used to control domestic animal rabies, transmission to man is by wild mammals. The species differ in various parts of the world with wolves, foxes, raccoons, skunks, and bats all important.

Travellers are most at risk of rabies in India, Africa, South America, and the Philippines. Most cases result from bites but licks of wounds or mucous membranes are also recorded as leading to rabies. Very occasional cases have occurred in cave explorers, after inhalation of aerosols of virus in bat habitats.

Clinical features

The incubation period of rabies varies from a few days to 3 months, although rare cases have occurred up to 5 years after exposure. The first symptoms are often tingling or pain at the site of inoculation, associated with non-specific malaise, fatigue, headache, and fever. Neurological features begin after a few days: they include apprehension, agitation, hyperactivity, bizarre behaviour, and hallucinations. Hydrophobia occurs in about half the patients. Most patients become paralysed and comatose before death. Even with the most expert intensive care only three people have been known to survive rabies.

Treatment

Because the management of rabies is so unsatisfactory, the correct use of post-exposure prophylaxis is vitally important. It is mandatory that a GP faced with a traveller with potential rabies exposure should obtain specific current recommendations from a centre of expertise, and follow them *to the letter.* The general principles include immediate scrubbing of the wound with soap or detergent and water, removal of foreign material (this is obviously of less importance to the GP but should be included in the advice to travellers), and consideration of active immunization with human diploid cell vaccine.

The decision whether to use this or not will depend on when and where exposure occurred, the site and severity of the bite (or lick), and the species, behaviour, and fate of the animal involved.

In the UK, expert advice regarding the need for post-exposure prophylaxis is available from departments of tropical medicine (see vaccination section for telephone numbers) and the Central Public Health Laboratory, Colindale. If used, it is given as 1 ml intramuscular (IM) injections into the deltoid region on days 0, 3, 7, 14, and 28. A single dose of human rabies immunoglobulin, half infiltrated around the wound and half given IM into the gluteal region may also be advised.

Case history

A young woman who had just returned from backpacking in India presented to her GP on Christmas Eve. She had been bitten slightly by a dog in a rural village about 7 days previously and had been advised by a friend to see a doctor on return to the UK. Fortunately, she was seen at Colindale that day, provided with supplies of human diploid cell vaccine, which was administered by the GP despite the holiday season.

Myalgic encephalomyelitis and chronic fatigue syndrome

This puzzling disorder is also known as epidemic neuromyasthenia, Iceland disease, Royal Free disease, and post-viral fatigue syndrome.[13] None of these names is strictly suitable since the condition occurs in sporadic as well as epidemic form, does not always follow a viral infection, and was described many years before the outbreaks in Iceland and the Royal Free Hospital, London. Myalgic encephalomyelitis is the term used more commonly by the media and patient self-help groups than by the scientific press, which tends to favour the term 'chronic fatigue syndrome' (CFS)[14] to describe the condition.

The term 'CFS' encompasses a clinical entity characterized by a sudden onset; followed by at least six months duration of fatigue, often exacerbated by exertion; myalgia; impaired memory and concentration; depressed mood; chronic and recurrent perception of changed body temperature; recurrent pharyngitis; adenopathy; and sleep disorders. The diagnostic criteria published by the Centers for Disease Control in the USA require the exclusion of numerous medical conditions.[15] Many sufferers date the onset of their symptoms to an acute 'flu-like' illness. Fatigue of short duration is a common accompaniment to such illnesses but recovery within a few weeks is generally the rule: in patients with CFS the symptoms persist or relapse for many months or years. Physical examination and routine blood tests are usually completely normal.

There is a continuing, and often heated debate as to the cause of the condition and opinion tends to be polarized into the 'organic disease' and the 'psychological disease' camps. Fatigue of some degree for six months or longer is a common complaint in young and middle-aged adults in UK surveys, and CFS may represent the morbid end of a statistically normal distribution of fatiguability.[16] Furthermore, such symptoms are highly correlated with emotional distress and are often attributed by the sufferer to social or psychological factors; self-declared CFS is very uncommon even among those with fatigue. There is a greater incidence of the disorder among women and in those of high socioeconomic status. The strong correlation of CFS symptoms with psychological symptoms has led to the suggestion that it is a psychological illness. Indeed, application of increasingly rigid criteria for the diagnosis of CFS (duration and severity of fatigue, percentage of time fatigued, muscle pains) strongly enhanced the association with psychological morbidity in the UK study reported by Pawlikowska *et al.* (1994).[16]

On the other hand, proponents of an organic cause of the illness point to studies showing that CFS is associated with high concentrations of antibodies to Epstein–Barr virus and human herpesvirus type 6, or those finding evidence of enteroviral or retroviral RNA within the muscles of patients with CFS. Hence, the condition earned the alternative name of 'chronic glandular fever' or 'post-viral fatigue syndrome'. Subsequently, however, these findings have not been confirmed and there is no conclusive evidence of a common causative infectious agent in CFS. A number of subtle and diffuse immunological abnormalities have been described in CFS (e.g. changes in B-and T-cell subsets, immunoglobulin subclass abnormalities, activation of CD8 cells, decreased natural killer cell and macrophage function, elevated cytokines of various types), supporting the notion that the disorder represents a chronic immunological imbalance initiated and perhaps maintained by some form of infection. This hypothesis suggests that following a trigger (a virus or other challenge to the immune system) the immune system either fails to return to its normal resting state and continues to produce the cytokines that are responsible for many of the systemic symptoms (fatigue, myalgia, etc.) associated with illnesses such as influenza, or is depressed and allows reactivation of latent viruses, which themselves than lead to cytokine release. The persistent overactivation of the immune system is then believed to affect function of the brain, particularly the hypothalamus, and to produce the associated symptoms of sleep disturbance, temperature control, and mood. However, other studies of immunological parameters have produced conflicting reports and randomized trials of immunological treatments have been disappointing.

The categories of physical and psychological illness are, of course, not mutually exclusive and the relationship between the two would be described by sociologists in terms of illness behaviour. Inappropriate illness behaviour does not indicate that there is no illness (physical or psychological) present, but merely indicates that the illness behaviour is perceived by the clinician as disproportionate to that illness. Most patients with CFS improve over time but only a small minority (6%) of a group of Australian patients followed prospectively had fully recovered after three years.[17] Immunological abnormalities and virological measures do not predict outcome; the only prognostic predictors for poor outcome in that study were a primary psychiatric diagnosis and a strong conviction that the illness represented a physical disease. Such convictions, together with psychological denial, prevents self-help and deters sufferers from dealing with their personal difficulties. The worst outcomes are reported by those who view their illness as of completely infectious aetiology and who advocate complete rest. Such attitudes are reinforced by much of the media coverage of the condition, which tends to stress a medical model of illness and stigmatizes psychological illness. A cognitive–behavioural model for the development and persistence of chronic fatigue has been proposed.[18] In this model, avoidance of activity during an acute illness is followed by (perfectly normal) fatigue upon exertion, but this produces a belief in the continuation of the original illness, further avoidance of activity, expectations of failure, decreased physiological and psychological tolerance, and feelings of helplessness and loss of control. A vicious circle is created with increasing avoidance of exercise, inactivity, and fatigue. In order to overcome this it is necessary for the patient to be provided with a sympathetic and problem-oriented approach to their illness. In patients with CFS, with evidence of a psychological disorder, immunological dysfunction and, perhaps, a 'chronic' viral infection, there may be little purpose in determining which came first. To the practising doctor the more important question is what form of therapy will be most effective.

It is an understatement to say that the treatment of CFS is disappointing. Antiviral drugs such as acyclovir and amantadine, immunoglobulin infusions, immune stimulators such as transfer factor, mismatched double-stranded RNA (ampligen), interferons, inosine pranobex and corticosteroids, magnesium injections, zinc supplements, vitamin preparations, essential fatty acids, etc., have all been tried but no specific therapy has consistently proved effective and many have been associated with serious adverse events. A large number of 'alternative' therapies have also been advocated. Some patients have been subjected to colonic lavage, gluten-free diets, total exclusion diets, and antifungal therapy, or extraction of dental fillings despite a complete lack of scientific rationale for such potentially hazardous and ineffective therapy.

The patient should be told that there is great uncertainty about the condition, that there is no threat to life and that the patient needs to take back control of his/her life—with clear-cut realistic goals. They should have an individualized behavioural programme with agreed lifestyle and exercise limits. Setting these limits is often the most difficult process for the patient; many have never had to do it before. These limits are not static, however, they will change from day to day and month to month. In addition to explanation, support, an agreed gradual increase in the exposure to exercise, and cognitive strategies,[19,20] patients also need symptom relief.

Many patients with chronic fatigue syndrome, or myalgic encephalomyelitis, do have psychiatric morbidity, and appropriate management of this would ameliorate at least some of their symptoms. The problem is that many patients with this syndrome have been convinced by media and self-help organizations that there is a clear distinction between physical and psychological illnesses and that exploration of psychological factors somehow implies that they are not genuinely ill. The use of antidepressant medications is viewed with particular distrust by many patients. In fact, however, they are one of the few therapies that appear to provide some symptomatic relief, particularly upon the sleep disorder that is associated with CFS. If it is explained that secondary depression is an almost inevitable consequence of their prolonged illness or, if they do not accept that they are clinically depressed, that the therapy is intended to correct biochemical imbalances in the hypothalamus and produce an improvement in their sleep pattern, then many will be willing to take tricyclic antidepressants with considerable improvement in their condition. Despite this, however, it is fair to say that no randomized, double-blind studies of antidepressants have been reported in patients with CFS and reassurance and understanding remain the most important aspects of therapy for those with this controversial condition.

Space-occupying lesions

Suppurative infections develop within the central nervous system in one of four situations:

(1) from an adjacent site of infection, particularly the paranasal sinuses, middle ear, or mastoids;

(2) following a traumatic or surgical wound;

(3) after haematogenous spread from a distant site; and

(4) cryptogenic, where no source of infection is ever determined.

Infection within the sinuses can readily spread into the cranial fossae. The anterior fossa forms the roof of the frontal and ethmoidal sinuses, and the sella turcica (and laterally the middle fossae) the roof of the sphenoid sinuses. Similarly, infection of the middle ear or mastoid air cells extends either anteriorly into the middle fossa or posteriorly into the posterior fossa, and hence the cerebellum or brainstem. Metastatic brain abscesses in children are frequently associated with congenital heart cyanotic disease, and in adults are often secondary to suppurative pulmonary infections.

Brain abscess

The brain parenchyma is very resistant to infection and some degree of ischaemia is probably necessary to provide a suitable environment for the development of an abscess. Although there is an extensive collateral circulation within the central nervous system, there are certain parts of the brain that are 'watershed areas'. These areas, such as the junction between the parietal, temporal, and occipital lobes, are supplied by terminal

Table 8.4 *Aetiology of a Brain Abscess*

Otitis media or mastoiditis
- *Site of abscess.* Temporal lobe or cerebellum
- *Usual bacteria.* Mixed (particularly *Bacteroides fragilis*, streptococci, and Enterobacteriaceae)

Sinusitis
- *Site of abscess.* Frontal lobe
- *Usual bacteria.* Streptococci (aerobic and anaerobic), particularly *Strep. milleri, Staph. aureus,* and *H. influenzae*

Lung infection
- *Site of abscess.* Anywhere
- *Usual bacteria.* Very mixed, often streptococci and anaerobes

Congenital heart disease
- *Site of abscess.* Anywhere
- *Usual bacteria.* Usually streptococci

Trauma or surgery
- *Site of abscess.* Anywhere
- *Usual bacteria. Staph. aureus*

Immunocompromised
- *Site of abscess.* Anywhere
- *Usual bacteria.* Fungi or *Toxoplasma gondii*

Neonatal meningitis
- *Site of abscess.* Anywhere
- *Usual bacteria. Citrobacter diversus*

---

branches of two or more arteries. Such areas are particularly likely to become ischaemic and hence sites for cerebral abscesses to develop. Inflammation begins with cerebritis, and over a period of 10–14 days the necrotic area becomes encapsulated and surrounded by further cerebritis and cerebral oedema.

The organisms most commonly isolated from brain abscesses are anaerobes, often several species mixed with aerobic bacteria, although the likely aetiology of an abscess depends to some extent on the underlying cause (Table 8.4). The predominant features of a brain abscess are due to the expanding mass and raised intracranial pressure: fever is often not striking. Headache, altered consciousness, and vomiting are present in most patients and seizures occur in about one-third. Focal neurological signs, related to the site of the abscess are found in three-quarters of cases. If brain abscess is suspected then lumbar puncture is contraindicated and a CT scan should be performed. If CT is not available, isotope brain scan is the best non-invasive technique.

Therapy of a brain abscess generally involves a combination of intravenous antibiotics and surgical therapy. Now that CT scanning allows effective monitoring of progress, surgery is often limited to aspiration of pus rather than complete excision of the abscess. Antibiotics are often started, empirically based on the likely precipitating cause: combinations of penicillin, or a third-generation cephalosporin, such as cefotaxime, with chloramphenicol or metronidazole are usually recommended. Once the responsible bacteria have been identified therapy can be tailored accordingly. Therapy should be continued for six weeks. The use of dexamethasone is controversial but other measures to control cerebral oedema and the control of seizures are important.

The prognosis of brain abscess is now quite good with mortality generally less than 10% and more than half the survivors showing no neurological sequelae.

Subdural empyema

This accounts for about one-fifth of cases of intracranial suppuration. It is more common in males and most cases occur in young adults. Sinusitis is the most common source of infection although in children it often follows meningitis, particularly that due to *H. influenzae.* The pus may remain localized in the subfrontal or parafalx region but the arachnoid and dura are not firmly attached to one another and so subdural infection usually spreads over the cerebral convexities. Thrombophlebitis of the venous sinuses and cortical veins often complicates subdural empyema, thrombosis and purulent meningitis or brain abscess may also occur.

Symptoms and signs usually develop acutely and may rapidly progress. Headache is prominent and most patients are febrile. The other symptoms reflect raised intracranial pressure, meningitis, and focal cortical damage, resulting from pressure or thrombophlebitis. Focal neurological signs are the rule and seizures are more frequent than with a brain abscess.

The diagnosis is best made by CT scanning that classically shows a extracerebral collection of reduced density. Lumbar puncture carries considerable risk. Where CT scanning is not available arteriography is probably the most useful alternative. Treatment requires a combination of surgical drainage, antibiotics, oedema-reducing agents and anticonvulsants. Antibiotic selection should be guided by the Gram-stain and culture but the likely pathogens can be empirically covered by the same combinations as for a brain abscess (see above).

Extradural abscess

This is a much less common condition, unless there is an associated brain abscess or subdural empyema. Infection outside the dura does not spread very extensively intracranially since the dura mater is firmly attached to the periosteum of the skull. A spinal epidural abscess, on the other hand, does spread since there is a fat-filled epidural space between the dura and the periosteum of the vertebrae. Major neurological signs are infrequent. Headache and signs of the primary focus of infection in the sinuses or ears may be the only features. The diagnosis is therefore often delayed but can be made by CT scanning or angiography. Once confirmed, neurosurgical intervention is necessary. Antibiotic therapy is similar to that for other forms of intracranial sepsis.

Neuritis

Inflammation of the peripheral nerves is very occasionally caused by micro-organisms directly. The best examples are leprosy and South American trypanosomiasis, which are both dealt with in Chapter 15. Lyme disease is another infection where painful radiculoneuritis occurs. The effects of infections upon peripheral nerves are, however, generally caused either by bacterial toxins (tetanus and botulism) or a result of a post-infectious demyelinating process (Guillain–Barré syndrome). Neuropathies are also associated with human immunodeficiency virus infection. The clinical features and pathogenesis of these various infectious and parainfectious phenomena are distinct and will be described separately.

Tetanus

This is caused by the potent neurotoxin produced by *Clostridium tetani*. In many parts of the world tetanus is an important and avoidable cause of death. Probably half a million people die each year from tetanus and up to 90% of these are new-born infants. The prevalence of tetanus is high in hot, moist, tropical areas such as Africa. In the UK, most parts of Europe and North America, vaccination programmes have largely eliminated the risk.

Clostridium tetani lives in the intestinal tract of man and of animals where it causes no disease. However, the bacteria produce spores which are passed in the faeces and hence are widespread in the environment. Under anaerobic conditions in contaminated wounds, tetanus bacilli germinate from the spores and produce the neurotoxin, tetanospasmin. Deep, penetrating, dirty wounds are the most likely to be responsible but other sources of tetanus are compound fractures, animal or human bites, operations, tattooing or ear piercing, and infected umbilical stumps in neonates.

The incubation period of tetanus varies from 1 day to several months but in most cases it is from 4 to 14 days. During this time tetanospasmin is produced locally and is avidly bound to neuromuscular junctions. The toxin then migrates within the axon to the central nervous system where it blocks inhibitory transmitters and causes the symptoms of tetanus.

Most tetanus is generalized and is characterized by muscular rigidity and painful muscle spasms precipitated by a variety of stimuli. These symptoms often start in the bulbar muscles with masseter spasm, causing lockjaw (trismus), and risus sardonicus. These painful spasms may involve the paraspinal muscles, causing opisthotonus, those of the extremities, or larygeal or pharyngeal muscles, producing respiratory embarrassment. Instability of temperature control and other autonomic nervous system functions also occurs.

Occasionally, purely local tetanus occurs with episodes of spasms and repetitive sustained contractions in the wounded limb, but without rapid evolution to generalized disease.

Treatment of tetanus involves surgical debridement of the wound, antibiotic therapy, neutralization of circulating toxin with human tetanus immune globulin, and sedation and supportive measures during the period of neurological and autonomic dysfunction. All patients with tetanus should be given a course of active immunization with tetanus toxoid, since the amount of toxin present in an attack of clinical tetanus is insufficient to induce immunity against re-infection.

Tetanus can be prevented by active immunization with tetanus toxoid, which is usually administered combined with either diphtheria toxoid and pertussis vaccine (as DPT) for primary immunization in childhood, or with reduced dose diphtheria toxoid (Td) for immunization of older children and adults (see Chapter 2).

Botulism

In the UK, botulism is an extremely rare form of food poisoning: it results from the production of botulinum toxin by the anaerobic bacterium *Clostridium botulinum.* Notorious small clusters of cases have occurred in recent years from the ingestion of tinned salmon and hazelnut yoghurt. Food contaminated by toxin may appear and taste normal and the toxin is so potent that even a tiny nibble of contaminated food can be life-threatening. The toxin binds to the neuromuscular junction and prevents acetylcholine release, leading to a flaccid paralysis. The symptoms begin between 12 and 36 hours after toxin ingestion with severe dryness of the mouth and dizziness and then within a few more hours with diplopia, blurred vision, dysphagia, and muscular weakness. The patient remains afebrile. Sensation is normal but the descending weakness causes bulbar or respiratory failure requiring admission to an intensive care facility. It is a condition that is almost always initially misdiagnosed unless there are other cases in the vicinity or a public health alert has been issued about a particular foodstuff.

Guillain–Barré syndrome

The Guillain–Barré syndrome (GBS) is an acute symmetrical polyradiculopathy with predominantly motor dysfunction. It characteristically follows within 4 weeks of a viral illness, but it can also follow immunization and a number of other infectious agents (e.g. *Mycoplasma* or *Campylobacter jejuni*). The cardinal feature is segmental demyelination of peripheral nerves and dorsal nerve roots which is believed to be caused by immunological sensitization to a myelin antigen.

The first symptom of GBS is often weakness of muscles, although some individuals have pain or paraesthesiae beforehand. The weakness is progressive and usually ascends proximally. Cranial nerve involvement may also occur. The paralysis is flaccid and the tendon reflexes are lost. Most patients reach the point of maximal disability within 10 days, but in some the symptoms progress for up to a month. A variety of autonomic nerve dysfunctions are common. The diagnosis of GBS can usually be made on clinical grounds. The typical feature seen in the CSF is dissociation between the protein level (which is usually elevated) and the cellular response, which is absent or minimal.

Patients with suspected GBS should be admitted to hospital. Most will benefit from plasmapheresis, especially when it is performed early in the course of the syndrome. The mortality of CBS is only about 5% and the vast majority of individuals make a full recovery; improvement from GBS can, however, be very slow, sometimes continuing for up to a year. During this time intensive support is required.

References

1. Office of Population Censuses and Surveys. *Communicable disease statistics: England and Wales* (no 15) London: HMSO (1988)

2. Sorensen H T, Neilson J O, Neilson B. Problems in diagnosing meningitis in general practice. *J Internal Med* (1990) **228**: 199

3. Jones D M, Kacsmarski E B. Meningococcal infections in England and Wales: (1991). *Communicable Disease Report* (1992) **2**: R61–3

4. Cartwright K, Reilly S, White D, Stuart J. Early treatment with parenteral penicillin in meningococcal disease. *BMJ* (1992) **305**: 143–7

5. Strand J, Pugh E. Meningococcal infections: reducing the case fatality rate by giving penicillin before admission to hospital. *BMJ* (1992) **305**: 141–3

6. Begg N. Reducing mortality from meningococcal disease. *BMJ* (1992) **305**: 133–4

7. Havens P L, Garland J S, Brook M M *et al*. Trends in mortality in children hospitalised with meningococcal infections, 1957–1987. *Ped Infect Dis J* (1989) **8**: 8–11

8. Howard A J, Dunkin K T, Millar G W. Nasopharyngeal carriage and antibiotic resistance of Haemophilus influenzae in healthy children. *Epidemiol Infect* (1988) **100**: 193–203

9. Cartwright K, Begg N, Hull D. Chemoprophylaxis for *Haemophilus influenzae* type b: Rifampicin should be given to close contacts. *BMJ* (1991) **302**: 546–7

10. Kennedy C. Acute viral encephalitis in childhood. *BMJ* **310**: 139–40

11. Will R, Zeidler J, Cousens M *et al*. A new variant of Creutzfeld–Jacob disease in the UK. *Lancet* (1996) **347**: 921–5

12. A panel of experts responds to: Creutzfeldt-Jacob disease and bovine spongiform encephalopathy: any connection? *BMJ* (1995) **311**: 1415–21

13. Jenkins R, Mowbray J F (Ed.) *Postviral fatigue syndrome.* Chichester: Wiley (1991).

14. Holmes G P, Kaplan J E, Gantz N M *et al.* Chronic fatigue syndrome: a working case definition. *Ann Intern Med* (1988) **108**: 387–9.

15. Fukada K, Straus S, Hickie I and the International Chronic Fatigue Syndrome Study group. The chronic fatigue syndrome: a comprehensive approach to its definition and study. *Ann Intern Med* (1994) **121**: 953–9

16. Pawlikowska T, Chalder T, Hirsch S R *et al.* Population based study of fatigue and psychological distress. *BMJ* (1994) **308**: 763–6.

17. Wilson A *et al.* Longitudinal study of outcome of chronic fatigue syndrome. *BMJ* (1994) **308**: 756–9

18. Wessley S, Powell R. Fatigue syndromes: a comparison of chronic 'postviral' fatigue with neuromuscular and affective disorder. *J Neurol Neurosurg Psych* (1989) **52**: 940–8

19. Wesseley S, David A, Butler S, Chalder T. Management of chronic (post-viral) fatigue syndrome. *J Roy Coll Gen Pract* (1989) **39**: 26–9

20. Sharpe M *et al.* Cognitive behaviour therapy for the chronic fatigue syndrome: a randomised controlled trial *BMJ* (1996) **312**: 22–6

CHAPTER NINE

Infections of the gastrointestinal tract

Infections of the gastrointestinal tract are common and important problems in general practice. As well as the everyday event of patients presenting with diarrhoea and vomiting, newer infections such as hepatitis-C or *Helicobacter pylori* infections require attention and increasingly, imported infections and infestations must be dealt with by the GP.

Acute gastroenteritis

Acute gastrointestinal infections are common in Britain. Figures from general practice suggest that more than 2 million individuals (of whom two-thirds are adults) visit their family doctor each year with presumed infectious diarrhoea.[1] Most GPs consider many of these infections to be viral and very few patients have microbiological investigations performed. Of those that are investigated bacterial pathogens account for more than 50% of the confirmed cases in adults. There were about 40 000 cases of gastrointestinal infection due to Campylobacter and 30 000 due to *Salmonella* species (see Fig 9.1) reported in England and Wales in 1994.[2]

Microbial diarrhoea

Diarrhoeal infections are the leading cause of childhood death worldwide and, although the major burden of these diseases is borne by the developing world,[3–5] there are still a number of deaths from diarrhoea in Britain. Those that are reported are particularly likely to occur among the children of young, socially deprived, often single, mothers. There is an important role for the primary health care team in prevention and management of these infections where the aims are to provide appropriate advice which supports self-care and to reduce inappropriate prescribing while ensuring early diagnosis of dangerous infections.

Pathogenesis

There are two pathogenic mechanisms for microbial diarrhoea and they lead to different clinical pictures. Most cases are the result of interference with the absorptive function of the small bowel villi. This can be due to the effects

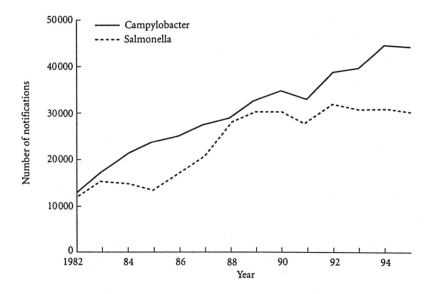

Fig 9.1 *Laboratory reports of campylobacker and salmonella in England and Wales 1982 to 1994.*

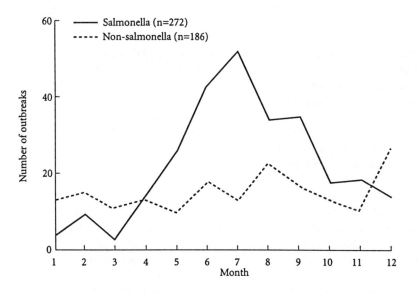

Fig 9.2 *Seasonal distribution of outbreaks of infectious intestinal disease, 1992 and 1993 (n = 458).*

Table 9.1 *Clinical features and mechanism of microbial diarrhoea*

Clinical presentation	Absorptive dysfunction	Invasion and cell damage
Fever	No	Yes
Systemic toxicity	No	Yes
Abdominal pain	Mild	Severe
Tenesmus	No	Sometimes
Stool	Watery	Small volume
Blood in stool	No	Yes
Polymorphs in stool	No	Yes

of an bacterial enterotoxin or to viral or protozoal damage to the mucosal cells. The second type of enteric infection is inflammatory and results from either invasion of the intestinal mucosa (such as occurs in *Shigella, Salmonella, Campylobacter*, and amoebic infections) or damage caused by a cytotoxin (as is seen in *Clostridium difficile* infection). The clinical pictures that result are summarized in Table 9.1.

1. Absorptive dysfunction of the small bowel villi. The classical toxins involved in infective diarrhoea are the so-called enterotoxins which bind to intestinal cells and then act on the biochemical mechanisms of the small bowel as a result of activation of the enzymes adenylate cyclase and guanylate cyclase. The result of activation of these intracellular 'second messengers' is an increase in fluid secretion by the small bowel and a loss of sodium, chloride, and bicarbonate. This presents as a severe watery diarrhoea with no morphological damage to the intestinal mucosa and no features of inflammation. There is, therefore, none of the cardinal symptoms of inflammation; no fever or systemic toxicity, little abdominal pain and no blood or polymorphs in the stool. Toxins of this type are widespread among the bacterial species that cause enteric infections, but are particularly important in *Vibrio cholerae* and the strains of *Escherichia coli* that cause much of travellers' diarrhoea.

Watery diarrhoea can also be caused by reversible damage to the small intestinal villi such as that induced by rotaviruses and *Cryptosporidium parvum*. The diarrhoea is due to both a lack of surface area for absorption (with no reduction in secretion from the intestinal crypt cells) and also to osmotic changes consequent upon impaired carbohydrate absorption.

2. Invasion and inflammation of the bowel wall. There are two ways in which invasive bacteria damage the cells of the intestinal mucosa:

(1) invasion of the mucosa, and

(2) cytotoxin-induced cell death.

These mechanisms cause ulceration and an intense acute inflammatory response in the bowel wall. There is fever and systemic toxicity, together with severe abdominal cramps. Blood, mucus, and polymorphs are found in the stool, which is usually of small volume, and oedema of the rectal mucosa causes tenesmus. Severe forms of the disease may cause acute colonic dilatation and occasionally bowel perforation.

Clinical features

Certain features in a patient's history provide important clues to the aetiology of acute gastroenteritis. The duration of illness, whether the symptoms are predominantly those of upper or lower gastrointestinal (GI) tract infection, the presence of fever and/or blood in the stools, geographical considerations, the age of the patient, and a history of travel are useful pointers to the type of infection. A history of recent antibiotic administration may suggest pseudomembranous colitis.

Certain infections need to be particularly considered in the immunocompromised host. Patients with agammaglobulinaemia or IgA deficiency are prone to chronic or recurrent infection with *Giardia lamblia*. Those with defects in cellular immunity, particularly people with AIDS, are susceptible to infections with a number of protozoan infections. Cryptosporidiosis is particularly common but *Isospora belli*, *Entamoeba histolytica*, and *Giardia* also occur more frequently and assume a prolonged and severe course. Mycobacteria, particularly *M. avium-intracellulare*, cytomegalovirus, and herpes simplex can also affect the GI tract of these patients.

Investigation, referral, and treatment

Patients with diarrhoea experience considerable morbidity with restriction of activity and time off work. Nevertheless, most adults do not consult the GP and when they do it is because of fever, restriction of activity, and the severity and duration of the diarrhoea.[6] The patient wishes to recover quickly and in addition the doctor must decide if further investigation or referral are indicated before recommending treatment. In a study of 235 adults with diarrhoea seen in general practice, frequent, bloody diarrhoea, signs of dehydration, a fever and tenderness on abdominal examination (particularly occurring in an older person) were very important in the decision to refer to hospital.[7] Of patients that were not referred to hospital, 36% had a stool specimen sent for culture of which one third were positive. The most frequently isolated pathogen was *Campylobacter jejuni*.

Oral rehydration therapy. The basic principle of treatment for acute diarrhoea is rehydration and this can almost always be achieved by the oral route. Effective oral rehydration therapy revolves around the critical physiological process of coupled transportation of sodium and glucose or other small organic molecules in the small bowel. The maximal absorption of water and electrolytes occurs when the rehydration fluid contains a ratio of carbohydrate to sodium less than about 2 or 3:1. Commercial oral rehydration fluids also contain potassium, chloride, and bicarbonate ions and have an osmolarity of 250–300. Other fluids such as fruit juices or carbonated drinks, such as cola, are unsuitable for rehydration because of their high osmolarity or an inappropriate carbohydrate to sodium ratio.

Many patients (and some doctors) believe that compounds such as kaolin, charcoal, or pectin are helpful in the management of diarrhoea—presumably on the grounds that they bind to bacterial toxins or absorb water. None of these agents have been shown to reduce either the stool weight or volume in controlled trials and their use is unjustified. Antimotility drugs, including agents containing synthetic opiates and atropine, can slow the intestinal transit time but rarely can cause paralytic ileus or toxic dilatation of the bowel in individuals with inflammatory diarrhoea. Bismuth, which acts as an antisecretory agent can reduce the severity of diarrhoeal infections but has to be given in very high dosage.

The role of stool culture and the use of antibiotics.   Empirical antibiotic therapy is not recommended for most patients with acute enteric infections. There are a number of reasons for this:

(1) until the 1990s, there was no single antimicrobial that was active against all the potential pathogens;

(2) adverse effects may result from disturbance of the normal bacterial flora of the bowel; and

(3) the emergence of resistant isolates.

On the other hand, routine collection of stool specimens and the institution of antibiotic therapy only after the aetiological agent is identified is expensive and there would be an unavoidable delay of two to three days while the cultures were processed. It seems sensible to limit the microbiological examination of stool specimens to cases of diarrhoea that have persisted for several days and to illnesses that are accompanied by fever, bloody diarrhoea or tenesmus or to those cases in which empirical antimicrobials are started. An illness that has lasted for more than week, particularly in a homosexual man or following travel abroad, should prompt the examination of a stool specimen for parasites.

For certain types of diarrhoeal infection, there is a clear benefit from early antibiotic treatment. Travellers' diarrhoea is one example (see Chapter 15).[8] Another is acute dysentery; an effective absorbable antibiotic can reduce the duration and severity of *Shigella* infection. The newer quinolone antimicrobials have *in vitro* activity against all the common bacterial pathogens that cause enteritis and recent studies have shown that empirical antibiotic therapy with a quinolone does reduce the duration of acute diarrhoea in ambulatory adults. Furthermore, these antibiotics do not cause profound changes in the normal bacterial flora of the bowel and hence overgrowth of other organisms after treatment is not a problem. From these data, a case can be made for giving empirical quinolone therapy to those patients with non-travellers' diarrhoea who are moderately or severely ill with symptoms indicative of an invasive pathogen (fever, abdominal pain, blood or pus in the stool). It is fair to say, however, that the effects of widespread implementation of such a policy in terms of cost and spread of bacterial resistance have not been comprehensively assessed. In addition, these antimicrobial agents are not recommended for use in children and growing adolescents because of their toxic effects on cartilage in young animals.

Gastroenteritis in children

Gastroenteritis is still one of the major causes of death in children in the developing world and even in Britain it is one of the ten most common causes of hospital admission in children. Viruses are now known to be the most common cause of severe diarrhoea in infants and young children, accounting for 40% or more of cases.[3] The viruses responsible are rotaviruses, adenoviruses, astroviruses, Norwalk virus, and other small, round viruses. In UK children the other pathogens are campylobacters (about 5% of specimens from children with diarrhoea contain this pathogen), *Cryptosporidium* (4%), *Salmonella* (2.5%), and *Shigella* (>1%).

Each day an infant has a fluid intake that represents 10–15% of their body weight and hence any fluid deficit resulting from vomiting and diarrhoea is of great consequence. In further contrast to adults, almost any infection in infancy can present with diarrhoea and/or vomiting. Some infections need particular consideration: urinary and respiratory tract infections, otitis media, osteomyelitis, meningitis can all present in this way.

The major danger of gastroenteritis in an infant is dehydration. The degree of this is usually described in terms of the percentage of total body weight that has been lost. If less than 5% of the body weight has been lost then the child looks well and the only clinical abnormality is dryness of the mucous membranes. Between 5% and 10% dehydration causes loss of interstitial fluid, and hence sunken eyes, loss of skin elasticity, and sunken fontanel, together with acidosis and oliguria. When dehydration increases beyond 10% of body weight there are signs of shock and circulatory failure, and the child is critically ill.

The majority of children with gastroenteritis can be managed in general practice. Oral rehydration of the infant with a mild degree of dehydration should be with a solution of the correct osmolarity and containing carbohydrate and sodium in a ratio not exceeding 2:1. There are several oral rehydration solutions available in Britain and no one formulation is better than any other. Home-made salt and sugar solutions are of extremely inaccurate and inconsistent concentration and should not be used. Neither should soft drinks which are usually hyperosmolar and low in electrolytes. Generally, feeds are withheld during the first 24 hours of illness, when vomiting and diarrhoea are at their peak, and during this time the infant should be given about 200 ml/kg body weight oral rehydration fluid. This may need to be given initially from a spoon if vomiting is severe.[9]

Most children with uncomplicated gastroenteritis can be managed at home with oral rehydration solutions. Hospital admission should be arranged for those with persistent vomiting, hypothermia, reduced consciousness, abdominal distension, and more than mild dehydration (e.g. reduced urine output). Infants from deprived social backgrounds are particularly vulnerable.

There is no harm in discontinuing bottle-feeding for 24 hours at the onset of gastroenteritis and some authors have reported that immediate modified feeding with rice or cereal does not affect the severity of the diarrhoea and may be beneficial in malnourished children.[10,11] After 24 hours, immediate reintroduction of normal full strength feeds is usually satisfactorily tolerated in infants over 6 months old.[12] In those bottle-fed infants younger than 6 months, however, and those whose symptoms relapse after reintroduction of full strength feeds, the usual infant formula or cows' milk is reintroduced gradually over 3 to 5 days. This process of regrading is done by diluting the usual feed with rehydration solution firstly to quarter strength, then to half strength, then to three-quarter strength and, finally, to full strength at intervals of 12–24 hours. There is no need for special infant formula or foods in the routine management of gastroenteritis and whole protein milks such as goats' milk or ewes' milk should never used in infants. Breast-fed babies can be fed as normal after the first 24 hours with supplementary rehydration solution as necessary. Recurrent or persistent diarrhoea and vomiting after an initial episode of gastroenteritis should be an indication for hospital referral for further investigation.

None of the drugs used in adults for symptomatic relief, such as kaolin, diphenoxylate or codeine phosphate have a place in the treatment of childhood gastroenteritis. They are unhelpful and may be dangerous in infants. Antibiotics are only needed for certain specific infections identified by stool examination.

Stool examination should be undertaken for persistent or bloody diarrhoea, symptoms following foreign travel, high fever, and investigation of an outbreak in a nursery or school.

Food poisoning

There are numerous infections that can be acquired as a result of contaminated food or drink but the term 'food poisoning' is usually reserved for those that include GI symptoms. Some forms of food poisoning are chemical (from accidental contamination or from vegetable or animal toxins) but the majority are microbiological. Food poisoning is a statutorily notifiable disease in Britain but it is considerably under-reported, probably because sporadic cases of diarrhoea or vomiting tend not to be microbiologically investigated. Reports of cases peak during the summer and most of the nearly 60 000 cases reported in England and Wales between 1986 and 1988 (this does not include diarrhoea caused by *C. jejuni*) were caused by *Salmonellae*. A high proportion of the remaining cases were due to *Clostridium perfringens*, and reported cases caused by *Staphylococcus aureus* and *Bacillus cereus* were less common. Cases due

Table 9.2 *Differentiation of food poisoning syndromes*

Short incubation period: <8 hours
Staph. aureus: 2–7 hours
   Cream-filled pastries; milk products; unrefrigerated meat; custard
Bacillus cereus: 1–5 hours
   Rice; dried foods; dairy products; herbs and spices

Medium incubation period: 8–36 hours
Salmonella: 12–36 hours
   Raw meat and poultry; eggs; unpasteurized milk
B. cereus: 8–16 hours
   Vegetables; sauces; puddings
Clostridium perfringens: 8–24 hours
   Meat and poultry
C. botulinum: 12–36 hours
   Fish and home-canned products
Vibrio parahaemolyticus: 8–24 hours
   Raw fish and shellfish
Norwalk agent: 24–48 hours
   Shellfish; food-handlers

Long incubation period: >36 hours
Campylobacter: 2–5 days
   Raw meat or poultry; milk; water
Cryptosporidiosis: 4–12 days
   Water; milk

---

to *Vibrio parahaemolyticus* are extremely rare; infection is almost always associated with eating raw fish, a habit that only the Japanese seem to practice with enthusiasm.

The types of food poisoning can be divided into those with short, medium, and long incubation periods (Table 9.2).

Short incubation period

This type of food poisoning tends to be caused by toxins. Staphylococcal food poisoning is the result of ingestion of a preformed toxin that is heat-stable and hence is not destroyed by rewarming food. Severe nausea and vomiting are the predominant symptoms, although diarrhoea also occurs. In the most severe cases the individual can become prostrate but the symptoms normally remit spontaneously within 24–48 hours. *Bacillus cereus* emetic toxin can cause an identical illness, typically seen after consumption of precooked 'fried rice' from Chinese restaurants. There has been a great increase in the number of reported cases of vomiting due to *B. cereus* in recent years in the UK.

Medium incubation period

Salmonellas are one of the main causes of food-borne illness. *Clostridium perfringens* (type A strains) produce a heat-labile toxin when they sporulate. After ingestion of heavily contaminated food, particularly meat pies prepared well in advance and then reheated, the usual symptoms are diarrhoea and severe abdominal pain: fever and vomiting are unusual. *Bacillus cereus*, in addition to the short incubation vomiting illness described above, can also cause a diarrhoeal form of food poisoning caused by a different toxin that is produced when the bacteria multiply in proteinaceous foods. Botulism is extremely rare and is a neuroparalytic illness rather than a cause of GI disease.

Long incubation period

Although campylobacter enteritis is frequently transmitted from food or drink, it is not usually regarded as a cause of food poisoning since most cases are sporadic and their source unknown.

Food-handlers and food poisoning

A question often asked is how long food-handlers need to be excluded from employment if they are excreting pathogens. There is certainly good evidence that food-handlers who are symptomatically ill present significant risk of transmission but only with *Salmonella typhi* and *S. paratyphi* is there any evidence that asymptomatic excreters present a risk. For all other pathogens there is no reason to exclude food-handlers from work once they are free of symptoms and have normal formed stools. There are, however, public concerns that need to be allayed and the Public Health Laboratory Service suggests that food-handlers whose work involves touching unwrapped foods that will be consumed without further cooking should be followed microbiologically until the pathogens have been cleared.

Viral gastroenteritis

Rotavirus

Rotaviruses are named after their resemblance to a wheel when viewed under an electron microscope. Rotavirus is responsible for about half the cases of watery diarrhoea in infants and young children worldwide. Its real incidence is in infants between 3 and 15 months old: younger babies are protected by maternal antibody. Rotavirus infections can affect the parents of infected children and outbreaks have also occurred in geriatric wards.

The peak prevalence of rotaviral infection in Britain is in the winter and early spring. The infection is very contagious with attack rates in closed communities (nurseries, etc. approaching 100% of susceptibles. The virus multiplies within the cytoplasm of the cells of the small intestine and there is villous blunting.

Clinical features

In many cases the initial symptoms are those of a respiratory tract infection with cough and runny nose. Following this there is a fever and then there is vomiting and watery diarrhoea that is free of blood. Vomiting lasts for 1–3 days and the diarrhoea may persist for 5 days or so.

Investigation and treatment

Diagnosis is fairly easy since the virus is found in large quantity in the faeces and can be readily detected by electron microscopy. A number of antigen assays are also available. Treatment is symptomatic. An oral rotaviral vaccine is under development but is not in immediate prospect.[13]

Norwalk virus

This agent is a small, round RNA virus with an amorphous surface on electron microscopy. It is the cause of many outbreaks of gastroenteritis that occur in all age groups in closed communities (cruise liners, holiday camps, etc.), or as a result of eating inadequately cooked shellfish harvested from sewage-polluted water. Person-to-person spread may occur by the airborne route (probably from aerosols generated by explosive, projectile vomiting). Over 90% of adults are seropositive with infection early in life common in the UK.[14]

Clinical features

The incubation period is 12–48 hours and then there is malaise, anorexia, abdominal cramps, and headache. Vomiting, often copious and projectile, and/or watery diarrhoea lasts for 1–2 days. Virus shedding can continue for up to 6 days even in subclinical infections.[15]

Other enteric viruses

A number of other viruses are now recognized as causing diarrhoea, particularly in childhood. They are all diagnosed from electron microscopical examination of the stools. Enteric adenoviruses (types 40 and 41) are the second most common cause of viral gastroenteritis, predominantly in children aged less than 2 years old. The illness is typically longer lasting but milder than that caused by rotaviruses and respiratory symptoms are probably rare.

Caliciviruses and astroviruses are both RNA viruses that cause non-specific watery diarrhoeal infection in preschool children.

Bacterial gastroenteritis

Campylobacter enteritis

Campylobacters are spiral Gram-negative bacteria that have been recognised as a cause of acute enterocolitis for about 15 years. They have now emerged as the most frequent cause of bacterial gastroenteritis in humans with laboratory reports in England and Wales showing an annual incidence of about 85/100 000 (the true rate is likely to be about 1100/100 000). The strain that is principally responsible is *C. jejuni* (*C. coli* also causes some infections) which is found in the gut of many animals and birds. Most human cases are transmitted via undercooked meat or poultry, and milk or water. Epidemiological studies have shown a significant correlation between handling and consuming chicken; barbecues present a special hazard because they allow easy transmission of the bacteria from raw meat to hands and other foods.[16] Milk- and water-borne infections occur in outbreaks but most cases are sporadic and occur in infants or young adults.

Clinical features

The incubation period ranges from 1 to 7 days and there may be a non-specific prodrome for a few hours before diarrhoea and vomiting start. The clinical features of infection are generally indistinguishable from those of *Salmonella* food poisoning or *Shigella* dysentery, indicating mucosal damage, although there is a tendency for the abdominal pain to be more severe and prolonged in *Campylobacter* infections. Almost all cases resolve within a week although excretion of the organism in the faeces can persist for several weeks.

Treatment

If therapy is commenced early enough, erythromycin or ciprofloxacin can shorten the duration of diarrhoea. While bacterial cure can be achieved with both of these agents the clinical benefits are less clear.[17] The emergence of resistant organisms to both quinolones and ciprofloxacin is of great concern[18] and reminds the GP that most patients should be encouraged to weather the infection with rest and oral rehydration with antibiotics reserved for proven and severe cases. Septicaemia is rare and complications infrequent: reactive arthritis (as with all forms of infective colitis) and the Guillain–Barré syndrome (GBS) are exceptions that may occur a week or two later and some patients endure unnecessary surgery for appendicitis. A strong association between *C. jejuni* infection and GBS has emerged in the literature in the 1990s although the mechanism is not yet understood.[19]

Shigellosis (bacillary dysentery)

There are four species of *Shigella* (*Sh. sonnei*, *S. flexneri*, *Sh. boydii*, and *Sh. dysenteriae*). The infective dose is very small and infection is usually spread from person-to-person by faecal contamination of hands in crowded communities and institutions with poor hygiene.[20] Houseflies are mechanical vectors for *Shigella* organisms.

Clinical features

The bacteria multiply throughout the bowel and invade the epithelium particularly that of the colon. There are features of systemic toxicity and in young children febrile convulsions may occur. The mucosa is ulcerated and bleeding but infection does not usually involve the entire thickness of the bowel wall and septicaemia is very rare.

The severity of the disease is very variable: *Sh. sonnei* infection is generally very mild and settles within a few days, *Sh. flexneri* and *Sh. boydii* cause moderately severe illnesses lasting for a week or 10 days, and *Sh. dysenteriae* causes epidemics of dysentery with an appreciable mortality.

Organisms may be excreted in the bowel for a few weeks after recovery.

Treatment

Treatment for confirmed cases is with well-absorbed oral antibiotics to which the organism is sensitive *in vitro*. Appropriate therapy shortens the duration and reduces the severity of the illness. Treatment can also be used to eradicate the organisms from the bowel in order to minimize the potential for spread of infection in conditions of poor hygiene. Resistance is now very commonly seen to ampicillin and tetracyclines and quinolones are probably the best first-line agents in adults. Antimotility agents should not be used as they prolong the illness.

Salmonellosis

There are more than 2000 different strains of *Salmonella*, Gram-negative bacteria that are ubiquitous intestinal parasites of most domestic and wild animals. Most are strains of *S. enteritidis* that cause a self-limited enterocolitis after accidental transmission to man, usually as a result of poor food hygiene. The bacteria are killed by adequate cooking so that *Salmonella* infection often results from inadequate cooking of animal products containing salmonellas, or follows cross-contamination (during animal slaughter or food preparation by food-handlers) of foods that are to be eaten without further cooking. The infective dose of salmonellas is quite high so that there is usually a need for the contaminated food to be held for a period at a temperature suitable for the multiplication of salmonellas prior to it being eaten. Poultry and egg products account for the majority of cases of salmonellosis in man and the number of cases has grown steadily with the increased consumption of frozen poultry. There has also been a significant epidemic of infection in Britain in recent years caused by a particular strain of *S. enteritidis* that is able to spread trans-ovarially in chickens and is hence present within egg yolks. One raw, infected egg is capable of contaminating large batches of mayonnaise or similar uncooked egg-based products.

The increased frequency of *Salmonella* infections has had a significant impact. In a UK study of 1482, cases time lost from work averaged 13 days, the cost to individual families was estimated at £70, and to the health care system £280 per case, including the costs of investigation.[21]

Clinical features

Symptomatic infection with salmonellas usually causes diarrhoea, abdominal pain, fever, nausea, and vomiting usually starting between 12 and 36 hours after infection. Generally, these symptoms settle within 4 or 5 days although in a significant number of individuals the organism continues to be asymptomatically excreted in the stools for several months. Illness is more severe in very young or elderly persons and septicaemia is not uncommon in these groups. It is also a particular problem in individuals with AIDS, in whom recurrences of septicaemia are likely to occur. These illnesses are similar to typhoid (see below). Following blood-borne spread the salmonellas may cause focal infections including osteomyelitis, meningitis, and abscesses.

Treatment

Antibiotic therapy has traditionally not been used in *Salmonella* enterocolitis, since it has not influenced the acute illness and may have prolonged the period of chronic carriage of salmonellae. This was probably related to the relative inability of the older antibiotics to penetrate to the intracellular sites of bacterial replication. The quinolone antibiotics do penetrate readily into cells and recent data suggest that these drugs are beneficial in treating *S. enterocolitis* and do not lead to increased carriage (indeed they may reduce the frequency of chronic carriage).

Typhoid

Salmonella typhi is different from other salmonellae in that it is an exclusively human pathogen. It causes typhoid fever, which is not really a diarrhoeal infection but presents as enteric fever. It is therefore described elsewhere (see generalized infections). An effective oral vaccine composed of a live-attenuated strain of *S. typhi* is now available and is free of many of the systemic side-effects that are seen with the parenteral vaccine.

Antibiotic-associated colitis: Clostridium difficile[22]

Antibiotic-associated colitis (AAC) has been associated with almost all antibiotics and in about 90% of instances is due to a cytotoxin produced by *C. difficile*. In the more severe cases there is formation of a pseudomembrane over the colonic mucosa. *Clostridium difficile* is a sporing Gram-positive rod that is found in the stools of 30% or so of adults not receiving antibiotics. Damage to mucosa is associated with the presence of a cytotoxin (toxin B) and an enterotoxin which are produced in increased amounts when antibiotics are administered.

Clinical features

Antibiotic-associated diarrhoea (AAD) typically starts 4–10 days after commencement of antibiotic administration with the sudden onset of watery, foul-smelling, green, non-bloody diarrhoea, associated with abdominal cramps, leucocytosis, and fever. If the antibiotic is stopped then the illness usually settles within a week. More severe cases, and particularly those that first start after antibiotic therapy has been stopped, have mucosal oedema and necrosis, a polymorph infiltrate, and a pseudomembrane comprising yellowish plaques of debris and exudate over the colonic mucosa. Toxic megacolon and perforation may occur.

The diagnosis is made by culture of the organism and cytotoxin assay from the stools. Sigmoidoscopy or colonoscopy may show the pseudomembrane.

Treatment

These patients can become very ill and if the GP suspects AAD it is wise to discuss the patient with a specialist colleague. Although most cases have been reported in hospital patients there are certain to be occurrences in practice as the same antibiotics are used in the community setting, and indeed a few cases have been reported.[23] Specific treatment is needed for the more severe cases and the treatment of choice is oral vancomycin 125 mg, 4 times a day for 7–14 days: this gives an initial cure rate of more than 90%. Metronidazole 500 mg orally, three times a day, seems to be equally effective and is less expensive: however, metronidazole itself has sometimes caused AAD. Relapses are not infrequent—possibly due to sporolation and persistence of the bacteria throughout therapy—and these should be treated with oral vancomycin.

Yersinia infections

Most human infection with the zoonotic pathogens *Yersinia enterocolitica* and *Y. pseudotuberculosis* follow ingestion of contaminated food (particularly undercooked pork), water, and milk.

Clinical features

The incubation period is a few days. In young children, the illness is an enterocolitis lasting for 1–2 weeks, whereas in older persons there is terminal ileitis and mesenteric adenitis with symptoms similar to acute appendicitis. Erythema nodosum may occur. Bacteraemia and focal abscesses may complicate the illness in adults. Enterocolitis does not require antibiotic therapy, settling spontaneously in 1–2 weeks.

Protozoal gastroenteritis

Giardiasis

Giardia lamblia is a major cause of diarrhoeal infection in the world and is acquired from faecally contaminated water (the cysts can survive chlorination of drinking water). In the UK, infection is particularly common among children in daycare and homosexual men. Following ingestion of viable cysts the trophozoites adhere to the mucosa of the small bowel and after an incubation period of 1–3 weeks may produce illness. Asymptomatic infection is very common but a minority of persons develop chronic diarrhoea, flatulence, bloating, and malabsorption. Several stools should be sent for microscopical examination if the diagnosis of giardiasis is suspected and even after three specimens the detection rate is not 100%; duodenal aspiration or biopsy may be needed.

Therapy for giardiasis is with metronidazole.

Cryptosporidiosis

This protozoan infection is now known to be a relatively common cause of transient watery diarrhoea, especially in young children and visitors to countries with water supplies contaminated from animal sources (*Cryptosporidium parvum* is a zoonosis of many domestic and wild mammals). In a study of 62 421 patients in England and Wales with presumed acute infectious diarrhoea 4 775 (2%) were excreting cryptosporidia with the highest positivity rate (5%) in children aged 1–4 years.[24] It is also a major cause of progressive relentless watery diarrhoea in persons with AIDS. Diagnosis is made by visualization of the cysts in the stool but, unfortunately, there is still no effective therapy for this infection.

Gastrointestinal infections from outside the UK

Cholera[25]

Although cholera has been known in Asia since ancient times, pandemic spread to Europe and other parts of the world first occurred at the beginning of the nineteenth century. The geographical distribution of the disease has waxed and waned at intervals over the past 200 years. At the moment, the seventh recorded pandemic of modern times is in progress and has recently spread to cause large numbers of cases in South America.

Vibrio cholerae is a comma-shaped Gram-negative organism that only infects man. As the classical studies of John Snow demonstrated in the streets of London's Soho in the middle of the last century, the disease is primarily spread via contaminated water supplies. Spread by contaminated food and by the direct faecal-oral route also occur.

After negotiating the gastric acidity the cholera vibrios attach themselves to (but do not invade) the small intestinal mucosa and secrete cholera toxin. Cholera toxin binds to specific receptors on the cell surface and then activate adenylate cyclase leading to increased concentrations of cyclic-AMP. This results in an failure of absorption of sodium and water and increased secretion of chloride.

Clinical features and treatment

The massive increase in secretions from the small intestine as a result of cholera leads to large volume watery diarrhoea (rice water stool) and hence dehydration. If the dehydration becomes severe (and the patient with cholera can lose 10–20 litres of stool daily) then hypovolaemia, shock, renal failure, acidosis, and ultimately intracellular dehydration and death follow.

Rehydration is the mainstay of treatment of cholera. This can be achieved by intravenous administration but this is not usually necessary. In order to absorb sodium (and hence water) from oral rehydration solutions, glucose must be added. The glucose absorptive mechanism is not inhibited by cholera toxin and one molecule of sodium is absorbed for each molecule of glucose. An antibiotic such as tetracycline will deal with the vibrios but the toxin bound to the small bowel cells cannot be displaced and must await the natural death of these cells after a few days.

Other vibrios

Other water-borne vibrios can cause diarrhoea. The most important species is *Vibrio parahaemolyticus*. This organism is found in coastal waters and infection usually results from ingestion of inadequately cooked shellfish. It is a particularly troublesome cause of diarrhoea in Japan and outbreaks have occurred on the west coast of the USA and on cruise ships in the Caribbean. The organism produces an enterotoxin but also invades the bowel wall causing inflammation.

The incubation period is less than 24 hours and there is a sudden onset of watery diarrhoea and abdominal pain. Fever and chills can also occur. No specific therapy is normally required.

Enterotoxin-producing Escherichia coli

Enterotoxigenic *E. coli* (ETEC) are responsible for at least 50% of cases of travellers' diarrhoea but are uncommon causes of diarrhoea in industrialized countries. ETEC adhere to the mucosa of the small bowel and produce two distinct enterotoxins. One of these acts by activating adenylate cyclase (similar to cholera toxin) and the other by stimulating guanylate cyclase, and hence producing increased intracellular concentrations of cyclic guanosine monophosphate (cGMP). The result is the same: increased secretion of sodium and water.

Clinical features and treatment

The organisms are spread via faecally polluted food or water and the incubation period is from 12 to 72 hours. The illness consists of watery diarrhoea with some abdominal cramps and nausea but little or no fever. The illness is generally not severe and lasts for a few days only.

It is not easy to distinguish ETEC from other *E. coli* cultured from the stool: specialized techniques utilizing DNA probes are available in research laboratories.

Often, adequate intake of a glucose-containing oral rehydration solution is all the treatment that is needed. The more severe cases should be given antibiotic therapy and since antibiotic resistance is very common in many parts of the world, a quinolone is probably the best available choice.

Haemolytic–uraemic syndrome

Enterohaemorrhagic *E. coli* (EHEC), often the O157 strain, adhere to the mucosa of the distal ileum and proximal colon and produce a powerful cytotoxin similar to that originally described in strains of *Shigella dysenteriae* (the shiga toxin or vero toxin). These organisms produce a broad spectrum of disease—mild diarrhoea, acute haemorrhagic, colitis and the distinctive clinical picture termed the haemolytic–uraemic syndrome. The incubation period is longer than one week and then there is severe abdominal pain, abdominal distension, and tenderness associated with diarrhoea that may contain blood. The mucosa is oedematous and friable with haemorrhages and ulceration and this may be mistaken for ischaemic or ulcerative colitis. In about 10% of cases systemically absorbed toxin damages endothelium. This causes fibrin deposition and intravascular haemolysis, which in turn leads to deteriorating renal function and the haemolytic–uraemic syndrome. One large study of children with the syndrome demonstrated evidence of *E. coli* O157 infection in 86% of cases.[26] There is some evidence that these infections are associated with the consumption of poorly cooked beef (particularly hamburgers) but person-to-person spread also occurs.

Amoebiasis

Entamoeba histolytica lives in the wall and lumen of the human colon, particularly the ascending colon. As the faeces become more solid the vegetative forms encyst and the cysts are passed in the stool. The cyst is transmitted to a fresh host via contaminated water or vegetables (or occasionally by direct faecal–oral spread), and active trophozoites develop in the colon. Incidence of infection is very high in many areas of the world. In the UK it is particularly common in immigrants, homosexual men, and those in long-stay institutions.

Clinical features

Asymptomatic infection is common and even those with illness generally only have mild, chronic, intermittent diarrhoea, and abdominal pain. Severe infections, which may be precipitated by concomitant bacterial enteritis, produce dysenteric symptoms (which are often less florid than those in bacillary dysentery). Spread of infection to the liver may occur (see below).

Amoebiasis is diagnosed by finding cysts or trophozoites in the stools or in rectal mucus obtained at sigmoidoscopy. In those with asymptomatic cyst excretion the serological tests are often negative but the indirect fluorescent antibody test is positive in almost all cases of amoebic dysentery. Invasive colitis can be treated with metronidazole followed by diloxanide furoate to eradicate cysts. Diloxanide and tetracycline will cure asymptomatic intraluminal infections.

Tropical sprue

This inflammatory disease of the small bowel is probably caused by chronic contamination by toxigenic coliform bacteria following an initial episode of acute bacterial enteritis. It occurs in those who have lived in certain areas of the tropics for a year or two and produces chronic diarrhoea, abdominal distension, and folate malabsorption. Small bowel biopsy shows partial villous atrophy. Treatment is with tetracycline and folic acid.

Enterobiasis (threadworms)

Enterobius vermicularis, the common threadworm or pinworm, is the only helminth commonly found in the UK in those who have never been abroad. It is especially prevalent among children aged 5–10 years old in all socioeconomic classes. It has been estimated that up to a quarter of all primary schoolchildren may be infected. The adult worms live in the colon and the females migrate at night to lay eggs upon the perianal skin. The eggs are then transferred on fingers to the mouth to auto-infect the host or to transmit the infection to others. Adult threadworms do not proliferate in the large bowel and live only for six weeks. For the infection to continue the ova must be swallowed and exposed to the action of the digestive juices of the upper GI tract. Transmission is very common within families, especially to those who handle clothing or bedding of infected children.

Clinical features and treatment

The only symptom of threadworms is intense perianal itching, particularly at night. This can cause self-induced trauma to the skin and occasionally a vulvovaginitis if the adult worms migrate to the vagina of young girls. The adult worms can sometimes be seen in the stools and the diagnosis can be confirmed by applying clear adhesive tape to the perianal region and then examining the tape microscopically for adherent eggs. Treatment should be administered to the entire family. A single dose of mebendazole, pyrantel pamoate or piperazine, repeated 2 weeks later is effective.

Threadworm infections can be very upsetting to parents and clear information tactfully presented is necessary to prevent re-infection. Good personal hygiene, morning bathing if possible, and handwashing before eating are all important; understanding of the difficulties when small children are involved is essential.

Imported helminth infestations

Helminth infestations are extremely common in many areas of the tropics and subtropics and patients occasionally present in UK general practice.

Case history

A young Nigerian woman student attended with her 2-year-old son. She produced a jam-jar containing two 5-inch worms which she said the child had vomited up an hour before. The GP recognized *Ascaris lumbricoides* from textbook photographs seen when a student.

Most infestations are asymptomatic and cases are usually diagnosed accidentally when ova are seen in a stool specimen sent for investigation of diarrhoea of some other aetiology or when the passage of the whole or part of an adult worm causes the patient to seek advice (Table 9.3).

Ascariasis

Infection with *Ascaris lumbricoides* is the most common helminthic infection and is distributed world-wide, particularly in tropical countries. The adults live in the distal small intestine and the eggs are excreted in the faeces and develop in soil. After ingestion the larvae hatch in the jejunum, penetrate the bowel wall, and then migrate via the circulation to the lungs. From the alveoli the larvae ascend the trachea and are swallowed to complete

Table 9.3 *Helminth infections of humans*

Ascaris lumbricoides
- Roundworm eggs from soil; abdominal discomfort; rarely cause intestinal obstruction

Ancylostoma duodenale, Necator americanus
- Hookworm larvae in soil penetrate skin; anaemia; iron therapy needed

Enterobius vermicularis
- Threadworm eggs in environment; auto-infection; peri-anal itching; need to treat whole family

Trichuris trichiura
- Whipworm eggs in soil; abdominal discomfort; may cause bloody diarrhoea

Taenia solium, T. saginata
- Pork and beef tapeworms; cysts in meat; no symptoms; pork tapeworm may lead to cysticerscosis

Hymenolepis nana
- Dwarf tapeworm; auto-infection; eggs in faeces, abdominal discomfort

Diphyllobothrium latum
- Fish tapeworm from freshwater fish; no symptoms; Vitamin B_{12} deficiency rare

their development into adults. Infections are usually asymptomatic but large numbers of adult worms can interfere with small bowel absorption and a mass of worms can also cause intestinal or biliary obstruction. Large numbers of larvae migrating through the lungs can produce an allergic pneumonitis (Loeffler's syndrome).

Trichuriasis

Trichuris trichiura (whipworm) is a very common infection in tropical countries with poor sanitation. The adults live in the caecum and colon and the eggs are excreted into the faeces and thence reach moist soil where they develop further. Infective eggs are ingested by another human host and develop into adults in the large bowel. Most infections are asymptomatic but heavy infections can cause mucosal damage and bloody diarrhoea. Rectal prolapse occasionally results from very heavy infections.

Hookworms

Infection with one or other of the two species of human hookworm affects more than 25% of the world's population. The adults have specialized mouthparts by which they attach to the mucosa of the small bowel and ingest blood: heavy infections eventually lead to iron-deficiency anaemia. The eggs develop into larvae in the soil and these larvae live in the surface of the soil and are capable of penetrating intact human skin. Infection results from walking barefoot or working by hand in the soil. After penetration of the skin the larvae migrate through the circulation and lungs in a similar fashion to those of roundworms and pass to the small bowel.

The symptoms of hookworm infection correspond to the life cycle: intense pruritus (ground itch) can persist for 2 weeks after penetration of the skin, Loeffler's syndrome may accompany larval migration, and a variety of acute abdominal symptoms may follow initial infection. Chronic infection leads to iron-deficiency anaemia.

Tapeworms

These have both definitive hosts, in which the adult worms inhabit the bowel, and intermediate hosts, which harbour the larval forms. Humans are the definitive host for four tapeworms:

- *Taenia saginata* (beef tapeworm)
- *Taenia solium* (pork tapeworm)
- *Diphyllobothrium latum* (fish tapeworm)
- *Hymenolepis nana* (dwarf tapeworm)

Taeniasis is acquired by eating undercooked beef (*T. saginata*) or pork (*T. solium*) which harbours the encysted larvae. The adults are 2–12 metres in length. The head or scolex has four suckers by which they attach to the small intestine and the terminal segments or proglottides contain eggs which are shed in the faeces and are eaten by cattle or pigs, which serve as intermediate hosts. The pork tapeworm is particularly dangerous to man in that the eggs, after ingestion via the faecal–oral route, can develop into larvae and encyst, producing mass lesions in almost any part of the body (cysticercosis).

Diphyllobothrium latum requires three hosts. The intermediate hosts are freshwater crustaceans and fish, and human infection is acquired from eating raw or lightly pickled fish. Few symptoms result from infection although the adult worm competes with the host for vitamin B_{12}, and megaloblastic anaemia can occur. *Hymenolepis nana* is the smallest tapeworm to infect man, the adult being only 1–2 inches long. It also differs from other tapeworms in that no intermediate host is required and infection can pass directly from human to human. Few symptoms result.

Tapeworms are diagnosed by finding proglottides (segments of the adult worm) or ova in the faeces.

All the helminth infections shown in Table 9.3 can be treated successfully with a limited number of drugs. Mebendazole given twice daily for 3 days is effective for whipworm, hookworm and roundworm infestations, and as a single dose (repeated 2–3 weeks later) is a suitable treatment for threadworms. Piperazine given as two doses 14 days apart is also suitable for threadworms. The repeat dose is necessary to kill adults that may have developed from ova already in the bowel at the time of the first dose.

Expert advice should be sought before treating tapeworm infestations.

Strongyloidiasis

Strongyloides stercoralis is widely distributed in tropical countries. The adult female worms live in the mucosa of the duodenum and upper small intestine and produce larvae which burrow into the lumen. They are excreted in the faeces and may then develop into free-living adults or into filariform larvae which are able to re-infect humans by penetrating skin. The larvae travel throughout the venous system to the lungs, are coughed up and swallowed into the bowel, where they develop into further adults. Strongyloidiasis can also cause repeated auto-infections, since filariform larvae may develop within the lumen of the bowel, and hence infection can persist for decades after leaving an endemic area. These infections are still being seen in those who were Far East prisoners of war who worked on the infamous Burma–Thailand railway. Infections are often asymptomatic but can cause colicky epigastric pain similar to that of a peptic ulcer, diarrhoea, nausea, and weight loss. There is usually an eosinophilia. Severe bowel symptoms with malabsorption and sometimes disseminated disease can occur in the immunocompromised patient. As the larvae migrate through the body they can produce a characteristic, rapidly elongating (about 1–2 cm/hour) pruritic skin rash. This settles after a day or so, only to reappear elsewhere at intervals. An eosinophilic pneumonitis can develop as the larvae migrate through the lungs. Strongyloides infections can be diagnosed by finding larvae in the faeces or duodenal fluid or by serological tests for antibodies. Immigrants and others in whom infection is possible need to be carefully screened prior to organ transplantation or other forms of immunosuppression.

Oesophageal infections

Infections of the oesophagus are most unusual in immunocompetent individuals. In persons with defective immunity, however, infections caused by *Candida* species and herpes simplex virus are not unusual. This is particularly true of patients with leukaemia, lymphoma, or human immunodeficiency virus (HIV) infection.

Candida

Candida oesophagitis usually occurs in conjunction with severe oropharyngeal candidiasis (thrush), although sometimes patients do not have oral lesions. Oesophageal infection causes discomfort and difficulty in swallowing and sometimes retrosternal chest pain.

Most patients with this syndrome will already be under specialist supervision but those who are not need referral to hospital for a definitive diagnosis. This usually involves an endoscopic evaluation when oesophageal ulceration and the white plaques typical of candidosis can be seen extending the length of the oesophagus (and sometimes into the stomach and small intestine). Microbacterial or histological examination of biopsy specimens confirms the diagnosis.

Therapy with oral nystatin or amphotericin lozenges usually leads to relief of symptoms but the more severe infections or those that relapse should be treated with oral fluconazole or itraconazole. In patients with candidiasis associated with HIV infection permanent eradication of the organism is impossible; the best that can be offered is suppressive therapy.

Herpes simplex

Oesophagitis caused by herpes simplex virus is also seen almost exclusively in patients with defects of cellular immunity, whether as a result of malignancy, immunosuppressive therapy, or HIV infection. The symptoms are those of any oesophagitis and the diagnosis is made from biopsies taken during endoscopy. Acyclovir given intravenously is very effective in the treatment of this infection.

Gastritis

There is now convincing evidence that a bacterium termed *Helicobacter pylori* (formally *Campylobacter pylori*) is an aetiological agent in acute gastritis and chronic antral, type B ('idiopathic'), gastritis, duodenal, and gastric ulcers. An association with gastric carcinoma has also emerged.[27] The bacteria, which are curved Gram-negative rods, live in the mucous layer on the surface of the gastric epithelium and do not invade the mucosa. Although they are susceptible to acid, their ability to survive in the acid gastric environment probably relates to their production of an urease enzyme which catalyses the hydrolysis of urea to ammonia; this then neutralizes the gastric acidity.

The diagnosis of *H. pylori* infection is made by one of a number of methods; either by direct visualization or isolation of the organism from biopsy specimens, determination of serum antibodies, or by demonstration of urease activity. The latter is the basis of a rapid test on biopsy specimens and also a breath test with [^{14}C]-labelled urea; the patient ingests this and if *H. pylori* are present radiolabelled CO_2 is released by the urease and is detected in the exhaled breath.

The prevalence of *H. pylori* in asymptomatic individuals is less than 10% in those under 30 years but more than 50% in the over-60s. The prevalence is almost 100% in those with duodenal ulcer and about 80% in those with gastric ulcers. Transmission is probably from person-to-person and is associated with childhood overcrowding and poverty.[28,29] The incidence of acquisition is about 1% annually. The evidence that *H. pylori* is the primary pathogen in gastritis is not just epidemiological: there is a clear relationship between eradication of the organism and resolution of the symptoms.[30,31] Although there is a strong association between antral gastritis and duodenal ulcer, quite how infection with *H. pylori* predisposes certain infected individuals to develop duodenal ulcers is not clear. Whatever the pathogenesis the data now suggest that eradication of the organism will lead to prolonged cures of duodenal ulcer disease. There is no convincing evidence of an association for *H. pylori* infection with non-ulcer dyspepsia. The role of the organism as a factor in gastric carcinomas is the focus of considerable research.

Triple or double therapy for H. pylori-*associated duodenal ulcer disease*

The eradication of *H. pylori* from the stomach requires combination therapy but the ideal treatment is not yet clear. Triple therapy with bismuth salts, tetracycline and metronidazole for 2 weeks or omeprazole, amoxycillin (or clarithromycin) and metronidazole for 1 week is probably the first choice. Dual therapy (omeprazole and amoxycillin or clarithromycin) has less certain results.[32] Side-effects associated with broad spectrum antibiotic therapy may occur. Following eradication of the bacteria the symptoms and histological abnormalities of gastritis improve. Therapy results in a marked decrease in relapse of peptic ulcer disease.

A practice clinical meeting

Implications for general practice of the role of H. pylori *in peptic ulcer disease.*

A recent US National Institutes of Health consensus conference[32] came to several important conclusions:

1. Patients with peptic ulcers and *H. pylori* infection require antimicrobial

therapy in addition to other drugs at their first presentation or on recurrence.

2. The value of treating non-ulcer dyspepsia patients which *H. pylori* infections is not yet determined.

3. The association between *H. pylori* and gastric cancers requires further exploration.

The issue for the GP is to create a practice policy that reflects evidence-based practice but that is cost effective.[33]

Considerable costs are added if all patients under 45 years with dyspepsia and *H. pylori* infection require endoscopy to establish peptic ulcer disease before antimicrobial therapy is started. If, however, the possibility of preventing gastric cancer is added into the discussion how does that change priorities? This debate would be a good basis for a practice clinical meeting.

The liver

Hepatitis

Acute viral hepatitis is a common infectious disease characterized by liver inflammation and necrosis. There are a large number of different viruses that are known to cause hepatitis as part of a more generalized illness but there are five viruses that cause hepatitis as their major manifestation after infection. These are: (1) hepatitis A virus (HAV); (2) hepatitis B virus (HBV); (3) hepatitis C; (4) delta virus; and (5) hepatitis E. These five agents cause the vast majority of cases of acute hepatitis seen in the world but there are undoubtedly other viruses waiting to be discovered.

All five forms of acute hepatitis are very similar clinically but their epidemiology and incubation periods and the viruses that cause them are very different.

Clinical features

The icteric case of acute viral hepatitis is a very characteristic illness and should rarely present any difficulty in diagnosis. Most patients can date the onset of their illness quite well. The initial symptoms are usually non-specific malaise and anorexia followed soon after by nausea, vomiting, and right upper quadrant pain. This pain usually takes the form of a dull aching discomfort. A minority of patients have fever and headache at this stage and describe their symptoms as influenza-like. These non-specific symptoms last for a few days and then the patient, or one of his relatives, notices that he is jaundiced. The urine becomes dark. As the jaundice appears most patients feel better with return of their appetite for food (and cigarettes if they are a smoker), and loss of nausea. The jaundice lasts for 1–3 weeks on average and with clearance of the jaundice the lingering malaise also resolves. It is worth remembering that, in fact, most cases of acute viral hepatitis are non-icteric or even totally asymptomatic and it is only about 30% of cases overall that fit well into the description given above.

The patient with hepatitis is, by the time medical advice is sought, afebrile and does not appear very ill. There is a variable degree of scleral icterus and often little else to find. The liver may be enlarged and somewhat tender and in a small number of cases there is also splenomegaly. Otherwise, examination is usually unhelpful. A tiny minority of patients with acute hepatitis will develop fulminant infection due to massive hepatic necrosis: such patients will have the signs of hepatic encephalopathy (flapping tremor, mental changes, and a sweet-smelling foetor).

The most dramatic biochemical abnormality in acute hepatitis is elevation of the aminotransferase enzymes (AST or ALT) and very much less marked elevation of alkaline phosphatase and lactic dehydrogenase levels. The only other conditions that cause a similar pattern of laboratory abnormalities are hepatitis caused by anoxia or non-specific injury (shock), toxins (alcohol), or hepatotoxic drugs (paracetamol; isoniazid). These non-viral causes can usually be ruled out by a careful history and some straightforward laboratory investigations. Distinguishing each of the five viral causes of hepatitis depends upon certain epidemiological features together with some specific serological tests (see below).

Treatment

There is no specific therapy for acute viral hepatitis. Most patients do not require hospitalization: those who do are those who have no one to care for them at home, those with persistent vomiting, and those with evidence of hepatic failure. Most patients with icteric hepatitis should be advised to take things easy during the acute phase; this does not mean that they should be put on strict bed rest—although there are some who will feel so rotten that they will not want to be up and about during the early illness. Once the symptoms have improved there is no evidence that exercise affects the speed of recovery or predisposes to chronic liver disease (Table 9.4).

There is little evidence that any specific dietary limitations should be advocated during hepatitis. Most patients will not wish to eat much fat but if they do it will not affect the speed of recovery. Medications are best avoided altogether while the liver is inflamed, but some patients will ask

Table 9.4 *Advice for patients with viral hepatitis*

- *Rest*: only while symptomatic
- *Exercise*: normal when symptoms resolved
- *Diet*: unrestricted
- *Medications*: contraindicated
- *Alcohol*: prohibited during the acute phase only
- *Hospital admission*: for intractable vomiting or signs of liver failure

for symptomatic therapy for severe pain, nausea, or insomnia. Sedatives and hypnotics should be discouraged; paracetamol is probably the least hazardous of the analgesics and any anti-emetic other than chlorpromazine can be given in a small dosage.

Alcohol only needs to be prohibited during the acute phase: total abstinence for six months or even one year does not influence the risk of relapses and is unnecessarily harsh advice.

Patients should be informed about the mode of spread of their form of hepatitis and should be asked to pay particularly attention to careful hand-washing and personal hygiene for the period of infectivity. The prolonged cholestatic illness that can occur after acute viral hepatitis (particularly with HAV infection) is accompanied by fatigue and pruritus. These symptoms can be helped by a course of corticosteroids but this should only be undertaken once this form of hepatitis has been confirmed. Giving steroids to those with hepatitis B or C virus still in their liver could increase the risk of further liver damage.

Hepatitis-A

Infection with hepatitis A (formally infectious hepatitis) occurs world-wide. The causative agent is an enterovirus which is present in the faeces during the late incubation period and first few days of the acute illness. There is no animal reservoir and HAV is spread predominantly by the faecal-oral route. It is highly contagious and patients are most infectious during the late incubation period. Most cases occur in young children, those living in crowded settings, homosexual men and those who travel to countries where housing and sanitation are inadequate.

Clinical features

The incubation period of HAV is 2–6 weeks. Almost 90% of cases of hepatitis A are asymptomatic and those who become ill usually have an acute self-limiting disease. It often begins suddenly and the time course of the illness is relatively short. In some patients there is a relapsing course of acute hepatitis and, although chronic hepatitis is not caused by HAV, a cholestatic phase lasting for several months is not uncommon. During this phase there is prolonged jaundice, dark urine and pale stools, an elevated alkaline phosphatase level and no evidence of dilated bile ducts on abdominal ultrasound.

Infection with HAV is followed by lifelong immunity to reinfection. IgM antibodies to HAV (anti-HAV) appear in the serum during acute infection and persist for few months. Specific IgG antibodies appear during early convalescence and persist for life. The easiest way of diagnosing hepatitis A is detection of the specific IgM antibodies.

Normal human immunoglobulin can provide effective pre- or post-exposure prophylaxis against hepatitis A. After exposure, a single intramuscular injection of 0.02 ml/kg body weight given within the first 2 weeks of the incubation period will reduce the risk of clinical hepatitis A by about 90%. It is widely given to household contacts of hepatitis A in some countries but this is not the practice in the UK. Prevention of hepatitis A in travellers has been dealt with elsewhere (Chapter 15).

Hepatitis-B

Hepatitis B (formerly serum hepatitis) is a more serious disease than hepatitis A. It is the most prevalent form of acute hepatitis world-wide, has a propensity for chronicity, and is a risk factor for hepatocellular cancer of the liver. The virus is a DNA virus with two major components, a core containing the c-antigen (or HBcAg), and the surface component HBsAg. It is spread predominantly by transmission from carrier mothers to their new-born infants, by sexual contact and by the parenteral route (from intravenous drug abuse, contaminated blood, tattooing, acupuncture, etc.). Man is the only reservoir of the virus which is found in high amounts in the blood of an infected individual and is also present in a number of other body fluids.

Clinical features

The usual incubation period of acute hepatitis B is between 2 and 6 months and 10% or so of patients suffer a serum-sickness-like syndrome with fever, urticarial rash, and arthralgia during the pre-icteric phase.

Diagnosis

The acute illness is indistinguishable from other forms of viral hepatitis and the diagnosis depends upon specific serological testing. During the acute phase both HBsAg and the core associated e-antigen (HBeAg) can be detected in the blood. Antibody to core antigen (anti-HBc) also appears at the same time as the symptoms; initially this is of IgM type. As the illness improves HBsAg and HBeAg disappear and antibodies to them appear and persist for many years, together with IgG anti-HBc. Once these antibodies have appeared the patient is no longer infectious and is immune to further infection. About 5–10% of adults and almost all neonates with HBV infection become persistently infected. These patients typically have a mild acute illness but HBsAg, with or without HBeAg, persists indefinitely and no anti-HBs develops. Those with HBeAg are likely to develop chronic liver disease and possibly hepatocellular carcinoma. No therapy has been shown to influence acute hepatitis-B although corticosteroid therapy and human interferon-alpha have produced benefits in the treatment of patients with chronic hepatitis. Pre- and post-exposure prophylaxis against hepatitis B with specific immunoglobulin or vaccination is dealt with in Chapter 2.

Hepatitis C

Hepatitis C virus was discovered in 1988–9 and is now known to be the cause of most cases of classic (parenterally spread) non-A, non-B hepatitis. This is the most common form of post-transfusion hepatitis and is also frequent among intravenous drug users and haemophiliacs. The virus is an RNA virus which seems to be closely related to arthropod-spread encephalitis viruses. Only a quarter of infections are icteric.

Clinical features

The clinical illness is very similar to hepatitis B, although the illness has a relapsing course with transaminase enzymes often fluctuating for several months. Although the illness may be benign and asymptomatic it may cause progressive liver disease, cirrhosis, and primary liver cancer. The ultimate prognosis for patients with chronic disease is difficult to predict.

Hepatitis C infection can be diagnosed by detection of antibody to the virus. Interferon-alpha therapy has been of limited use in the treatment of chronic hepatitis although the indications for treatment are not yet defined and it is uncertain whether patients who have a good response have a better long-term prognosis. The treatment is given subcutaneously and is associated with possible unpleasant side-effects.

Implications for general practice

Patients with chronic disease should be referred for specialist opinion on the need to start interferon and for counselling about the implications of the diagnosis.[34] They should avoid alcohol and should be counselled about the parenteral route of transmission. The risk of sexual transmission is low and patients in long-standing monogamous relationships should avoid sex during menstruation but need not start to use barrier contraception after the diagnosis is made. Condoms should be used for all casual sexual contacts.

Delta hepatitis

The hepatitis delta virus (HDV) is unusual: it is a defective RNA virus that can only replicate when HBsAg is present. Delta infection thus only occurs in those with concomitant acute or persistent hepatitis B infection. Delta virus is common in the Mediterranean and in the Middle East, occurs in epidemic form in some parts of South America, and causes sporadic infection among drug addicts in Europe and North America. If acute delta infection is a co-infection with acute hepatitis B, then the illness is of little consequence and the virus is cleared as the HBsAg disappears. If acute delta infection occurs in a patient with chronic hepatitis B, however, then chronic co-infection results and many patients develop cirrhosis. Diagnosis is made by detection of anti-HDV. There is no treatment for delta hepatitis but immunization against hepatitis B can provide immunity against delta virus.

Hepatitis E

Infection with hepatitis E is very similar to hepatitis A. It is faecally transmitted and usually causes an acute self-limiting illness with no chronic after-effects.

However, there are important differences: hepatitis E mainly affects young adults and can have a high mortality in pregnancy, especially in women in lesser developed countries.[35]

Amoebic abscess

Intestinal infections with *Entamoeba histolytica* in travellers and those who have lived abroad is described in Chapter 15. Infection is sometimes complicated by spread of amoebic trophozoites into the liver via the portal vein. The organisms multiply and may form single or multiple abscesses, usually in the right lobe of the liver. This may occur in the complete absence of intestinal symptoms but usually becomes clinically obvious some time after an episode of diarrhoea.

Clinical features and treatment

These are fever (sometimes with rigors), pain in the right upper abdomen or lower chest, tenderness of the liver, and a neutrophil leucocytosis. Sometimes, the patient has diarrhoea and other symptoms of intestinal amoebiasis. Rapid weight loss is common.

The usual laboratory findings are mildly abnormal liver function tests (with an elevated alkaline phosphatase being the most prominent), a neutrophil leukocytosis and, often, anaemia. The chest X-ray may show an elevated right hemidiaphragm and ultrasound or scan will confirm the presence of an abscess. Serological tests for amoebiasis are almost always positive in amoebic liver abscesses.

The treatment of an amoebic abscess is with metronidazole, given for one week and followed by diloxanide furoate to eradicate any amoebic cysts from the bowel. Aspiration of the abscess is usually reserved for those that may potentially rupture or those not rapidly responding to therapy.

References

1. Royal College of General Practitioners, Office of Population Censuses and Surveys, Department of Health and Social Security. *Morbidity statistics from general practice. Third National Study, (1981–2)*. MB5. No. 1. London: HMSO (1986)

2. The Chief Medical Officer. *On the state of the public health*. Department of Health. London: HMSO (1995)

3. Huilan S, Zhen L, Mathan M *et al*. Etiology of acute diarrhoea among children in developing countries: a multicentre study in five countries. *Bull WHO* (1991) **69**: 549–55

4. Wanke C, Schoring J. Barret I *et al*. Potential role of adherence traits of *Escherichia coli* in persistant diarrhea in an urban Brazilian slum. *Ped Infect Dis J* (1991) **10**: 746–51

5. Ferreccio C, Prado V, Ojedo A *et al*. Epidemiologic patterns of acute diarrhea and

endemic shigella infections in children in a poor periurban setting in Santiago, Chile. *Am J Epidemiol*, (1991) **134**: 614–27

6. Thoren A, Lundberg O, Bergdahl U. Socioeconomic effects of acute diarrhoea in adults. *Scand J Infect Dis* (1988) **20**: 317–22

7. Nathwani D, Grimshaw J, Taylor R. Factors influencing general practitioners' referral to hospital of adults with presumed infective diarrhoea. *Brit J Gen Pract* (1994) **44**: 171–4

8. Farthing M. Traveller's diarrhoea: mostly due to bacteria and difficult to prevent. *BMJ* (1993) **306**: 1425–6

9. Fox R. Pre-hospital management of infantile gastroenteritis. *Brit J Gen Pract* (1990) **40**:

10. Hoghton M, Mittal N, Sandhu B, Effects of immediate modified feeding on infantile gastroenteritis. *Brit J Gen Pract* (1996) **46**: 173–5

11. Gore S, Fontaine O, Pierce N. Impact of rice base ORS on stool output and duration of diarrhoea: meta-analysis of 13 clinical trials. *BMJ* (1992) **304**: 287–91

12. Wharton B, Pugh R, Taitz L *et al.* Dietary management of gastroenteritis in Britain. *BMJ* (1988) **296**: 450–2

13. Research priorities for diarrhoeal disease vaccines: memorandum from a WHO meeting. *Bull WHO* (1991) **6**: 667–76

14. Gray J, Jiang X, Morgan-Capner P *et al.* Prevalence of antibodies to Norwalk virus in England: detection by enzyme-linked immuosorbent assay using baculovirus-expressed Norwalk virus capsid antigen. *J Clin Microbiol* (1993) **31**: 1022–5

15. Graham G, Jiang X, Tanaka T *et al.* Norwalk virus infection of volunteers: new insights based on improved assays. *J Infect Dis* (1994) **170**: 34–43

16. Skirrow M. Epidemiology of Campylobacter enteritis: a review. *Int J Food Microbiol* (1991) **12**: 9–16

17. Petrucelli B, Murphy G, Sanchez J *et al.* Treatment of travelers' diarrhea with ciprofloxacin and loperamide. *J Infec Dis* (1992) **165**: 557

18. Nachamkin I. Campylobacter infections. *Curr Op Infect Dis* (1993) **6**: 72–6

19. Rees J, Soudain S, Gregson N. *Campylobacter jejuni infection* and Guillan–Barré syndrome. *N Engl J Med.* (1995) **333**: 1374–9

20. Lee L, Shapiro C, Hargrett-bean N *et al.* Hyper-endemic shigellosis in the United States: a review of surveillance data for 1967–88. *J Infect Dis* (1991) **164**: 894–900

21. Sockett P, Roberts J. The social and economic impact of salmonellosis: a report of a national survey in England and Wales of laboratory-confirmed *Salmonella* infections. *Epidemiol Infect.* (1991) **107**: 335–47

22. Mitty R, LaMont T. *Clostridium difficile* diarrhoea: pathogenesis, epidemiology, and treatment. *Gastroenterologist* (1994) **2**: 61–9

23. Habib F *et al. Clostridium difficile* after antibiotic therapy. (Letter) *Brit J Gen Pract* (1994) **44**: 331

24. PHLS Service Study Group. Cryptosporidiosis in England and Wales: prevalence and clinical and epidemiological features. *BMJ* (1990) **300**: 774–7

25. Moreira Lima A. Cholera: molecular epidemiology, pathogenesis, immunology, treatment, and prevention. *Curr Op Infect Dis* (1994) 7: 592–601

26. Bitzan M, Ludwig K, Klemt M *et al.* The role of *Escherichia coli* O157 infections in the classic (enteropathic) haemolytic uraemic syndrome: results of a central European multistudy. *Epidemiol Infect* (1993) **110**: 591–600

27. Rathbone B, Heatley R, (ed.) *Helicobacter pylori and gastroduodenal disease.* 2nd ed. Oxford: Blackwell (1992) 124–7

28. Webb P, Knight T, Greaves S *et al.* Relation between infection with *Helicobacter pylori* and living conditions in childhood: evidence for person to person transmission in early life. *BMJ* (1994) **308**: 750–3

29. Patel P, Mendall M, Khulusi S *et al. Helicobacter pylori* infection in childhood: risk factors and effect on growth. *BMJ.* (1994) **309**: 1119–23

30. Hosking S, Ling T, Chung S *et al.* Duodenal ulcer healing by eradication of *Helicobacter pylori* without anti-acid treatment: randomised controlled trial. *Lancet* (1994) **343**: 508–10

31. Logan R, Gummett P, Misiemicz J *et al.* One week's anti-*Helicobacter pylori* treatment for duodenal ulcer. *Gut* (1994) **35**: 15–18

32. *Helicobacter pylori* in peptic ulcer disease. NIH Consensus Statement (1994) Feb 7–9 **12**(1) National Institutes of Health: 1–23

33. Briggs A, Sculpher M, Logan R *et al.* Cost effectiveness of screening for and eradication of *Helicobacter pylori* in management of dyspeptic patients under 45 years of age. *BMJ* (1996) **312**: 1321–5

34. Dusheiko G, Khakoo S, Grellier L. A rational approach to the management of hepatitis C infection. *BMJ* 1996 **312**: 357–64

35. Skidmore S. Hepatitis E (editorial). *BMJ* (1995) **310**: 414–15

CHAPTER TEN

Infections of the urinary tract

Urinary tract infection is one of the commonest conditions seen in general practice and about 3% of consultations are for related symptoms.[12] Indeed, infections of the urinary tract are among the most common of all bacterial infections, with schoolgirls, sexually active young women, men with prostatic hypertrophy, and the elderly being the groups principally affected. The vast majority of these infections occur in women, where the shorter urethra allows easier access into the bladder for microorganisms present on the perineal surface. About 25–35% of women have experienced urinary tract infection (UTI) symptoms at some time, with many having repeated infections leading to substantial morbidity, and increased use of health care resources.[3] In all about 50% of women experience 'dysuria', defined as burning pain on micturition, at some time in their lives.[4] While women with symptoms suggestive of UTI may or may not have bacteriuria, studies have shown that 5% of sexually active women have asymptomatic bacteriuria. There is a substantial rise in the elderly, and in geriatric units the figure may be as high as 30–50%. Although these figures relate to asymptomatic infections, symptomatic UTIs follow the same trends. Peaks occur in neonates, women in late adolescence, early adult life, and in old age.

Men experience UTI much less commonly and when they do it is usually related to some anatomical abnormality.[5] Urinary tract infections are frequently seen in childhood and account for 4–10% of febrile children admitted to hospital: 3% of girls and 1% of boys have a symptomatic urinary infection before the age of 10. Children rarely experience symptoms but when they do, investigation is of increased importance, particularly in boys.

The term 'urinary tract infection' refers only to the presence of 'significant bacteriuria' defined as 10^5 colony-forming units per millilitre of urine, and may or may not be accompanied by clinical symptoms. It is also usual to indicate whether infection involves only the bladder (cystitis) or may include the renal parenchyma as well (pyelonephritis).

With the exception of the distal urethra of both sexes which may be colonized by a variety of organisms, the normal urinary tract is bacteriologically sterile. The most important route of urinary infection is the ascent of urethral organisms into the bladder and up into the ureters to the renal pelvis and parenchyma. Blood-borne spread of infection to the renal parenchyma does occur but this usually results in abscess formation.

Table 10.1 *Urinary tract infection (UTI): risk factors and the characteristics of common causative organisms*

Intrinsic risk factors
- Turbulent urethral flow in the shorter female urethra
- Urinary obstruction, stasis and reflux
- Pregnancy and old age
- Persons with B or AB blood groups
- Hyperosmolarity of the renal medulla
- Host defences (humoral and cellular factors)
- Vaginal colonization with *E. coli*

Extrinsic risk factors
- Catheterization or instrumentation
- Surgery
- Indwelling catheter
- Sexual activity in women
- Poor urinary flow
- Use of diaphragms for contraception

Virulence factors in causative organisms
- Fimbrial adhesins allowing adherence to uroepithelium
- Production of haemolysins
- The quantity of K-antigen
- Ability to resist serum killing

Aetiology

The faecal flora, particularly *Escherichia coli*, is the principal source of the bacteria that cause UTI. In women, the organisms first colonize the perineum, introitus and distal urethra, and then ascend to the bladder. Men are protected from infection by the longer male urethra. Although almost any bacterium can cause a UTI, some bacterial strains possess a number of virulence factors which make them more likely to do so. Risk factors for urinary tract infection and the characteristics of the organisms most likely to cause it are shown in Tables 10.1 and 10.2.

Clinical features

Urinary tract infections present to the general practitioner in many different ways and current terminology can be confusing: in addition, presentation varies in the extremes of age, different body build, in the sexes, and in pregnancy. The terms 'chronic cystitis' and 'chronic urinary tract infection' are unhelpful when used to describe patients with recurring infections. It is clinically impossible, for example, to distinguish between cystitis and urethral syndrome, and diagnoses of cystitis or pyelonephritis are not mutually exclusive. Equally, 'chronic pyelonephritis' is another confusing term and

Table 10.2 *Mechanical factors that predispose to UTI*

Poor urinary flow
- low intake
- bladder residual
- Hot climate

Malfunctioning bladder
- neuropathic
- diverticulum

Reflux nephropathy

Outlet obstruction
- calculi
- prostatic enlargement
- Urethral stricture
- congenital anatomical abnormalities
- constipation
- cystocoele

Spread from bowel
- diverticulitis
- appendix abscess
- enterovesical fistula

Instrumentation
- catheter
- urological surgery

Renal pelvis obstruction
- calculi
- post-surgery damage
- stricture
- papillary necrosis

should be restricted to those patients with a radiologically proven diagnosis. The term 'pyelitis' is inaccurate and should not be used as no UTI remains confined to the renal pelvis.

Further confusion results from the way in which patients present with a UTI. When individuals use the word 'cystitis' they usually mean a symptom complex called the 'frequency dysuria syndrome'. This syndrome variously includes: frequency, discomfort or pain on passing urine, nocturia, haematuria, lower abdominal or loin pain, and fever, etc. Significant bacteriuria, may however, be present in only some 50% of such cases. In many women, the underlying problem is a vaginitis with external dysuria or pain caused by urine flowing over an inflamed perineum. The confusion can be limited by a careful history in which the patient is encouraged to describe the problem in detail rather than using the shorthand phrase 'cystitis' and the careful use of medical terms by the GP.

In this chapter the presentation, clinical course, diagnosis, investigation and treatment of UTI will be discussed under the headings:

- Acute cystitis
- Recurrent acute cystitis
- Acute urethral syndrome
- Acute pyelonephritis
- Chronic pyelonephritis
- Urinary tract tuberculosis
- Prostatitis
- Epididymitis
- Orchitis

Diagnosis

As 2–3% of consultations in general practice are due to symptoms suggestive of urinary infection it is important to develop a clinically correct and economic policy for investigation and management. The diagnosis of UTI in general practice has been the subject of much debate. Is it justifiable to always send mid-stream specimens of urine (MSUs) to overworked microbiology laboratories? It has been found that when tests for nitrite, blood, and protein, using reagent strips, are all negative in a clear urine the absence of bacteriuria can be predicted with a predictive value of 98.5%.[6] Ditchburn and Ditchburn[7] found that simple low power microscopy is more accurate than a reagent strip which measures nitrite and pyuria. These authors compared three diagnostic techniques in practice

(1) drop method microscopy,

(2) cytometer count,

(3) dipstick.

They concluded that it is not normally necessary to send urine samples that do not have sufficient pyuria for culture. The majority of lower UTIs seen in general practice are in non-pregnant women with the frequency dysuria syndrome, only half of whom have significant bacteriuria. To prescribe an antibiotic at the initial consultation means that half receive antibiotics unnecessarily. General practice studies of sideroom prediction of UTI and simple scoring systems further substantiate the claim that in the interests of economy and expediency laboratory urine specimens are not always necessary. Each practice must decide its policy in relation to urine culture in UTI, the use of reagent strips to screen urines is a reasonable alternative in uncomplicated situations,[8] particularly when accompanied by a detailed history and attention to the risk factors discussed above.

If urine culture is considered necessary it is important to differentiate between a true UTI and contamination by organisms that accidentally enter the urine from the perineum during voiding.[9] Assuming a clean, voided (MSU) specimen, the diagnosis of bacterial UTI is based upon the presence of the number of bacteria needed to meet the criterion of 'significant bacteriuria'. There is no absolute value for this concept which depends on the patient's sex and the presence of symptoms of UTI. A concentration of >100 000/ml of bacteria of a single type in pure culture (usually expressed as colony-forming units, CFU/ml) has a predictive accuracy of bladder bacteriuria of 80% in asymptomatic women and about 95% in women with symptoms of UTI. Two consecutive positive cultures of >10^5 CFU/ml increase the predictive accuracy to 95% in asymptomatic women. It is now accepted that lesser bacterial concentrations are meaningful in symptomatic women: only concentrations <10^2 CFU/ml should be disregarded. Some authors have reported data which suggest that low-count bacteriuria may represent the early phase of a UTI.[10] In contrast, colony counts of 10 000–100 000 CFU/ml without associated signs and symptoms of UTI are almost always due to contamination. The likelihood of contamination is much less in men than in women and colony counts of >10^2 CFU/ml should be taken to indicate infection whether or not the individual is symptomatic.

The isolation of more than 10^2 CFU/ml from a suprapubic aspiration of the bladder is significant. Specimens from patients with indwelling urinary catheters are best obtained by direct puncture of the catheter and aspiration with a sterile needle rather than by opening the closed drainage system or culturing the urine from the bag. If samples are taken in this way, contamination is most unlikely and a concentration of >10^5 CFU/ml is 95% predictive of true bladder infection.

Some of the reasons for adopting numbers of CFU/ml in men and women in the presence or absence of symptoms are summarized as follows:

- Different species of bacteria multiply at different rates
- Frequency of micturition can interfere with the result
- In some women, bacteria may be involved in a urethral lesion and may not get an opportunity to multiply in bladder urine.
- In men, bacteria may multiply in prostatic fluid where counts may be low because of the presence of prostatic antibacterial factor

Some GPs use a microscope for screening urines. A standard technique for urinalysis is recommended. Microscopic examination of the sediment from approximately 5 ml of centrifuged urine may permit a presumptive diagnosis. The presence of more than 20 white blood cells per high power field (hpf) of the sediment is correlated with a bacterial colony count >10^5 CFU/ml in most cases. The presence of bacteria in each hpf of a Gram-stain of uncentrifuged urine also correlates with significant bacteriuria. Negative urine microscopy does not, however, rule out significant bacteriuria.

Table 10.3 *Clinical features that indicate the need for investigation of an adult with UTI*

- Second infections in women
- Single (debatable) infection in males
- History of childhood infections in an adult
- Persistent haematuria following appropriate anti bacterial treatment
- History of renal colic or passage of urinary calculus
- History of pyelonephritis
- Coexistence of hypertension
- Enuresis
- Urinary retention
- Loin tenderness

Investigations

Further investigation of a single proven UTI in a healthy younger woman is unnecessary if she is symptom-free, and the urine is free of blood, protein, and nitrites on completion of treatment. Situations requiring investigation and sometimes referral are summarized in Table 10.3. The purpose of the investigations is to identify:

(1) anatomical predisposing factors,

(2) damage resulting from chronic infection,

(3) physiological dysfunction,

(4) obstruction from calculi or prostatic enlargement,

(5) associated clinical conditions,

(6) fistulae, pelvic, or intra-abdominal disease, malignancy,

(7) tuberculosis of the urinary tract.

The nature and extent of the investigations carried out in practice will depend on local facilities and the interest and experience of the GP. Most GPs will wish to get as far as possible in finding an underlying cause before or while awaiting referral. Investigations may include the following:

- *Available to all general practitioners*
  - Simple biochemical tests of renal function

- *Available to many general practitioners*
  - Intravenous urogram (IVU)
  - Ultrasound
  - Three consecutive and complete early morning specimens of urine for acid-fast bacilli

- *Specialist investigations*
  - Urodynamic studies
  - Micturating cysto-urethrography (MCU)
  - Cystoscopy and urethroscopy
  - Renal biopsy
  - MRI scan

Radiographic examination of the urinary tract is not indicated in all patients with cystitis, but should be performed in groups with a high risk of renal parenchymal damage. As there is a strong possibility of renal scarring in young children if infection is accompanied by vesico-ureteric reflux, they should be referred for voiding cystourethrography. Recurrent attacks of cystitis may lead to the finding of a thickened bladder wall with irregular mucosa on intravenous urography and occasionally vesico-ureteric reflux and residual urine on voiding cysto-urethrography. Some of these findings are temporary and, where possible, radiographic studies should be delayed for at least six weeks after resolution of the infection.

Asymptomatic bacteriuria

Screening programmes have shown bacteriuria in a significant proportion of the population, particularly women: 1–3% of preschool or school-age girls[11] and 0.03% of boys[12] are affected. The prevalence is 1–3% in non-pregnant younger women and 0.1% in younger men. The prevalence increases sharply in the elderly to 10% of men and 20% of women. The majority of these asymptomatic patients have infection of the lower urinary tract only. In pregnancy, however, there is a greater than 20% risk of asymptomatic bacteriuria leading to acute pyelonephritis, which is a risk factor for prematurity or stillbirth. Asymptomatic bacteriuria in pregnancy requires therapy and regular review with all pregnant women screened during the antenatal period. Otherwise, asymptomatic bacteriuria in women only needs to be treated when there is obstruction present. The urine cannot be sterilized in the catheterized patient because the catheter acts as a foreign body. The only consequence of treating asymptomatic bacteriuria in these patients is the selection of resistant organisms in the bowel flora (which subsequently cause further UTIs).

The consequences of urinary tract infection

Apart from the distress that the frequency dysuria syndrome causes many women, serious consequences are likely where chronic urinary tract infection occurs in the presence of a pre-existing renal abnormality. Unrecognized, untreated infection particularly in infancy and particularly if ureteric reflux is present, may lead to renal scarring and damage.[13] The other sequaelae include:

- Papillary necrosis
- Stone formation
- Chronic pyelonephritis
- Chronic pyelonephritis and septicemia
- Hypertension
- Decreased renal function and eventual renal failure

The GP should be aware that a raised plasma urea or creatinine, moderate proteinuria (>1 g/day), and an IVU appearance of loss of renal substance all indicate a poor prognosis in this situation.

Acute cystitis

Aetiology

The presence of significant numbers of bacteria in the bladder leads to inflammatory changes in the bladder wall. In mild cases, the mucosal oedema and cellular infiltrate may be largely superficial, but in severe cases this may involve the entire bladder wall. Occasionally, severe mucosal hyperaemia and petechiae results in haemorrhagic cystitis, seen particularly in catheterized patients.

Escherichia coli is responsible for more than 90% of episodes of acute bacterial cystitis (see also table 10.4).

Viruses can cause cystitis and the adenoviruses are particularly likely to cause haemorrhagic cystitis. This is much more common in schoolboys than in girls.

Clinical features

The symptoms of acute cystitis in adults usually include dysuria, frequency (sometimes more pronounced after voiding), urgency, and less reliably, nocturia. Frequently, there is associated suprapubic discomfort and haematuria. This symptom complex does not exclude subclinical pyelonephritis.

Table 10.4 *Organisms responsible for acute cystitis*

- *Escherichia coli*
- *Staphylococcus saprophyticus*
  (coagulase-negative staphylococcus)
- Enteric bacteria
  - *Klebsiella*
  - *Proteus*
  - *Enterobacter* species

- *Pseudomonas aeruginosa*
- Yeasts (*Candida* and *Torulopsis glabrata*)

Fever in excess of 38°C is unlikely if the infection principally affects the lower urinary tract. Haematuria is usually very alarming for the patient who will need an explanation and reassurance. The infection spreads by the ascending route: in women the route may be from the rectum to the vagina and urethra with bacterial entry to the bladder facilitated by sexual intercourse. While the ascending route is the most usual portal of entry of infection, haematogenous spread may occur infrequently. Acute cystitis is not usually associated with any anatomical or functional abnormality of the urinary tract with predisposing factors present in only 5% of women. The infection may present in a variety of ways:

- Acute urinary symptoms
- Post-coital urinary symptoms
- Acute retention in men
- Failure to thrive in infants
- Chronic debility in the elderly
- Acute pyelonephritis in pregnancy
- Asymptomatic bacteriuria

Empirical management

Cure rates of 85–90% are expected in the general practice treatment of UTI. Although there is debate about the need to send an MSU to the laboratory for every patient there is no debate about confirming cure if the cure is symptomatically in doubt. As patients with occult upper tract infection will not be cured or will relapse after short courses of antibiotics, and as differentiation of upper from lower UTIs is not possible clinically, follow-up cultures should be taken 1–2 weeks after stopping therapy. It is sensible to continue follow-up for children for at least 2 years and the GP should ensure that this happens. The parents will usually act as a good spur to excellent practice if given the responsibility in parallel.

When treating cystitis the GP should take into consideration the prognosis of the infection in different individuals, the presence or absence of symptoms, and the inconvenience and side-effects of the various antimicrobial agents. Symptomatic patients are usually treated, but in asymptomatic patients, bacteriuria has been shown to have serious consequences only in preschool children and pregnant women. Many patients are in extreme discomfort and they require rest and advice to drink copious amounts of clear fluids and to take paracetamol, which has a helpful effect on the dysuria and suprapubic ache. The choice of antibiotic will depend on the patterns of resistance among the locally prevalent urinary pathogens and can be adjusted or stopped when the result of the MSU is known. The agents used for UTI in general practice are all well absorbed from the GI tract, are of low toxicity, concentrated in the urine, and relatively cheap. Conventional therapy has always been for 7–14 days but it is now considered

Table 10.5 *Antibiotics for general practice treatment of UTI*

- Trimethoprim (avoid in pregnancy)
- Co-amoxiclav
- Nitrofurantoin
- Quinolones (e.g. ciprofloxacin)
- Cephalosporin

Note: Co-trimoxazole is best avoided. Amoxicillin and sulphonamides are no longer recommended because of widespread resistance. Quinolones should be reserved for special circumstances, such as bacterial resistance to other antibiotics and for use in *Pseudomonas* infections.

safe to use very short (i.e. 3-day) or 1-dose regimes for uncomplicated cystitis.[14,15]

If infections occur repeatedly or the underlying cause for a relapsing infection cannot be eradicated, then chronic suppressive therapy with daily trimethoprim or nitrofurantoin (which have little effect on the bowel flora) can be used. Similar prophylactic antibiotics can be given to women in whom UTI frequently follows sexual intercourse.

Recurrent acute cystitis

The presentation is essentially similar to that for acute cystitis, although the severity of symptoms may be less, usually because the patient increases fluid intake at the first sign of a problem. It is important to distinguish between relapse and re-infection. A *relapsing infection* is a recurrence (usually within 2 weeks) with the original infecting organism. Common reasons for failure of cure are non- or poor compliance, occult upper UTI, inappropriate choice of antibiotic, or variance in the *in vitro* and *in vivo* sensitivity patterns. A *re-infection* is the recurrence of bacteriuria with a new organism. Recurrent infections may eventually lead to pyelonephritis, hence careful investigation, treatment and follow-up is important as underlying urinary tract pathology may be present (Table 10.5).

Treatment

Some of these patients will be managed by specialists but where no underlying pathology is identified treatment may be approached in two ways:

1. Each time the patient reports symptoms of a UTI the infecting organism should be identified and treated with the correct antibiotic according to *in vitro* sensitivity. The patient should be followed up with an MSU at 1 and 6 weeks.

2. Treat with daily low dose prophylactic antibiotics for some months. The

Table 10.6 *Pointers to recurrent UTI*

---

1. Organisms resistant to three or more of usually prescribed antibiotics
2. Repeated positive cultures after appropriate treatment
3. Mixed infection
4. Frequently varying pattern of bacteria
5. Recurrent *Proteus* infection
6. Persistent sterile pyuria

---

aims of prophylactic antibiotics are to keep the urine sterile, to render the patient symptom-free, and to prevent renal damage due to chronic infection (Table 10.6). Only a few antibiotics are suitable for long-term use. The most useful are:

– Nitrofurantoin (but not for *Proteus*)

– Trimethoprim (not in pregnancy)

– Amoxycillin (*Candida albicans* infection a high risk)

– Cefaclor (occasional use in some circumstances)

The dosage for prophylactic antibiotic treatment is one-quarter the usual treatment dose and the drug is best taken at night after voiding to ensure adequate concentration.

Acute urethral syndrome

The 'urethral syndrome' is the name given to the common situation where a woman with symptoms of frequency and dysuria but without fever and systemic symptoms, is not found to have 'significant bacteriuria' (greater than 10^5 CFU/ml).[16] The frequency dysuria syndrome is a persistent problem for about 4% of women who are usually young and sexually active.[17] It is now recognized that many of these patients do have acute cystitis but with low counts of bacteria in the urine (10^2–10^4 CFU/ml).[18] These women usually have pyuria and respond to antimicrobial therapy. Urethritis caused by sexually transmitted agents such as *Chlamydia trachomatis*, herpes genitalis, or the various forms of vaginitis may also cause similar symptoms. Women with the frequency dysuria syndrome and a sterile urine should be examined vaginally and swabs taken, as prompt treatment for a vaginal infection will resolve the situation. Other women have frequency and dysuria but no infective cause can be determined although many patients recognize a connection between the symptoms and sexual activity. This impression has been supported by research which showed that 75% of cystitis episodes occurred within 24 hours of intercourse.[19] These women often develop ways of coping with recurrent symptoms: commonly a high fluid input, simple analgesia, heat, and rest are effective. The frequency of attacks may be reduced by voiding before and after intercourse, washing if convenient, and avoiding sexual positions, such as vaginal penetration from behind, which some women associate with attacks of 'cystitis'. Other women find that the use of a diaphragm for contraception exacerbates the situation a finding that has been confirmed in recent studies.[20]

Acute pyelonephritis

Inflammation of the kidney parenchyma, calices, and pelvis, commonly due to bacterial infection, is known as pyelonephritis. Infection usually reaches the kidney by ascending via the ureters from the lower urinary tract, although blood-borne infection can also occur. The classical presentation is of acute loin pain associated with high temperature (usually > 38.5 °C). Additional constitutional symptoms may include myalgia, headache, nausea, and rigors. Patients may become acutely ill very quickly and the condition may, if not treated promptly and energetically, lead to Gram-negative septicaemia with metastatic infection involving endocardium, meninges, or bone. Up to 40% of patients with acute pyelonephritis have bacteraemia. The presentation may present a broad differential diagnosis to include, lobar pneumonia, herpes zoster, cholecystitis, myocardial infarction, pulmonary embolus, appendicitis, and pelvic inflammatory disease. Pathological changes are most prominent in the renal medulla, with multiple micro-abscesses present in severe cases. Occasionally, a large intrarenal abscess (renal carbuncle) may occur.

At the other end of the spectrum, it is also recognized that many patients with symptoms suggestive only of lower UTI do in fact have subclinical pyelonephritis. The presence of casts containing white blood cells in the urinary sediment, formed in the renal tubules and collecting ducts, signify involvement of the kidney. Fungal pyelonephritis is usually due to C. *albicans* and results from systemic infection rather than ascending UTI. It is particularly likely to occur in immunosuppressed individuals. Rarely, magnesium ammonium phosphate stones occur in association with infection due to *Proteus* species. Bladder stones are nearly always found in men in association with an obstruction due to an enlarged prostate or urethral stricture (Tables 10.7 and 10.8).

Table 10.7 *Risk factors for developing acute pyelonephritis*

1. Ureteric reflux
2. Renal calculi
3. Recurrent urinary tract infections
4. Pregnancy
5. Neuropathic bladder
6. Indwelling catheter
7. Neglected or poorly managed urinary infections

Table 10.8 *Indications for long-term prophylaxis in UTI*

- Children with recurrent infections or reflux
- Some pathological urinary tract abnormalities
- Very frequent symptomatic infections
- Pregnancy with a history of recurrent symptomatic infections

Treatment

The diagnosis is confirmed by the history, clinical assessment, and examination of the urine. The patient may be extremely ill and treatment should
commence empirically with a suitable antibiotic such as co-amoxiclav
accompanied by adequate analgesia. Admission to hospital for parenteral
treatment may be required but in any event blood cultures should ideally
be taken before antibiotic treatment is started. Those who are severely ill or
who have bacteraemia will need parenteral antibiotics: an aminoglycoside,
cephalosporin, or quinolone for those with community acquired infections
and imipenem or ceftazidime for those with possible *Pseudomonas* or
highly resistant Enterobacteriaceae infection (nosocomial or catheter-
associated infections). Those who are less unwell can be managed at
home with oral trimethoprim, co-amoxiclav, or ciprofloxacin. Therapy
should be given for 10–14 days. Relapse occurs in 10–50% of patients
after 2 weeks of therapy: these should be treated again with a 4-week
course of antibiotics. Whether patients with symptomatic pyelonephritis
should be treated in hospital or in general practice depends largely on
clinical judgement. In any event, radiological investigation should be
undertaken and follow-up urine cultures should be arranged in children, pregnant women, and those with obstruction of the urinary tract.
These patients should also have their blood pressure checked at regular
intervals.

Complications of pyelonephritis

Renal abscess

In the past, intrarenal abscesses usually arose as a complication of staphylococcal infection elsewhere in the body. Nowadays, they are principally seen
as complications of acute pyelonephritis and are caused by Gram-negative
organisms. These patients usually present with acute symptoms suggestive of
acute pyelonephritis; those with renal abscesses secondary to haematogenous
spread may sometimes present more chronically with symptoms of malaise
and weight loss. Urine culture is often normal if *Staphylococcus aureus* is the
causative organism, but when Gram-negative bacteria are responsible urine
culture usually shows the same organism. The presence of gas within the
renal shadow on a plain abdominal X-ray is suggestive, but the diagnosis is

usually made by intravenous or retrograde urography and ultrasonography. An intrarenal abscess is best managed with empirical parenteral antibiotic therapy directed against the likely pathogens and ultrasound-guided percutaneous aspiration. Pus can then be cultured, decompression may be possible, and surgery avoided.

Papillary necrosis

Severe pyelonephritis may lead to papillary necrosis, especially in diabetics and in individuals with urinary tract obstruction, sickle-cell disease or trait, or analgesic abuse. A characteristic radiographic appearance may be seen on intravenous pyelography, consisting of collections of contrast material outside the caliceal system in cavities produced by the necrosis and sloughing of the papillary tissue.

Perinephric abscess

If renal infection extends through the capsule of the kidney into the perinephric fat, an abscess may result. These patients usually have severe pyelonephritis associated with obstruction of the urinary tract, renal calculi, or diabetes. The infecting organisms are typically Gram-negative bacteria or, in the case of perinephric abscess secondary to bacteraemia, *Staph. aureus*. The patient complains of fever and chills associated with abdominal and flank pain, often of several days duration. Examination may or may not reveal a mass in the flank. Urine culture is generally positive. Treatment consists of drainage of the abscess after starting parenteral antibiotic therapy. Antibiotic choice may need to be empirical but is usually governed by the urine culture results. Drainage can often be undertaken percutaneously.

Chronic pyelonephritis

The term 'chronic pyelonephritis' is poorly defined but is generally used to describe a cluster of pathological findings associated with chronic inflammation and fibrosis of the kidney. Although these changes may be due to infection they can result from analgesic nephropathy, urinary tract obstruction, vascular disease, and urate nephropathy. Many of these patients do not have bacteriuria and the response to antimicrobial therapy is poor. The process leads to asymmetric contraction and distortion of the kidney with deep cortical scars overlying dilated and blunted calices. Chronic infection and scarring is important because the loss of renal substance compromises function.

The condition characteristically follows recurrent childhood infections associated with reflux and early identification of these patients is vital. Unfortunately, the initial presentation may be with early renal failure, hypertension, or both, with subsequent progress to end-stage renal failure, dialysis, and transplantation. Pyelonephritis is the primary cause of renal failure in about 20% of patients requiring dialysis.

Treatment

Patients with chronic pyelonephritis are usually cared for by renal physicians. The chronic nature of the disease, which may lead to death at an early age, inevitably leads to the need to develop a shared approach between primary and secondary care for management. The prime responsibilities of the GP are:

- Identification of those at risk
- Prevention by correct treatment
- Diagnosis of patients with chronic pyelonephritis
- Early referral to a specialist
- Hospital liaison
- Family support
- Involvement with any subsequent home dialysis programme

Urinary tract tuberculosis

Any part of the genitourinary system may be affected by tuberculosis. The first lesion is most commonly in the kidney from which infection may extend to the bladder, prostate, and seminal vesicles. Ascending infection also occurs and, in the male, tuberculous epididymitis is a common feature of genitourinary tuberculosis. About 50% of cases have evidence of extrarenal disease (usually inactive) and genitourinary tuberculosis often only emerges into clinical significance at a very late stage in the natural history. It may be seen in elderly patients in whom tuberculosis has remained latent for many years or even decades. Inner city GPs need to maintain a high level of suspicion for renal tuberculosis which is more common in recent immigrants from S. Asia.

Most of these patients do not have constitutional symptoms and many are truly asymptomatic. Usually, there is pyuria or haematuria and culture of three early morning urine specimens confirms the diagnosis in almost all cases. Most patients are tuberculin-positive. The IVU is frequently abnormal, usually unilaterally.

Treatment with chemotherapy regimens containing rifampicin and isoniazid is usually sufficient alone to cure urinary tract tuberculosis. The minimum necessary duration of therapy has not been determined but it seems that short courses (6 months), similar to those required for pulmonary disease, are adequate. Surgery may be needed if scarring produces obstruction.

Tuberculous epididymo-orchitis

Male genital tuberculosis is usually present concurrently with renal tuberculosis (see above). Epididymitis generally follows prostatic infection and presents as a palpable painful scrotal swelling with a 'bead-like' feel to the vas deferens. Chronic infection can result in scrotal sinuses. The tuberculin skin test is usually positive and the diagnosis can be confirmed by biopsy and culture. Standard antituberculous therapy is effective.

Prostatitis

The term 'prostatitis' is used as an explanation for a wide range of lower abdominal or perineal complaints in men. Often, the diagnosis is based on poor evidence and it is important to distinguish the several different forms of prostatic infection so that management can be correct.[21] As the prostate enlarges during the second half of life it can cause obstruction to bladder emptying with urinary stasis and predisposition to urinary tract infection. However, the prostate itself, with the posterior urethra may become involved in infections of the male genital tract. The diagnosis of prostatitis should only be given if:

(1) there is a history of recurrent UTI in an otherwise normal urinary tract,

(2) there is high pressure in the prostatic urethra during voiding, usually in patients with a neurogenic bladder,

(3) there is long-term symptomatic bacteriuria following resection of the prostate.

Infection in the prostate may be acute or chronic and patients present with a wide variety of symptoms (Table 10.9).

Acute bacterial prostatitis

Acute prostatitis is relatively uncommon. When it occurs it may present with severe rigor, malaise, dysuria, and frequency. Suprapubic or rectal discomfort may be present and on occasion retention of urine may result. Rectal examination reveals an exquisitely tender enlarged prostate. Prostatic massage is not advised because of the risk of bacteraemia. Complications include prostatic abscess, pyelonephritis, and epididymitis, and in the past it was a much feared complication of gonococcal urethritis and had a high mortality. Most cases are caused by Enterobacteriaceae or *Pseudomonas*,

Table 10.9 *Symptoms of prostatitis*

- Frequency, dysuria, and haematuria
- Perineal pain radiating to lower back and inner thighs
- Haematospermia
- Urethral discharge
- Painful ejaculation

---

although a few are due to *Staph. saprophyticus* or *Enterococcus faecalis.* Examination of a routine urine specimen demonstrates pyuria and culture is positive. Antibiotic therapy, even with agents that do not penetrate well into the uninflamed prostate, readily cure the infection although ill patients may well require admission for parenteral treatment in the early stages of the infection. Suitable agents for empirical therapy are the quinolones, such as ciprofloxacin or norfloxacin.[22]

Chronic bacterial prostatitis

Chronic prostatitis is rather more common. Symptoms are much less severe but none the less debilitating, consisting of dysuria frequency and urgency. The condition usually affects men over the age of 35 and some may complain of suprapubic, testicular or loin pain. Sexual activity may pre-cipitate urinary symptoms or even a rigor. Organisms responsible may include *E. coli* and *E. faecalis.* Anaerobic infections have been suggested and there is an account of long-term cure of a patient with a 20-year history of prostatitis when incidentally treated with metronidazole for amoebic dysentery.

The diagnosis of chronic prostatitis can only be confirmed by microscopy of expressed prostatic secretions (EPS) together with quantitative bacteriological cultures of first and mid-stream urine specimens, and of prostatic secretions. The EPS will have more than 10 white blood cells per high power field (hpf), plus occasional lipid-laden macrophages.

Chronic bacterial prostatitis is an important cause of relapsing lower UTI in men. The patient is well between episodes of symptomatic urinary infection, and examination of the prostate is generally entirely normal. The only means of confirming the diagnosis is by localization studies which involve examination of urine collected at different stages of micturition and of expressed prostatic secretions obtained by prostatic massage. Antibiotic therapy is not always successful. Tetracyclines have been commonly used, ciprofloxacin and several other quinolones have shown excellent results in chronic prostatitis due to Enterobacteriaceae but are of less value when pseudomonads or enterococci are responsible.

Non-bacterial prostatitis

This condition is very common. Patients experience a range of lower abdomi-nal and perineal pain or discomfort, but there are no abnormal signs. There is no evidence of bacterial infection on careful localization studies (see above) but expressed prostatic secretions show an excess of white cells. The aetiology of this condition is unclear,[23] and opinion is divided over the role of *C. trachomatis* and *Ureaplasma urealyticum.* A small number of cases do improve with tetracycline or erythromycin therapy, but most are not helped. These men are often younger and may become extremely distressed by their continuing symptoms, particularly the continuous perineal aching that may be the major complaint. Long-term antibiotic courses of 3–6 months may help but in any case they require encouragement, and joint management between the GP and urologist or genitourinary physician. Transurethral microwave thermotherapy has shown promise in reducing symptoms.[24] The choice of specialist will be determined by the interest that the consultant is known to have in the condition, as the patient will become distressed if their symptoms are not taken seriously in the wake of normal investigations. These men are no more likely to develop prostatism in later life, and may be reassured that the situation will eventually resolve.

Epididymitis

Inflammation of the epididymis is common. It may be acute or chronic and either sexually transmitted or related to urinary tract problems. It produces a painful swelling of the scrotum, often associated with dysuria and/or a urethral discharge. Initially, the inflamed epididymis is felt as a tender swelling in the posterior scrotum; later the testis often becomes inflamed and it can be difficult to determine the anatomical limitation of the inflammatory mass. A hydrocele is commonly present. An important differential diagnosis for the GP is a torsion of the testicle and if there is any doubt a second opinion should be sought at once.

In young men, epididymitis is usually sexually transmitted and caused by *C. trachomatis*[25] or *Neisseria gonorrhoeae*. There may not be a history of urethral discharge but diagnosis depends on appropriate cultures of urethral swabs. Although therapy should be with drugs appropriate for both pathogens, in practice it is usual to refer these men to the genitourinary physician for investigation, treatment, and follow-up of sexual partners. The implications of a sexually transmitted infection should be explored with the patient and the GP must be ready to support the patient in informing sexual partners if appropriate. In older men, epididymitis is usually caused by coliforms, other Gram-negative bacilli, or Gram-positive cocci. It commonly follows urinary tract surgery or instrumentation in the presence of bacteriuria, or accompanies prostatitis. Medical management with antibiotics for both Gram-negative bacilli and Gram-positive cocci is usually effective.

Orchitis

Infection of the testis, without prostatitis and epididymitis, is nearly always due to viral infections, although blood-borne bacterial infections can occur.

Viral orchitis

The most common cause of orchitis is mumps. Orchitis occurs in about 20% of postpubertal males who develop mumps, but is very rare in the prepubertal.

The typical clinical picture is abrupt onset of unilateral testicular swelling starting during the first week of the parotitis. This is accompanied by a variable degree of testicular pain and, in the severe cases, by high fever, vomiting, and constitutional symptoms. The testis is tender and warm and the scrotum erythematous. In about one-third of cases the other testis becomes involved a few days later. Resolution can take anything from a few days to several weeks. Following resolution, there is testicular atrophy of variable severity but, contrary to popular belief, sterility seldom results. Bed rest, analgesia and support of the affected testis make the patient more comfortable. High dose steroid therapy during the acute phase seems to reduce the symptoms of mumps orchitis but has no effect on the subsequent testicular atrophy. Acute orchitis has also been recorded in infections due to coxsackie viruses (particularly coxsackie B) and echovirus 6. The disease is clinically identical to mumps orchitis.

Bacterial orchitis

Epididymo-orchitis is described above. Occasionally, orchitis can follow haematogenous spread. The patient is acutely ill with high fever, severe pain, marked testicular tenderness, and often an acute hydrocele. The testis is swollen and large areas of necrosis and abscess may form. These patients should be admitted urgently to hospital as parenteral antibiotic therapy is needed and surgical drainage may be necessary if an abscess or pyocele develops.

Special situations in urinary tract infections

In some situations commonly encountered in general practice there are special considerations either in the early diagnosis or management of UTIs.

Catheters

Patients with indwelling urinary catheters frequently develop cystitis. In addition, UTIs account for up to 40% of hospital-acquired infections, mostly associated with urinary catheters and mostly due to E. coli.[26] When prolonged catheterization is needed, prophylactic systemic antibiotics only prevent infections for about four days, after which there is no reduction in the infection rate as compared with controls and there is an increased risk of development of resistant organisms. Careful use of closed systems and aseptic techniques are the most important aspects of indwelling bladder catheterization.

The risk of infection following in and out catheterization in a healthy female is in the order of 1% but may be as high as 20% in hospital. The source of infection is mainly from periurethral spread of bacteria up the outside of the catheter. Infection may also be introduced by poor technique during insertion.

Table 10.10 *General indications for catheterization*

1. Collection of urine specimens when contamination is a problem
2. Urinary retention
3. Management of urinary incontinence
4. Fluid balance assessment in the acutely ill
5. Following certain surgery
6. Investigative procedures (e.g. measurement of residual volume)
7. Cystourethrography

Table 10.11 *Managing patients with catheters: important considerations*

Short-term catheterization
1. Is catheterization really necessary?
2. Precede with mid-stream urine (MSU) or catheter-specimen urine (CSU) to laboratory
3. Send CSU if pyrexia occurs while catheter *in situ*
4. Always remove as soon as possible
5. MSU 2–3 days following removal
6. Prophylactic antibiotics if history of rheumatic heart disease

Indwelling catheter
1. Is it really necessary?
2. Is it for patient or carer benefit?
3. Are additional 'infection risk factors' present?
4. Is intermittent self-catheterization an option?
5. If pyrexia occurs send CSU, blood culture
6. Mixed infection common
7. Discuss antibacterial management with local microbiologist
8. Monitor renal function
9. Abdominal X-ray at regular intervals to check for stone formation
10. Routine prophylactic antibiotics have no place in management
11. Routine bladder wash-outs of doubtful value. Instillation of chlorhexidine into bladder does not reduce the bacterial count
12. Change catheter regularly
13. Remove as soon as possible
14. Check MSU a few days following removal

Suprapubic catheterization carries less infection risk but is not usually carried out in the home or surgery but may be appropriate in a GP-run community hospital (Table 10.10).

If catheterization is contemplated in the practice setting the GP should bear in mind the points summarized in Table 10.11.

Diabetes

The widespread belief that diabetic patients have an increased susceptibility to UTI is not completely supported by research findings, and may have resulted from the fact that diabetics are subject to more frequent urine testing than non-diabetic patients. If, however, neurological problems affect correct bladder function then infection is more likely to supervene. This provides the basis for annual urine cultures as part of good care for diabetics within general practice. Acute or chronic urinary infection will, as is true for any infection, alter insulin requirements.

Pregnancy

Although the prevalence of asymptomatic bacteriuria in pregnant women is about 5%, similar to the rate in non-pregnant women, UTI is the most common medical complication of pregnancy. Within the 5% of women with bacteriuria in the first trimester it is likely that 1–2% will have had infection dating from childhood with the possibility of reflux nephropathy. Over 30% of women with reflux nephropathy present clinically for the first time during pregnancy.[27]

The complications of reflux nephropathy during pregnancy may be serious and include:

- Pre-eclampsia
- Hypertension
- Fetal loss
- Urinary infection
- Infected calculus
- Decreased renal function

In addition to the significant problems for pregnant women with reflux nephropathy, 30–40% of women with bacteriuria in early pregnancy will go on to develop acute infection later on. Screening for bacteriuria in early pregnancy is therefore an essential part of antenatal care and is conveniently arranged as part of the booking consultation. All pregnant women should be screened again in the third trimester. Both those GPs who undertake antenatal care and those who do not should ensure that the early pregnancy MSU result is recorded in the patient's record and that follow-up is undertaken for women with bacteriuria. The hospital cannot always be relied on to monitor this aspect of care unless the patient and her midwife are aware of the finding and its implications.

Acute urinary tract infection in pregnancy may present in several different ways:

- Pyrexia of unknown origin (PUO)
- Acute pyelonephritis
- Abdominal pain
- Hypertension
- Premature labour
- Urinary symptoms
- Vomiting

Treatment

If asymptomatic bacteriuria is detected it should be confirmed by repeating the MSU and consideration given to low dose antibiotic prophylaxis for the entire pregnancy. This decision will be taken with the consultant obstetrician and these women should probably receive shared care even if they are otherwise defined as low risk. Follow-up after pregnancy is important, starting with an MSU at the postnatal examination and referral if bacteriuria persists.

Women with a history of chronic pyelonephritis or reflux nephropathy (even if the urine is sterile) will require specialist supervision of their pregnancy. They are likely to be given low dose prophylactic antibiotics throughout the pregnancy. Acute pyelonephritis in pregnancy should be managed in hospital. All of these women will need careful monitoring and follow-up during and after pregnancy with regular checks of blood pressure and renal function.

Antibiotic treatment of UTI in pregnancy will depend on the results of the MSU. If blind initial therapy is deemed necessary it must take account of the sensitivities of local organisms and should ideally be discussed with the local microbiologist. Antibiotic dose must be reduced if renal impairment is present. Tetracyclines must not, of course, be given in pregnancy because of the effect on the developing teeth of the fetus.

Children

Urinary tract infections are common in childhood and account for 5–10% of febrile children admitted to hospital. Infection is by the ascending route, except in the newborn where haematogenous spread may occur from *E. coli* in the gut. In girls, infection is most frequently due to *E. coli*, whereas in boys *Proteus* is more likely. The diagnosis is important, but in very young children is not always considered due to the absence of symptoms relating to the urinary tract. The collection of urinary specimens in the very young adds to the difficulty.[28]

Although in adults infection may be confined mainly to the lower urinary tract, infants under 2 years may very rapidly develop an acute systemic illness with jaundice, fits, electrolyte imbalance septicaemia, and even acute renal failure. This is a particular risk in the neonate.

Studies of the incidence of UTI before the age of 10 years confirm the generally agreed incidence figures of 5% for girls and 1–2% for boys. Of children with UTIs approximately 11% of boys and 3% of girls develop the infection in the first decade. The commonest age for the first UTI is the first year of life. Infection is more likely in boys in the first month, but by the age of six months girls predominate. Unlike boys, re-infection in girls may occur many times right into adult life. The factors that predispose children to UTI are:

- Vesico-ureteric reflux

- Poor fluid intake

- Congenital abnormalities of urinary tract or adjacent structures

- Delayed bladder emptying: sometimes due to constipation

The long-term effects of undiagnosed UTI in children depend on the presence of vesico-ureteric reflux (VUR). Both infection and reflux are necessary for renal scarring to occur and in most cases the renal damage is already done by the age of 5 years.[29] In contrast, children with uncomplicated UTI have an excellent outlook and develop renal damage rarely. Children with VUR who are treated and investigated at their first infection have half the risk of renal scarring than children with VUR and recurrent infection.

The long-term consequences of renal scarring in early childhood are a decline in renal function up to 20 years after the scarring occurred: some of the women present in pregnancy. Others present with end-stage renal failure which is 100 times commoner in the this group than in the general population. Also, some 25% of children with renal scarring will develop hypertension during childhood demonstrating the overall importance of early diagnosis and investigation of childhood UTI.

General practitioners should always have the possibility of a UTI in mind when caring for sick children.[30] The non-specific presentation commonly includes unexplained fever, failure to thrive, abdominal pain, and diarrhoea and/or vomiting. However inconvenient, positive steps to obtain a urine sample (including referral) must be taken if these symptoms are not adequately explained by other causes. While the classical symptoms of UTI such as loin pain, haematuria, frequency, and dysuria, are associated with a higher likelihood of infection they are not diagnostic and UTI must be confirmed by culture. Nocturnal enuresis is more common in boys and is rarely associated with UTI; in contrast, nocturnal enuresis in girls is an important symptom of UTI. The onset of recent wetting or daytime wetting in either sex may indicate infection and should be investigated. Urinary microscopy and culture is mandatory in any situation where the diagnosis is suspected and should precede antibiotics. Even at the weekend a specimen should be taken, refrigerated, and sent for microbiology at the earliest possible moment. Children who are unwell should be referred or admitted to hospital as appropriate. It is important to identify the infecting organism. *Proteus*, in particular, has been associated with a high incidence of underlying kidney disease.

A clean-catch mid-stream urine specimen will be possible in the older child but 'bag' or suprapubic aspiration is necessary for infants.

Treatment

It is important that treatment is commenced as soon as possible particularly in infants. A sick infant should be admitted to hospital. If the child is managed at home, care will include good fluid intake, paracetamol, and appropriate antibiotic therapy to be commenced while awaiting the results of urine culture. This is a situation which is best discussed with the local microbiologist who will advise on local patterns of antibiotic resistance. The choice of antibiotic should be determined by culture and sensitivity as blind treatment of childhood UTI is not to be encouraged. The first-line antibiotics for oral treatment are usually

- trimethoprim
- co-amoxiclav
- nitrofurantoin
- nalidixic acid

Nitrofurantoin is best avoided in boys as they are more likely to have an infection due to *Proteus*. Both nitrofurantoin and nalidixic acid have poor tissue penetration and should be avoided if the patient has systemic symptoms. Cephalosporins should be held in reserve.

A first infection should be treated for 7–10 days and followed by prophylactic trimethoprim 1–2 mg per kg body weight per day until the urinary tract has been radiologically investigated. It is particularly important to carry on with an evening dose of trimethoprim if vesico-ureteric reflux is present. The blood pressure should be taken using a paediatric cuff and urine culture should be taken after 48 hours by which time the urine should be sterile. The MSU should subsequently be cultured at regular intervals which will depend on the results of any investigations and the long-term follow-up plans. The child should be followed up carefully. In particular, it is important that referral and long-term follow-up arrangements are explained to the parents so that they act to remind the practice if administrative arrangements should fail.

Indications for referral

It is essential that the GP carefully considers the need for specialist referral in every child where the diagnosis of UTI is suspected or documented. A child who is referred may well be subjected to unpleasant investigations with the attendant anxiety for the family only for no infection or abnormality to be found. Equally, failure to refer and follow-up may lead to irreparable renal damage and its appalling consequences. It is widely accepted in hospital practice that every child with a documented first UTI should be investigated, and as the incidence of abnormalities in primary care series that have been reported in the literature is not markedly different, a similar policy should be adopted within general practice. Guidelines from the Royal College of Physicians (RCP) underline this recommendation,[31] while studies within general practice have demonstrated a widespread failure to act in accordance with best practice thereby denying some children the investigation and follow-up they require.[32, 33] This is an issue that might well form the basis for a clinical audit within the practice, starting with the use of the RCP guidelines to set criteria for optimum management of UTI in children.

Although all children should be referred after the first documented UTI, absolute indications for specialist referral include:

1. Recurrent urinary tract infections.

2. Infection with associated fever

3. Failure to thrive.

4. Hypertension with urinary tract infection.

5. Enuresis + urinary tract infection.

6. Family history of congenital urinary tract abnormalities.

7. Persistent unusual organism or frequently changing organism.

8. *Proteus* infection (associated with high incidence of underlying abnormality).

Investigation

Although investigations will take place in hospital, the GP must be familiar with the likely sequence of events and be prepared to spend time talking to and reassuring parents.

Many specialists recommend a renal ultrasound, which is useful in detecting anatomical abnormalities and hydronephrosis, in conjunction with an IVU with limited exposure, which provides information on the renal size and structure as well as outlining the ureters and bladder. DMSA (dimercaptosuccinic acid) scanning is the most useful investigation for the identification of renal scars in a child under 2 years of age and its use has diminished the role of the IVU in investigating childhood UTI.[34] A micturating cystogram will demonstrate VUR and should be carried out in all children under 5 years, children over 4 years with recurrent infection, children with a positive family history of VUR, and those with other urinary tract abnormalities demonstrated during investigations. As new methods of radiological investigation evolve so local practice will change. The GP should be informed about the approach adopted locally, and check that it conforms to national guidelines. This then enables informed discussion with parents and sensible choice of place of referral.

Long-term follow-up

The GP has a central role in organizing the follow-up of children with UTI and the medical records and information to the parents should be designed to ensure that the process is not neglected. A shared approach with the paediatrician is ideal but should not allow a false sense of security to develop, particularly in deprived families who may not keep out-patient appointments. The records of children who have a history of UTI should be constructed to alert any clinician seeing the child subsequently so that the possibility is always considered. The parents should be instructed to refuse antibiotic therapy without prior urine culture being performed. Some children, principally those with VUR, will be on long-term, low dose prophylaxis and breakthrough infection in these children will need careful selection of an antibiotic if resistant infections are not to become a problem.

Children with normal intravenous urography and micturating cysto-urethrography should be followed up until the age of five, or until two years after the last infection, whichever is the latest. Children with reflux but with normal kidneys must be followed up until the reflux resolves. Patients with pyelonephritic scarring must be followed up indefinitely. Their renal function should be reviewed annually and a biannual blood pressure check and urine test for proteinuria recorded as the effects of renal scarring may not manifest for many years.

The elderly

The prevalence of urinary tract infection increases with age beyond 65 years, and is reported as high as 20% and 15% in women and men over 75 years, respectively (Table 10.12). While a UTI in an elderly person may present in the same way as in a younger individual non-specific presentations are common and the diagnosis should always be considered in the following circumstances:

- Frequency, dysuria, loin pain, haematuria
- Incontinence
- The smell of stale urine
- Confusion
- Weight loss

Table 10.12 *Predisposing factors to UTI in the elderly*

- Catheterization
- Decreased mobility
- Poor fluid intake
- Faecal incontinence
- Poor, or difficult to maintain, personal hygiene
- Ageing changes in bladder epithelium
- Long-standing infection
- Prostatitis
- Any outflow obstruction
- Drug-induced urinary retention (tricyclic antidepressants and anticholinergic drugs)
- Neurological bladder control problems

- Malaise
- Anaemia
- Pyrexia of Unknown Origin (PUO)
- Falls, dizziness

Treatment

Management can be difficult, particularly in the presence of a catheter. Care must be taken in selecting an antibiotic, as toxic effects are more pronounced and renal function will be reduced necessitating careful assessment of dosage and frequency. It is sensible to perform renal function tests at the same time as the initial MSU so that an informed choice can be made. Drug interactions are more likely as polypharmacy is common in this age group. Compliance may be difficult or impossible if the patient lives alone, and it is important to enlist the help of family, neighbours, or home helps in these circumstances. It is also important to discuss with the patient the need for a high fluid intake as many patient are so upset by incontinence that they restrict their drinking and make the infection worse. Help with bathing and incontinence aids will restore confidence and improve compliance but may need patient and regular visiting by GPs and nurses before it can be achieved.

Tetracycline should be avoided when there is evidence of impaired renal function; trimethoprim may accentuate any folate deficiency. Elderly women with recurrent infection are likely to benefit from intravaginal oestrogen cream.[35]

Asymptomatic bacteriuria in the absence of structural abnormality is common in the elderly and appears to be a relatively benign condition that does not impair renal function or shorten life.[36] It is not therefore a proper use of resources to screen for it, rather, the GP must treat symptomatic infection vigorously and consider the diagnosis in patients who present with non-specific symptoms. Patients with renal or outflow abnormalities or neurological lesions should have urine cultures performed periodically.

Indications for referral

Most patients can be managed in primary care but in the following circumstances specialist advice is indicated:

1. Toxic patients who cannot take oral therapy.

2. Ill patients who do not respond to antibiotics within 5 days.

3. Patients with complicated infection (e.g. structural abnormalities, outflow obstruction, calculi, analgesic nephropathy, chronic pyelonephritis).

Overall, the quality of management for elderly people with a urinary tract infection will be maintained by a rigorous adherence to the clinical standards described above in the face of difficult social circumstances. In other words, a challenge for the primary health care team and the bread-and-butter of general practice!

References

1. Royal College of General Practitioners, Office of Population Censuses and Surveys, Department of Health and Social Security *Morbidity Statistics from General Practice-Third National Study*, 1981–2. MB5. No.1. London: HMSO (1986)

2. *OPCS Morbidity statistics from general practice*. Fourth national study. Department of Health. London: HMSO (1996)

3. Maskell R. Antibacterial agents and urinary tract infection: a paradox. *Brit J Gen Pract* (1992) **42**: 137–40

4. Brumfitt W, Hamilton-Miller J M, Gillespie W A. The mysterious urethral syndrome: a rapid and accurate test for bacteruria would improve its management. *BMJ* (1991) **303**: 1–2

5. Lipsky B. Urinary tract infections in men. Epidemiology, pathophysiology, diagnosis and treatment. *Ann Intern Med* (1989) **110**: 138–50

6. Shaw K N, Hexter D, McGowan K *et al.* Clinical evaluation of a rapid screening test for urinary tract infections in children. *J Ped* (1990) **118**: 733–6

7. Ditchburn R, Ditchburn J. A study of microscopical and chemical tests for the rapid diagnosis of urinary tract infections in general practice. *Brit J Gen Pract* (1990) **40**: 406–8

8. Hurlbut H, Littenberg B. The diagnostic accuracy of rapid dipstick tests to predict urinary tract infection. *Am J Clin Pathol* (1991) **96**: 582–8

9. Baerheim A, Digranes A, Hunskaar S. Evaluation of urine sampling technique: bacterial contamination of samples from women students. *Brit J Gen Pract* (1992) **42**: 241–3

10. Arav-Boger R, Leibovici L, Danon Y. Urinary tract infections with low and high colony counts in young women. *Arch Intern Med* (1994) **119**: 454–60

11. Kunin C. A ten year study of bacteriuria in schoolgirls: final report of bacteriologic, urologic and epidemiologic findings. *J Infect Dis* (1970) **122**: 382–93

12. Jodal U. The natural history of bacteriuria in childhood. *Infect Dis Clin N Am* (1987) **1**: 713–29

13. Smellie J M. Reflections on 30 years of treating children with urinary tract infections. *J Urol* (1991) **146**: 665–8

14. Stamm W, Hooton T. Management of urinary tract infections in adults. *N Engl J Med* (1993) **329**: 1328–34

15. Wilkie M, Almond M, Marsh F. Diagnosis and management of urinary tract infection in adults. *BMJ* (1992) **305**: 1137–41

16. O'Dowd T C, Ribeiro C D, Munro J *et al.* Urethral syndrome: a self limiting illness. *BMJ* (1984) **288**: 1349–52

17. Jolleys J. Factors associated with regular episodes of dysuria among women in one rural general practice. *Brit J Gen Pract* (1991) **41**: 241–3

18. Gillespie W A, Henderson E P, Linton K B *et al*. Microbiology of the urethral (frequency and dysuria) syndrome. A controlled study with 5 year review. *Brit J Urol* (1989) **64**: 270–4

19. Nicolle L, Harding G, Preiksaitis J *et al*. The association of urinary tract infection with sexual intercourse. *J Infect Dis* (1982) **146**: 579–83

20. Hooton T, Hillier S, Johnson C *et al*. *E.coli* bacteriuria and contraceptive method. *JAMA* (1991) **265**: 64–9

21. Weidner W. Prostatitis; Diagnostic criteria. Classification of patients and recommendations for therapeutic trials. *Infection* (1992) **20**: S227–31

22. Weidner W, Schiefer H G. Chronic bacterial prostatitis: therapeutic experience with ciprofloxacin. *Infection* (1991) **19**: S165–S166

23. Shortliffe L, Sellers R, Schacter J. The characteristics of non-bacterial prostatitis: Search for an etiology. *J Urol* (1992) **148**: 1461–6

24. Nickel J, Sorenson R. Transurethral microwave thermotherapy of nonbacterial prostatitis and prostadynia: initial experience. *Urol* (1994) **44**: 458–60

25. Oriel J D. Male genital chlamydial trachomatis infections. *J Infect* (1992) **25**: 35–7

26. Bronsema D, Adams J, Pallares R. Secular trends in rates and etiology of nosocomial urinary tract infections at a university hospital. *J Urol* (1993) **150**: 414–16

27. McGladdery A, Aparcio S, Verrier-Jones *et al*. Outcome of pregnancy in an Oxford-Cardiff cohort of women with previous bacteriuria. *Quart J Med* (1992) **303**: 533–9

28. Austin N, Maskell R, Hallett R J. Diagnosis of urinary tract infection in children. *Lancet* (1992) **339**: 65.

29. Smellie J, Poulton A, Prescod N. Retospective study of children with renal scarring associated with reflux and urinary infection. *BMJ* (1994) **308**: 1193–6

30. South Bedfordshire Practitioners Group. Development of renal scars in children: missed opportunities in management. *BMJ* (1990) **301**: 1082–4

31. Guidelines for the management of acute urinary tract infection in childhood. Report of a working group of the Research Unit. Royal College of Physicians. *J Roy Coll Physicians London* (1991) **25**: 36–42

32. Jadresic L, Cartwright K, Cowie N *et al*. Investigation of urinary tract infection in childhood. *BMJ* (1993) **307**: 761–4

33. Gennery A.(letter) Urinary tract infection in childhood. *BMJ* (1993) **307**: 1141–2

34. Rickwood A, Carty H, McKendrick T *et al*. Current imaging of childhood urinary infections: prospective survey *BMJ* (1992) **304**: 663–5

35. Raz R, Stamm W. A controlled trial of intravaginal estriol in postmenopausal

women with recurrent urinary tract infections. *N Engl J Med* (1993) **329**: 753–803

36. Abrutyn E, Mossey J, Berlin J *et al.* Does asymptomatic bacteruria predict mortality and does antimicrobial treatment reduce mortality in elderly ambulatory women? *Ann Intern Med* (1994) **120**: 827–33

CHAPTER ELEVEN

Infections of the genital tract

The infections of men and women are considered separately in this chapter, with the infections of the male genital tract, which are inevitably associated with urinary tract infections, discussed in Chapter 10.

Genital infections in women

Genital infections in women present frequently in general practice and are responsible for a significant amount of morbidity.[1] While infections of the lower genital tract involve the vagina and cervix with different organisms principally responsible in each site, the endometrium and fallopian tubes are the usual sites in the upper genital tract.

Normal vaginal flora

It is recognized that there are characteristic and unique patterns of organisms within the vaginal flora which are affected by age, menstruation, pregnancy, contraception, and sexual activity.[2] In addition, the differences in the pH and epithelium of the vagina and the endocervix make it likely that there are ecological niches within the lower genital tract which harbour distinctive populations of organisms. The organisms which are isolated most commonly are lactobacilli (usually the most prevalent), diphtheroidal forms including *Gardnerella vaginalis*, *Staphylococcus epidermidis*, and alpha and non-haemolytic streptococci. Most studies have found that nearly all healthy premenopausal women harbour some species of anaerobic bacteria. After the menopause, facultative lactobacilli can be cultured from 65% of women but they do not predominate on Gram-stained smears.

Diagnosis

The diagnosis of genital infections in general practice is of great importance because of the misery that undiagnosed or inadequately treated infection can bring.[3,4] Women may suffer chronic pelvic infection with pain and menstrual disturbances, an increased risk of an ectopic pregnancy or infertility, or harm to unborn children if chlamydial and gonococcal infections remain undetected. The odour associated with bacterial vaginosis and trichomoniasis may lead to an avoidance of sexual and social contact and the itching of recurrent *Candida* may be hard to endure. Genital infections require the identification of the causative organism(s) as the basis for management. The doctor then has responsibility to ensure correct management, patient follow-up, and treatment of sexual partners, if relevant. The process of diagnosis must not, however, harm the patient (e.g. by clumsy inquiry about the possibility of sexual transmission). Presentations of genital infections form a rich source for teaching and learning about consultation skills, particularly if standardized patients trained to give feedback are used as a resource.

General practitioners, like many other doctors, are often inhibited in discussing sexual matters with their patients. We frequently assume that if a patient thinks she might have a sexually transmitted disease she will attend a genitourinary medicine clinic. In fact women often bring their unspoken fears to the surgery. They may present in family planning or well-woman sessions and request a cervical smear. Doctors and nurses in these settings commonly collude with this behaviour and avoid discussing sexual lifestyle or anxieties. The patient may leave the consultation after being told her examination is normal, falsely reassured that she does not have a genital infection.[5] Women presenting to the GP with a new episode of vaginal discharge may also agree with the doctor that 'it's thrush again' and be happy to receive yet another prescription without discussion of other possibilities or a vaginal examination. While the patient may well be right about the nature of the problem, care should be taken to establish the diagnosis both by discussion of risk factors for a sexually transmitted infection, a careful history, and a vaginal examination which includes an inspection of the cervix. In any case, it is important to discover if the patient is expecting to be examined before deciding not to. If this standard of care cannot be offered within the practice then the woman should be referred to a genitourinary (GU) clinic. Some GU specialists believe that all women with genital infections should be referred to them but this demonstrates a profound misunderstanding of the work of a GP. Many women resist referral and the large numbers of women presenting with vaginitis alone would make it impractical to refer them all. If, however, care is to be practice-based the standards must be high and reflect a dialogue between clinicians locally which defines a proper role for all of the clinical settings in which the women may present.

A further dimension to the management of women with vaginal discharge is that 30% have normal vaginal flora.[6] These women will also need an opportunity to discuss alternative explanations such as the normal variation in the amount of discharge with the menstrual cycle or sexual activity.[7]

Lower genital tract infections

Vaginitis and cervicitis

Clinical features

Lower genital tract infections commonly cause vaginal discharge, and about 8% of women aged 16–45 registered with a GP present with a new episode

Table 11.1 *Complications of untreated cervicitis*

---

1. Ascending intralumenal spread of pathogenic organisms resulting in upper genital tract infection
2. Ascending infection during pregnancy leading to chorioamnionitis, premature rupture of the membranes, and infection
3. The possible promotion of cervical intra-epithelial neoplasia

---

each year.[8] Although vaginitis is usually caused by yeast infections (*Candida* spp.), trichomoniasis, or bacterial vaginosis, rarer causes include an ulcerative vaginitis resulting from a forgotten tampon or cervical cap. The vaginal discharge caused by different organisms may be typical and associated with symptoms and signs said to be characteristic, but frequently, symptoms are non-specific or the patient may be uncomplaining and the diagnosis made during screening. Infections of the cervix are another common cause of vaginal discharge in general practice, either alone or in association with vaginitis.[2]

Although *Candida albicans* and *Trichomonas vaginalis* can both cause exocervicitis, the major infectious causes of cervicitis are *Chlamydia trachomatis*, *Neisseria gonorrhoea*, and herpes simplex virus. Frequently, more than one of these organisms may be present in one patient. The diagnosis and treatment of cervicitis is important as it may result in the three types of complications shown in Table 11.1.

Table 11.2 shows the ideal clinical history and examination for women with a new episode of vaginal discharge presenting to the GP, derived from a review of the literature on upper and lower genital tract infections. A GP who is in possession of this information about the patient will be in a good position to weigh up the probabilities in relation to the presence of infection with one or more pathogens and the need for further investigation or referral.

Vaginal discharge in children, pregnancy, and older women. Occasionally, children present with a vaginal discharge and vulvitis. While the commonest reason is threadworms or, infrequently, a vaginal foreign body, this is a difficult consultation as the possibility of sexual abuse must always be considered and ruled out. If there is any doubt about how to manage the situation it would be appropriate to discuss the case with the local community paediatrician.[10]

While vaginal discharge is a common feature of normal pregnancy genital infections also occur, some of which (chlamydia, gonorrhoea, syphilis, herpes simplex) have major implications for the unborn child. Group B beta-haemolytic streptococci are also associated with vaginal discharge and are implicated in neonatal infection of babies born to mothers who harbour the organism during late pregnancy.[11]

Vaginal symptoms are also prevalent in postmenopausal women who may

Table 11.2 *The ideal clinical history and examination for women aged 16–55 presenting with a new episode of vaginal discharge*

Demography
Age
Ethnic group

Obstetric, sexual, and contraceptive history
Contraceptive method
Sexual activity during the last year
Lifetime number of partners
New sexual partner during past 3/12 months
Sexually transmitted disease
(STD) clinic contact
Last menstrual period
Parity
Primary infertility
Secondary infertility

Medication
Antibiotics last 3/12 months

Symptoms
Urinary frequency
Vulval or perineal pain
Vulval soreness or itch
Offensive vaginal discharge
Previous episode of discharge during last year

Signs
Vulval pustules or papules
Vulval oedema or redness
Vaginal odour
Excess discharge
Vaginal plaques or clumps
Adherent discharge
Bloodstained discharge
Cervical polyp
Cervix bleeds on contact
Vaginal pH

Note. Always consider whether the patient should be referred to a genitourinary physician.

experience all of the above infections. However, thinning of the vaginal epithelium due to oestrogen withdrawal leads to atrophic vaginitis which should be differentiated from the usual forms of infection. This is because the management is different and is principally directed towards restoring a healthy vagina through local or systemic hormone replacement.

Investigations

For many years, the investigation of vaginitis in general practice was limited to the taking of a high vaginal swab, sometimes obtained without the use of a bivalve speculum to ensure proper sampling of any discharge. While swabs were sometimes smeared on to a plain glass slide and examined down a microscope and sent dry or in transport medium to the laboratory, the majority of women were managed on the basis of symptoms alone. With the advent of better training in gynaecology and contraception, and increased patient expectations and awareness, management has changed. The investigation of genital infections requires every GP to be proficient in bimanual vaginal examination, including visualization of the cervix, and have the ability to take cervical and vaginal swabs and smears, which are then stored and transported appropriately.

Candida vulvo-vaginitis [12]

Candida infections have been reported in almost every human tissue except hair. The commonest sites are in the mouth and vagina where the lesions are known as 'thrush'. The origins of this term are unknown but the frequency of the condition is demonstrated by the fact that there are common words for it in most languages. *Candida* infections have been recognized since antiquity and are referred to in the writings of Hippocrates and Galen: the first attributable description of vaginal candidosis was reported in the *Lancet* in 1849 by J.S. Wilkinson.

Candida albicans is the principal cause of vaginitis in 30% of new cases seen in general practice. The organism is harboured by 15–20% of asymptomatic women, but when vaginitis is present, it is characterized by intense vulvo-vaginal itching, vulval oedema and fissuring, external dysuria, and a cheesy, white vaginal discharge which forms plaques on the reddened vaginal wall. The infection is commonly seen in pregnancy and may be the initial presentation of diabetes mellitus

Epidemiology

It is frequently stated that the incidence of all types of *Candida* infections has risen since the advent of antibiotics and recent increases in the number of immunocompromised individuals in the general population. Reliable data are not available in many countries and the situation is complicated by the effect of improved methods of diagnosis and increased interest in the condition. It is likely that the incidence is increasing; in any event, *Candida* infections will always rise when the proportion of the population that is debilitated by chronic disease rises. Studies which report the incidence of *Candida* vulvo-vaginitis, basing the diagnosis on both positive clinical and microbiological findings, have found the prevalence to be about 5–10%. Most of these studies were in GU clinics or gynaecological out-patient settings. In 1987, the incidence in four East London general practices amongst women aged 16–45 years with vaginal discharge and proven microbiological infection was 27%.

Aetiology

In clinical practice, the diagnosis of candidal vulvo-vaginitis may be based on a range of information: from a typical history without examination through to the finding that an asymptomatic woman harbours *C. albicans* in her vaginal flora. Both of these approaches may lead to a false positive diagnosis of a *Candida* infection: the problem may be due to a different and more serious cause in the first example, and *C. albicans* may be present as a vaginal commensal in the second. Recent evidence would suggest that women with infection, as opposed to healthy carriers, harbour greater numbers of the organism in their vaginal flora. In general practice it is better to define the infection as present if the woman has symptoms and signs and the organism is isolated from the vaginal flora.

The genus *Candida* comprises more than 150 species of yeasts of which the medically significant are in the a minority. The yeasts which are known to be principally responsible for human candidosis have essentially been found in association with humans and other mammals. It is unusual to isolate *C. albicans* from samples of water, soil, or plants. In contrast, it is frequently found in the hospital setting and the evidence suggests that carriers of *C. albicans* often contaminate their immediate surroundings but that the contamination does not spread very far. The organism survives on toothbrushes, underclothes laundered at temperatures below 50°C, and in cosmetics; and it seems likely that intimate contact with a carrier can result in spread.

Despite the wide occurrence of the yeasts which cause candidosis the primary source of the organisms which cause human disease is the endogenous flora of the affected individual. *Candida* species occur commonly as commensals in the gut, and less frequently in other sites. Few of the many studies of normal women record a prevalence of vaginal yeast carriage as greater than 20%; the isolation rate for *Candida* species amongst 324 healthy asymptomatic women in a study carried out by the author was 21%. The rate of isolation of *Candida* species from the skin of the penis is much lower (about 5–10%), except in the partners of women with vaginal thrush, where it rises to approach 30%. Studies which have reported the relative frequencies of yeast species in the vaginal flora of uncomplaining women and women with vaginitis have found that, overall, *C. albicans* was isolated in 69% and 84%, respectively. The only other species commonly found in vaginal samples were *Candida tropicalis* and *Candida glabrata*.

In his comprehensive monograph *Candida and candidosis*, Odds states that

'*Candida* species are strictly opportunistic pathogens that rarely or never cause clinically important disease in a host with intact antimicrobial defences'.[12] He emphasizes that *any* impairment of any of the body defences against microbial attack can compromise the host's ability to fight infection. In the case of vulvo-vaginitis the degree of host impairment may be very limited, and be local to the affected area rather than a general problem.

The fact that *C. albicans* is harboured in low concentrations by up to 20% of asymptomatic sexually active women, leads some authors to regard it as a vaginal commensal as well as a pathogen. Others hold the view that in the vagina, as elsewhere, the local host resistance to microbial attack must be impaired even in apparently healthy women. The nature of the local change is still not clear, although the frequently quoted explanation involving the breakdown of glycogen by *Lactobacillus* species with an overgrowth of vaginal yeast at the lower vaginal pH is no longer believed to be relevant to vaginal candidosis. Recent work has suggested that a temporary deficiency in the vaginal T-lymphocyte responses may be linked to acute infection but further evidence is needed.

Only two factors have been definitely shown to predispose a woman to vaginal thrush, namely pregnancy and diabetes. The use of oral hormonal contraceptives,[13] antibiotics, and changes in vaginal pH have not been shown to be related to the onset of the condition when the evidence is reviewed. Further work in general practice is needed to support the widely held view that many women experience a relapse after taking antibiotics.

The principal reservoir of the *Candida* species that invade the vagina is believed to be the gastrointestinal tract. Sexual transmission does occur but studies indicate that this is likely to be only to a maximum of 40% of infected women and is usually of a much lower order.

Clinical features

Most reviews of vaginal thrush contain similar descriptions of the clinical features associated with the condition. The woman experiences an increased vaginal discharge, usually thick, white and cheesy, associated with intense itching. She may also experience pain and burning on passing urine and if intercourse is attempted. The most consistent finding on examination is oedema and erythema of the labia minora, introitus, and lower third of the vagina. The lesions in the vagina are analogous to those seen in oral thrush and take the form of white plaques on the epithelium of the vulva, vagina, and cervix.

Diagnosis and investigations

Symptoms and signs in women with vaginitis are not specific for the presence of infection, let alone a specific organism. The patient should not be given a diagnosis of 'thrush' unless the clinical picture is consistent with the disease and yeasts have been shown to be present in her vaginal flora. A high vaginal swab should be taken at the start of each new episode and sent in transport medium to the local lab.

Treatment

Women presenting with an acute *Candida* vulvo-vaginitis are in some distress and it is reasonable to begin therapy while awaiting the result of the vaginal swab which should always be taken in a new episode. The infection is usually treated by antifungal cream or pessories inserted high into the vagina. There are a wide range of formulations used in this condition and several dosage schedules. The most widely used drugs are from the imidazole group (e.g. clotrimazole, econazole) and are increasingly used in short, high dose regimes which have been shown to be effective in clinical trials. More recently, orally active anti-fungal agents, such as fluconazole, have been introduced for women with thrush, but should not be used routinely as a first line as they are expensive and may lead to gastrointestinal side-effects. As with all new drugs, careful monitoring of cure rates and side-effects is mandatory and the drug should not be used as a first-line treatment until greater experience determines its use in the primary care setting. Ketoconazole should not be used in general practice because of reports of liver toxicity. Nystatin has been used for vaginal candidosis for many years. It is cheap but it is unpleasant to use and the cure rate is about 75–80% compared with 85–90% for the imidazoles.

All of the anti-*Candida* regimes have a failure rate of about 15–20% when estimated by the presence of the organism in the vaginal flora between one and three months after therapy. Not all of these women will be symptomatic and the infection is best regarded as recurrent when the patient has both physical and microbiological evidence of infection. Alternative regimes using intravaginal pessaries and creams are a matter of personal preference by the patient, who usually requests the treatment that worked last time!

Some imidazoles are now available without prescription enabling women with recurrent thrush to treat themselves. This welcome shift of responsibility to the patient carries with it the worry that some women with other genital infections may delay or avoid diagnosis and treatment. The answer lies in patient education, appropriate leaflets with the preparation, and available community pharmacists who can advise women sensitively.[14]

Prevention

All GPs will know women whose lives are made miserable by recurrent vaginal thrush. The definition of this condition is the occurrence of three or four clinically *and* microbiologically proven attacks in a year despite compliance with adequate therapy. A great deal of research has been directed at detecting differences between these women and those who do not have a recurrence. It seems likely that the main source of the recurrence is due to the endogenous vaginal yeasts rather than re-infection from external sources such as the gut or a sexual partner. The most likely reason that some women suffer a recurrence is a difference in their specific immune status.[15] Several authors have raised the possibility of a local allergic reaction to the presence of the yeast, and although others have found a reduction in the plasma zinc levels in these women, this hypothesis remains unproven.[16] Other studies have reported the presence of defects in cell-mediated immune responses in women with recurrent *Candida* vaginitis. The basis for this miserable complaint is still far from clear and although the GP can reassure the patient that major research efforts are taking place, her main hope of preventing a relapse is careful compliance with therapy.

Recurrent 'thrush' must be confirmed by the presence of *C. albicans* as many of these women have other infections. Treatment of the sexual partner with cream for his penis may improve cure in refractory cases. While there is a debate about the role of antibiotics, susceptible women receiving penicillin, tetracyclines, and cephalosporins should receive simultaneous antifungal therapy. In intractable cases, monthly treatment with a single pessary of clotrimazole 500 mg between days 7–11 of the menstrual cycle reduces recurrences. Some women find antihistamines helpful and others gain relief from a prostaglandin inhibiter such as ibuprofen.[17]

Bacterial vaginosis[18]

Bacterial vaginosis was first described in the 1950s when Gardner and Dukes reported a clinical syndrome which comprised a thin, grey adherent vaginal discharge, a vaginal pH greater than 4.5, a fishy odour, and the presence of 'clue cells' on examination of a wet mount of the discharge. (Clue cells are vaginal epithelial cells coated with vaginal coccobacillary organisms.) They asserted that *Haemophilis vaginalis* was the organism responsible; eventually the name of the organism was changed to *G. vaginalis* and the condition previously known as non-specific vaginitis became Gardnerella-associated vaginosis. The word 'vaginosis' was adopted because, unlike other forms of vaginitis, the increased vaginal discharge is not associated with inflammation of the vaginal walls. The condition has been widely researched and is now recognized as resulting from complex changes in the vaginal flora rather than from the presence of *Gardnerella vaginalis* alone. The modern name for the syndrome is bacterial vaginosis (BV).[19]

BV is characterized by vaginal overgrowth with *G. vaginalis*, anaerobic bacteria (*Mobilluncus* spp., *Bacteroides* spp.), and *Mycoplasma hominis* and the relative absence of lactobacilli. The reasons for the changes in the vaginal flora are not yet understood, although risk factors include the presence of an intra-uterine contraceptive device, and more than one sexual partner in the month before diagnosis. There are decreased rates in monogamous couples. The evidence for sexual transmission is conflicting.

Epidemiology

The syndrome is present in 15 – 25% of women presenting with vaginal discharge in general practice and has been reported to have a prevalence of between 15% and 33% in several Swedish studies within sexually transmitted disease (STD) clinic populations. It continues to be the leading form of vaginal infection in the USA, with different incidence rates reported from a variety of settings: family planning clinics 23–29%, private physician clinics 16%, and gynaecology clinics 15–23%. The natural history of the condition is not well documented although some studies have reported a spontaneous remission of the signs of bacterial vaginosis in 25–43% of adults.

Clinical features

Bacterial vaginosis is characterized by an offensive vaginal discharge, the smell being particularly strong after intercourse because of the release of amines by the action of seminal fluid on vaginal secretions. Many women are distressed and embarrassed by the odour which may be causing problems within their sexual relationship.

Clinical examination reveals a homogeneous, grey, uniformly adherent discharge. The vaginal pH is raised (5 or above) and addition of 10% potassium hydroxide to the discharge releases a fishy smell. Clue cells are present on the Gram-stained smear. The diagnosis is essentially a clinical one and is made if any three of the above criteria are present.

Diagnosis and investigations

The diagnosis of BV is based on the criteria described above: culture is not required for confirmation although it is advisable as other causes of vaginitis may coexist. The finding of G. vaginalis in the absence of the clinical picture is not a basis for diagnosing bacterial vaginosis. Regular measurement of the vaginal pH in women with a new complaint of vaginal discharge gives useful information; it is normally about 4.5 and is raised to between 5 and 7 in women with bacterial vaginosis and T. vaginalis.

Treatment

Symptomatic women require treatment and many authorities also rec-ommend treatment for asymptomatic women who are about to undergo gynaecological procedures such as intra-uterine devices insertion which breach the cervical barrier. The treatment of bacterial vaginosis in pregnancy is controversial but if a woman has a history of premature labour, or has premature rupture of the membranes then the risks from bacterial vaginosis are materially increased. The treatment of BV is metronidazole 400 mg orally twice daily for 7 days. Shorter and once-only regimes give lower cure rates. The manufacturers recommend that high dose regimes should not be used in pregnancy and that all patients taking the drug should avoid alcohol. As recurrent clinical disease is a major problem (up to 80% within 9 months of therapy) it would seem reasonable to treat sexual partners in refractory cases after good compliance with therapy. More recently, 2% clindamycin vaginal cream nightly for one week has been recommended. This is an effective but expensive alternative to metronidazole.

Complications and prognosis

Although bacterial vaginosis does not always cause symptoms it is associated with serious sequelae in some women. There have been many reports of an association with pelvic inflammatory disease, and the onset of premature labour, and chorioamnionitis.

Prevention

Proof of sexual transmission is still lacking although sexual transmission of associated microorganisms does occur. Prevention is therefore directed at preventing complications by adequate therapy, especially in those women about to give birth or undergo gynaecological interventions when pelvic inflammatory disease becomes a risk.

Trichomonas vaginitis

Epidemiology

The infection is not notifiable and many reports are from STD clinics which give a false picture of prevalence. The infection is relatively common with some reports suggesting that 1 in 5 sexually active women will be affected during their lifetimes. The prevalence in general practice populations is below 5%. Although the age of peak incidence is 16–35 there is a high susceptibility in postmenopausal women. Indeed, the symptoms often occur when there is a natural increase in vaginal pH at the menopause. An analysis of the pattern of visits to 2100 primary care physicians in the US has shown a 40% decrease in *T. vaginitis* between 1966 and 1988, reflecting trends reported world-wide.

Aetiology

Trichomonas vaginalis is a flagellated protozoan with optimal growth and motility at pH 5.5–6.5 (higher than the normal vaginal pH), which is almost always sexually transmitted. However, spread by towels used to wipe the genitalia has been documented among institutionalized populations. It is one of the commonest causes of vaginitis world-wide and is now universally accepted to be a pathogen.

Clinical features

The infection involves squamous and not columnar epithelium and is therefore not involved in infections above the cervix. The urethra and Skene's glands are infected in 90% of cases and the organism may persist in these sites for years. Symptoms and signs are very variable, but include a profuse, frothy, offensive discharge, and intense pruritis. On examination, the vaginal walls and the exocervix are erythematous and in severe cases cervical punctuate haemorrhages may be present. This unusual clinical sign (a 'strawberry' cervix) occurs in only 2–3% of patients but is specific for trichomoniasis when present. The vaginal pH is raised above and is characteristically higher than that found in bacterial vaginosis. Up to 50% of women who harbour *T. vaginalis* are asymptomatic, although 30% of these women become symptomatic within six months lending support to the contention that asymptomatic women and their sexual partners should be treated.

Diagnosis and investigations

Although the diagnosis is most easily made by visualizing the motility of unstained organisms in a wet preparation examined rapidly on a slide or as a hanging drop, evaluation has shown the method to be insensitive and most general practices do not use it. When performed, direct examination of vaginal discharge shows pus cells interspersed with the pear-shaped nucleated and flagellated protozoans. Cervical cytology is a less specific method and direct staining of smears with monoclonal antibodies is sensitive but costly. In practice, swabs may be taken from the cervix and high vagina and sent in Stewart's medium to the laboratory for examination.

Treatment

Systemic therapy is better than local applications and the preferred treatment is with a single dose of oral metronidazole (2 g). Alternative regimes can be given but in all cases the patient should avoid alcohol. High dose regimes should not be used in pregnancy and it is better to delay any treatment until after the first trimester. A second dose usually deals with those infections that fail to respond initially.

As T. *vaginalis* is usually sexually transmitted the discussion with the patient requires tact. Sexual partners should be treated and if the man is not a patient of the practice the diagnosis should be given to the woman in writing so that he can consult his own doctor. As the organism can be present for many years its presence does not necessarily imply recent intercourse with a different sexual partner. However, the presence of the infection does increase the likelihood of other STDs and consideration should be given to screening the woman, with her consent, for gonorrhoea and chlamydia.

Prevention

The infection is prevented by monogamy and compliance with therapy by the patient and her sexual partner(s).

Chlamydial cervicitis

Epidemiology

Chlamydial genital infections are the most common sexually acquired infections in the UK. The prevalence has been variously reported as 3–5% in asymptomatic women to 20% in women seen in STD clinics. In inner city general practice, 8% of women seen for vaginal examination for any reason harboured the organism.[20,21] There are some indicators of high risk which have been reported in both American and European studies: these women are younger, with a recent change of sexual partner (who may himself have urethral symptoms), use the combined oral contraceptive pill, and are of non-white race. However, most of the studies of female chlamydial infections have been carried out in inner city clinic populations or student health facilities. A stereotyped and stigmatizing picture of the woman likely to harbour *C. trachomatis* may have arisen as a result which may in turn lead to underdiagnosis in other populations with different socioeconomic characteristics. The infection is sexually acquired and sex is a universal human activity.

Aetiology

The frequency of non-specific or non-gonococcal cervicitis, like gonorrhoea itself, has shown a marked increase in the last two decades; *Chlamydia trachomatis* has emerged as the most important cause. The genus *Chlamydia* is divided into three species: (1) *C. trachomatis*; (2) *C. psittaci*, the cause of psittacosis; and (3) *C. pneumoniae*, a recently recognized respiratory pathogen. Different groups of serovars of *C. trachomatis* are found in non-gonococcal cervicitis and urethritis (serovars D–K), in lymphogranuloma venereum (LGV) (serovar L), and in endemic trachoma (serovars A–C). These organisms are obligate intracellular parasites and their cultivation in tissue culture has enabled their importance to be better defined. Strains of *C. trachomatis* have been isolated from many female patients with chronic pelvic sepsis and are an important cause of infertility. Asymptomatic women provide a reservoir of infection, transmitting the disease to their sexual partners and to their neonates, resulting in neonatal ophthalmia and pneumonia.[22]

Clinical features

Chlamydia trachomatis infects the columnar epithelium of the endocervix. Numerous studies have stressed the non-specific nature of the symptoms and signs associated with *Chlamydia* infection and the large number of silent infections which are found later during the investigation of chronic pelvic pain or infertility. Genital symptoms are unhelpful, although the woman may complain of increased discharge. Chlamydial cervicitis is associated with a mucopurulent cervical discharge, cervical friability, and hypertrophic ectopy (an area of ectopy which is oedematous). In some women this leads to irregular bleeding and bleeding after intercourse.

Investigations

Clinical examination alone is unreliable for diagnosis which should be confirmed by the methods locally available. Culture, generally considered the most sensitive and specific test and hence the 'gold standard', is expensive and time-consuming and requires laboratory expertise. Culture methods may be insensitive if the specimens are of poor quality (the sample must include infected endocervical cells) or the transport arrangements inadequate.[23] Non-culture methods rely on antigen detection and there are two general approaches. (1) The direct immunofluorescence test (DIF test) uses fluorescein-conjugated monoclonal antibodies to detect chlamydial elementary bodies in a smear prepared from an endocervical specimen. The performance of the DIF test in intermediate prevalence populations shows a sensitivity which ranges between 61% and 96%, and a specificity range of 94–99%. The sensitivity of the test is largely determined by the skill of the technician in staining and examining the specimen and is usually high in research settings. This is the only method that allows direct evaluation of the quality of the clinical specimen. (2) The alternative approach relies on the detection of chlamydial antigen eluted from an endocervical swab and measured by enzyme-linked immunoassay methods (EIA test). In an intermediate prevalence population the test has a sensitivity range of 60–96% and a specificity range of 93–98%. Research aimed at developing tests based on the polymerase chain reaction (PCR) is providing another approach to diagnosis. This method is highly sensitive but is still prone to false positives.[24]

The laboratory diagnosis of female genital chlamydial infections is a difficult area for GPs, many of whom now realize the disastrous effect on family life that an untreated infection can have. Accuracy in diagnosis is essential: the implications of a false positive or false negative test are immense as the condition is sexually transmitted and can cause permanent damage to health and fertility. This situation requires the highest skills of the GP, namely, the ability to apply an understanding of clinical epidemiology to the care of the individual and her family, combined with rigorous attention to the underlying ethical issues. The GP must therefore exercise extreme care in using chlamydia antigen detection tests which may give false positive or false negative results. The first priority is to listen to the patient and encourage her to express her anxieties and problems. A frank and sensitive discussion of her sexual behaviour and any difficulties in her relationships which may point to risky behaviour on her part, or that of her current or recent sexual partner(s) will build trust and enable the GP to estimate whether she is likely to belong to a higher or lower prevalence population. If the doctor and patient together agree that there is a possibility of a chlamydial infection and the patient is prepared for a positive test result then it is reasonable to use an EIA or DIF test. If, however, the patient does not believe that a positive result is possible the physician should explain that a negative result is reliable but that a positive result indicates only an increased chance of infection which must be confirmed. It is irresponsible practice to use a DIF or EIA test for *Chlamydia* diagnosis or screening unless these uncertainties have been fully explored with the patient first.

The results of tests for any sexually transmitted disease should be discussed in the context of prevention, health promotion, and enhancing the patient's self-esteem and autonomy: giving information but also listening carefully to the meaning of a positive test for that particular patient. If this is achieved then the patient will have a good understanding of the effects of an untreated infection and will be more likely to comply with therapy, avoid intercourse with infected partners, and ensure that partners receive treatment if needed. All women with genital chlamydial infections should be followed up and many GPs prefer to refer them to the GU physician for screening for other STDs and partner notification. Some patients, particularly women, decline referral. It is an important part of the management of the infection that GPs work with local GU specialists, to reduce the stigma of referrals.

Treatment

Chlamydial cervicitis is treated with doxycycline 200 mg daily for 7 days, or with erythromycin stearate 500 mg 4 times a day for 7 days. Uncomplicated genital chlamydial infections are as effectively treated by a single oral dose of 1 g azithromycin with the great advantage that a single dose regime can bring.[25]

Prevention

The infection is prevented by avoiding sex with infected individuals and by follow-up and treatment of sexual partners. There has been considerable debate about screening for genital chlamydia in some populations. It seems reasonable to exclude the infection in women about to undergo abortion,[26] IUCD insertion,[25] and in pregnancy. The prevalence among low–risk asymptomatic groups is of the order of 3% and the decision to screen or not must take into account economics and the sensitivity and specificity of the screening tests. It is sobering to read that genital and associated chlamydial infections and their complications presently cost Britain £50 million a year for diagnosis and management, whereas in Sweden, where they have a co-ordinated approach to education and diagnosis, the incidence of the infection has fallen dramatically.[22,27] The availability of tests based on urine examination will make the introduction of a UK screening programme possible.

Lymphogranuloma venereum

This condition is caused by the L-1, L-2, and L-3 serovars of *C. trachomatis*. Most cases arise in subtropical and tropical countries but it may be seen in the West in patients who have had intercourse while travelling abroad, or in immigrants. The primary endocervical lesion in women is painless and is followed by regional adenitis, constitutional symptoms follow after 1–2 more weeks. In women and homosexual men, the perirectal glands suppurate and may be associated with painful proctitis and bloody anal discharge. Unless treated, the inflammation becomes chronic leading to fibrosis and lymphatic obstruction. Rectal strictures, sometimes with the formation of perirectal abscesses and fistulas, and elephantiasis of the genitalia may follow.

Gonorrhoea

Epidemiology

A steady increase in the incidence of gonorrhoea was recorded between 1955 and 1985 in all countries that kept records. Although the number of new cases has declined since the AIDS epidemic led to changes in sexual behaviour, gonorrhoea remains one of the major uncontrolled epidemics of infectious disease. Studies in UK inner city general practice show the organism to be present in the cervix in about 1 in 200 women presenting with a new episode of vaginal discharge.[22] In Western Africa it accounts for one in three female surgical admissions.

Aetiology

Neisseria gonorrhoeae is a Gram-negative intracellular diplococcus which causes symptomatic, asymptomatic, and complicated infection of several anatomical sites in men and women. The organism is always sexually transmitted in adults; gonococcal ophthalmia neonatorum is acquired from the mother's birth canal. In women, the primary site of infection is the endocervix although the anorectal mucosa, the urethra, Skene's glands, and Bartholin's glands are also commonly involved.

Clinical features

Symptoms occur from 2 to 5 days after infection and comprise vaginal discharge, dysuria, intermenstrual bleeding, and menorrhagia which may occur in any combination and vary from very mild, to acute and severe. Some women may have a normal cervix on examination, in others, the signs of cervicitis are a mucopurulent discharge, cervical bleeding, and erythema. While subclinical infection has been widely recognized in up to 50% of women it is now clear that 5–25% of infected men are also asymptomatic. These individuals are the major source of disease transmission. The infection frequently coexists with the other sexually transmitted pathogens, *C. trachomatis* and *T. vaginalis*.

Investigations

The majority of patients with gonorrhoea should be referred to the genitourinary clinic for investigation. However, all GPs sometimes find themselves managing patients, particularly women, who refuse to be referred. Cervical, urethral, and anal swabs should be taken the situation having first been discussed with the STD physician.

Treatment

The development of antibiotic resistance in *N. gonorrhoeae* has complicated the treatment of gonorrhoea. Resistance to sulphonamides emerged rapidly after their introduction, and susceptibility to penicllin has decreased, leading to the need for increasing doses in treatment. The emergence of highly penicillin-resistant strains since 1976 created further problems. Some of these strains produce a penicillinase (beta-lactamase); in others the resistance is chromosomally mediated and is not due to beta-lactamase production. In general, the selection of therapy depends upon the site of infection, any history of penicillin allergy, and the prevalence of penicillin-resistant strains in the community where the infection was acquired. For uncomplicated gonococcal urethritis, cervicitis, or rectal infection, therapy is usually undertaken with a single dose regimen. If the organism is not resistant to penicillin either oral amoxicillin (3 g) with probenecid, or intramuscular procaine penicillin (2.88

g) with probenecid may be used. Otherwise, the recommended therapy is intramuscular ceftriaxone (25 mg) or spectinomycin (2 g), either of which will deal with penicillinase-producing strains. The treatment of penicillin-resistant infections should not normally be undertaken in general practice. If special circumstances require it, specialist advice should be sought.

Prevention

The prevention of gonorrhoea is that of any sexually transmitted infection: avoidance of infected partners, compliance with therapy, and follow-up and treatment of sexual partners.

Syphilis

Syphilis has become an uncommon disease in women: in 1991 and 1992 clinics in England and Wales reported 220 cases of infectious syphilis in women and 5 cases of congenital syphilis in children under 2 years old.

Pathology and clinical features

Syphilis is caused by the spirochaete *Treponema pallidum* and is principally spread by sexual contact although transmission may occur *in utero* and via blood transfusions. In early syphilis, the primary and secondary stages are characterized by mucocutaneous lesions. After a latent period the tertiary stage is characterized by chronic progressive lesions of the cardiovascular, nervous, and musculoskeletal systems.

Primary syphilis. This stage is characterized by the appearance of a dull red papule which breaks down to form a well-defined indurated ulcer or chancre. The lesion appears at the site of inoculation of the spirochaete and while it is usually on the external genitalia or cervix it may also occur in the anorectal area, in the mouth or on the lips or fingers. The chancre appears between 10 days and 2 months after the patient is infected and it is well for the GP to remember its existence when any patient presents with painless genital ulcers accompanied by regional lymphadenopathy. The ulcer heals over 2–8 weeks if untreated.

Secondary syphilis. This stage appears about 6–8 weeks after the primary chancre. It is famous for its infinite variety of symptoms and signs with gen-eralized non-specific presentation. However, most patients have a generalized rash, generalized lymphadenopathy, and sometimes mucosal lesions. This situation will be rarely encountered in general practice although it underlines that the comprehensive clinical history from an adult with an atypical rash and a febrile illness should include questions about new sexual partners and recent painless ulcers.

Antenatal screening for syphilis

Syphilis is still relevant to general practice in that all pregnant women are screened for it. As transmission from mother to child usually takes place after 16 weeks' gestation, screening in early pregnancy is effective. Although the prevalence of syphilis is low in the UK there is an epidemic in the USA, principally among those living in poverty and using drugs (especially crack cocaine). These factors are prevalent in the UK, as is the risk of imported infection from developing countries, leading many authorities to argue the case for continuing to screen pregnant women.[28] The tests used to screen can lead to false positives and do not always differentiate syphilis from the non-sexually transmitted infection, yaws. General practitioners are so used to negative results that they do not always handle a positive test with sensitivity, thus leading to devastating effects on the woman and her family. All positive results must be confirmed before the results are given to the patient: this news is best given by individuals who are knowledgeable about syphilis, who have excellent communication skill, and who can provide follow-up. The level of input from the family doctor will vary but at the very least it will be essential to remain informed as the situation unfolds.

Treatment

The treatment of syphilis is with intramuscular penicillin; tetracycline or erythromycin are recommended for allergic patients. The regime should be determined by a genitourinary physician, although injections may be administered in the practice by agreement if it is more convenient for the patient.

Genital herpes

Genital herpes is one of the most important sexually transmitted disease in the Western World, showing a marked increase in incidence over the 1970s and early 1980s.

Epidemiology

Herpes simplex virus infections are increasing: between the years 1977 and 1983 the number of women presenting annually to STD clinics had doubled. In 1977, 8400 cases of herpes simplex virus (HSV) infections were seen in these clinics, but by 1983 the numbers had risen to about 18 000, an increase of 100% in 6 years. Data from industrialized countries suggest that the disease is increasing in frequency, particularly among groups with a previously low prevalence. This appears to be the case for young middle and upper class adults, although it is difficult to separate the effects of a greater awareness and reporting, and different diagnostic methods. A recent study showed that about half of those attending a genitourinary clinic for a first episode were in stable relationships and and about half were due to HSV type 1, most commonly found in cold sores.[29] This is relevant to patients seen in general practice who may be distressed when the question of other sexual partners is discussed. Orogenital contact is a more likely explanation for some couples and one they can more easily accept.

Aetiology

Herpes simplex virus (HSV) is a DNA virus found in two serological forms HSV-1 and HSV-2. About 80% of genital herpes infections are caused by type 2, and this form recurs more frequently. The infection is transmitted during intercourse or other close physical contact. Following primary infection the virus establishes latency in neurones of the sensory or autonomic ganglia. The genital disease caused by HSV-1 and HSV-2 is identical in presentation and severity.

Clinical features

Primary infection produces lesions a few days after exposure. It results in multiple clusters of painful vesicles or ulcers on the skin or around the introitus. The first episode of genital herpes is characterized by a prolonged period of viral shedding, generalized constitutional upset, and a herpetic cervicitis accompanying the painful lesions on the external genitalia in 70–90% of women. The cervix is usually abnormal on examination in primary HSV cervicitis and may may show local or diffuse areas of friability, ulcerative lesions of the exocervix, or rarely an extensive necrotic cervicitis. The infection usually involves the squamous epithelium of the exocervix in contrast to the mucopurulent cervicitis of chlamydial or gonococcal infection.

Viraemia is common in primary infection with resulting fever, headaches, and myalgia. Inguinal lymphadenopathy, discharge from the vagina, cervix or anus, urinary retention, tenesmus, and constipation may also occur. Rarely, there is a true meningitis or meningomyelitis. The mean duration of viral shedding from both the cervical and external genital lesions is 11 days. Recurrent attacks are much milder, and of women with recurrent external genital lesions only 15–30% have HSV isolated from the cervix, which often appears clinically normal. About half of those with primary HSV-1 infection and in 80% of those with HSV-2 will experience a recurrence within the first year. The frequency of recurrences is very variable but some women have them every month. Some patients relate the recurrences to menstruation, sex, or stress; but, in fact, the precipitating causes are poorly understood. Many women can predict an attack from tingling or paraesthesiae in the area for 1 or 2 days before the lesions appear: recurrences are always less severe than the primary infection.

Since the late 1980s, it has been increasingly recognized that most people with genital HSV infection are asymptomatic, with asymptomatic infection and virus shedding, playing an important role in the transmission of infection.[30] This has important implications for the transmission of the infection to sexual partners and during childbirth.

Investigations

The diagnosis of genital herpes can often be made clinically but should be confirmed by viral isolation from swabs. These are taken by rubbing a cotton wool swab vigorously over several of the most recent lesions. The swab should be placed in viral transport media and swilled about rather than broken off at once. Rapid tests for diagnosis are available, and the GP should check with the virologist for their local availability. If the history indicates that the infection has been sexually acquired the woman should be tested for other STDs including the rare possibility that the genital ulcers may be due to primary syphilis.

Treatment

Women with a primary genital herpes infection feel very unwell and are often extremely upset when they are told the diagnosis as they are well aware of the implications. They need reassurance and explanation about the risks and consequences of the infection. General advice about steps to minimize the transmission of the virus and about personal hygiene during an attack is important. However, although some may derive a measure of symptomatic relief from salt baths, only acyclovir therapy has been proven to shorten the acute attacks, suppress recurrences, and to terminate viral shedding (and hence transmission). In primary episodes of genital herpes, all three preparations of acyclovir (topical, oral, and intravenous) have been shown to be of clear benefit in reducing the severity of the local disease but the systemic symptoms will not respond to topical therapy. Furthermore, topical therapy is often impractical in women when many of the lesions are within the vagina or on the cervix. Women treated for primary infections in general practice should receive oral acyclovir (200 mg, five times daily for 7–10 days) and advised to rest. Referral to the STD clinic should be discussed and encouraged. Intravenous acyclovir is reserved for those patients who need hospitalization because of severe symptoms or who develop complications such as urinary retention or nervous system involvement. The clinical benefits of therapy in recurrent genital herpes are less obvious. Specific therapy should be started as soon as possible, and as the best results are obtained if the patient can initiate a 5-day course of oral therapy as soon as she gets prodromal symptoms. A course of treatment (200 mg, five times daily for 5 days) should be given to anticipate this situation.

For the patient with recurrences every few weeks consideration may be given to prophylactic administration: optimal suppression can be achieved using acyclovir, 400 mg twice daily. The new antivirals, famciclovir and valaciclovir are now also available for treatment of genital herpes.

Prevention

Primary prevention of genital HSV is the same as for all sexually transmitted infections. In addition, the avoidance of orogenital contact between infected individuals reduces transmission. Partners of women who have recurrent infection should use condoms during the attacks.

Follow-up

Many women suffer profound emotional distress on hearing the diagnosis of genital herpes and studies have reported a high incidence of depression, fear of rejection, feelings of isolation and low self esteem.[31–33] The GP must be aware of this possibility and make arrangements for follow-up to enable the patient to express her reaction as it develops.

Neonatal herpes simplex

HSV infection of the neonate is usually acquired at the time of delivery. The infant may suffer generalized infection with involvement of the liver, lungs, and CNS, and some will have atypical vesicular rash. The risk of acquiring a neonatal infection from a recurrent maternal infection at term has been estimated to be less than 8%, although the risks from a primary infection at term is much higher at up to 50%.[34] Attempts to reduce the transmission from mother to baby have not been entirely successful: most cases result from asymptomatic viral shedding from the cervix at the time of delivery and there is no way of predicting this other than by viral cultures at term. If a women with previous genital herpes and an otherwise uncomplicated pregnancy is to be cared for in general practice the history must be discussed with the local virologist and obstetrician.

Caesarian section may be be the wisest decision if the mother has clear evidence of genital lesions at the time of delivery although this is controversial.[35]

Genital herpes and carcinoma of the cervix

The association between genital herpes and carcinoma of the cervix, whether as a cause or as a covariable with papilloma viruses is still uncertain but until the situation is clearer these women should have annual cervical smears.

Genital warts

Epidemiology

Genital warts are relatively common; human papillomavirus (HPV) is the commonest viral sexually transmitted infection. A review of seven studies of the detection of HPV DNA in cervical cells reported a prevalence of at least 6%: HPV types 16, 18, and 31 which have been associated with cancers of the genital tract and anus were identified in about 50% of these specimens. HPV DNA was detected more frequently in younger women and more frequently in women with evidence of intra-epithelial neoplasia (CIN).[36]

Pathogenesis and clinical features

Genital and anal warts are caused by papilloma viruses and are nearly always spread by sexual contact. Human papillomaviruses (HPV) are non-capsulated DNA viruses approximately 50 nm in diameter. There are at least 60 different HPV types, differentiated on the basis of analysis of their DNA. Some of these types are linked to premalignant and malignant transformation of cervical, penile, and anal cells. Two types of genital warts are seen: condylomata acuminata and sessile warts. The former are fleshy soft growths that often coalesce into large masses, frequently affecting areas traumatized during intercourse.

Genital warts may be solitary but are usually multiple; they may occur anywhere on the external genitalia, within the vagina and on the cervix. Genital warts may be so profuse as to interfere with sexual intercourse. It is now recognized that subclinical HPV infections of the cervix, penis, vulva, and anus are common: lesions may be seen as white areas after the application of 5% acetic acid. Cellular immunity is believed to play a role in the progression or resolution of genital warts: when cellular immunity is depressed (as in pregnancy or in HIV infection), *Condylomata acuminata* proliferate. HPV replicate in squamous epithelium and the histological features of *C. acuminata* are similar to those of other warts. There is hyperplasia of the epithelium and within the stratum granulosum there are large vacuolated cells whose nuclei contain inclusion bodies. In the cervix and within the anus, HPV infection does not cause warts but leads to characteristic cellular changes (cells with hyperchromic nuclei surrounded by a clear, cytoplasmic halo, surrounded in turn by peripheral dark cytoplasm and called koilocytes).

Human papillomavirus and anogenital neoplasia

An association between HPV, particularly types 16 and 18, and cervical or vulval neoplasia has been widely reported[37–39] and there is also a similar association in the male genital tract and in the anus. HPV DNA sequences are associated with both CIN and intra-epithelial neoplasia of the anus and the penis. They have been found in at least 90% of cervical carcinomas in most studies reported, with almost 100% of lesions positive in some studies.[40] HPV DNA is, however, also found in normal tissues from these sites and the oncogenic potential of HPV is the subject of intense research. While the detection of HPV 16 and 18 is not proof of a high risk for progression to cancer, it does, however, constitute the most important risk factor for the development of anogenital neoplasia and women with the infection should be made aware of the increased risk and advised to seek regular screening.

Treatment (Table 11.3)

Genital warts are usually sexually transmitted and the diagnosis can result in negative feelings such as fear of cancer, telling new sex partners, worries about pregnancy, and long-term condom use. Newly diagnosed patients need an opportunity to discuss these matters.[41] Doctors, seeing couples in a stable monogamous relationship, can assume that both partners will be infected and that the finding of HPV on a cervical smear does not mean that the couple are doomed to barrier contraception for ever after. Clinically obvious lesions in either partner should be treated. Children with genital warts may have been sexually abused. These cases should be discussed with the community paediatrician.

Case history

A woman of 21, a single parent, consulted the doctor for chest pain which seemed to be of musculoskeletal origin. On reading her records the GP noticed that the trainee was treating her for perianal and vulvar warts. Further conversation revealed that the patient's 4-year-old daughter also had warts around the anus and that the GP registrar had asked her to bring the child in for treatment. While alarm bells rang in the GP's mind she decided not to discuss further with the patient whom she knew slightly. The next day, she raised the case with the registrar and was relieved to discover that, with the guidance of his trainer, he had followed the local child protection guidelines and referred the child to the community paediatrician. The mother was co-operative, although she had denied that sexual abuse was likely as the child's father does not live with them.

Genital warts can be treated in the surgery with a 10% or 20% solution of podophyllin resin in tincture of benzoin, applied to the lesions once or twice a week for 3 or 4 weeks. It is not licensed for self-treatment in the UK. Indeed, there have been reports of patients who have treated themselves with inadequate instructions from their GP, and developed severe genital ulceration.[42] It should not be used for cervical or intra-anal warts as its effects cannot be controlled at these sites and severe systemic toxic reactions have been reported. Warts may become extremely florid during pregnancy; these women must be referred. General practice treatment should be confined to non-pregnant women with minor external lesions or undertaken as shared care with the GU physician.

Table 11.3 *Recommendations for the management of Condyloma acuminata in women.*

The patient
- Refer all pregnant women
- Treat visible warts
- Test for and treat other sexually transmitted diseases[*]
- Exclude cervical dysplasia
- Use condoms with new sexual partners
- Annual cervical smear
- Allow time for the patient to express worries

Sexual partners
- Trace, examine, and treat visible warts[*]
- Test for, and treat other sexually transmitted disease

Note. Always consider whether the patient should be referred to a genitourinary physician.

Alternative therapies with systemic or intralesional interferon or topical 5-fluorouracil cream are similarly successful. Physical therapies, such as cautery, cryotherapy, and diathermy or laser therapy (under general anaesthetic), are suitable for internal or extensive lesions.

Regular cervical smears are mandatory. The increased risk for developing cervical cancer can be discussed in the knowledge that most genital squamous cell cancers take 20 or more years to develop and that regular screening will ensure early treatment and cure.

Upper genital tract infection

Salpingitis

Aetiology and epidemiology

Salpingitis is a common problem, with an estimated incidence in industrialized countries of 10–14 cases per 1000 women in the age-group 15–45, and a peak incidence at age 15–24. New cases typically occur in younger, sexually active women who are not in long-term mutually monogamous relationships. Most cases are caused by organisms which ascend from the lower genital tract; principally *N. gonorrhoea*, *C. trachomatis*, and microorganisms which are part of the normal vaginal, vulval, or bowel flora and which may cause infections in fallopian tubes already damaged by the sexually transmitted agents mentioned above. Susceptibility to ascending infection is increased during ovulation and menstruation and decreased when taking both combined and progesterone-only oral contraceptives. All of these factors influence the state of the cervical mucous plug. IUCD insertion, termination of pregnancy, dilation and curettage, and insufflation of tubes breach the cervical barrier and may be complicated by upper genital tract infection. Twelve per cent of women who develop salpingitis have been reported as undergoing such a procedure during the preceding four weeks. The risk of salpingitis is 7–9 times greater for nulliparous women using the IUCD compared with non-users, probably due to easier upper genital spread of chlamydial infections in these women rather than the presence of the device itself.

Clinical features

Women with acute salpingitis present with lower abdominal pain, metrorrhagia, deep dyspareunia, and purulent vaginal discharge. Chlamydial perihepatitis may be present in 5% of patients who may complain of right upper quadrant abdominal pain. On examination, the patient may have a temperature higher than 38°C, tender lower abdomen, cervical excitation, purulent discharge, and tender fornices, with or without a palpable mass. The identification of the responsible organism(s) is difficult, as cultures from the lower genital tract do not establish with certainty the cause of the tubal infection. In general, chlamydial PID runs a milder course than gonococcal PID or that due to anaerobic organisms. These features are not very specific and the diagnosis of acute salpingitis ought to be confirmed by isolation of pathogens from specimens taken at laparoscopy, although a minority of patients do in fact come to this procedure. The differential diagnosis includes ectopic pregnancy and appendicitis.

The most serious immediate complication is a tubo-ovarian abscess. These are usually the result of recurrent episodes of acute salpingitis but may also occur without prior pelvic infection, especially if an IUCD is used. The organisms responsible are similar to those causing salpingitis with the exception of the gonococcus and *Chlamydia*, which are only rarely isolated from abscesses. The symptoms and signs are similar to those of salpingitis except that a mass is often found on pelvic examination. If the abscess ruptures then acute peritonitis and shock develop very rapidly.

The long-term effects of salpingitis are devastating: 1 in 5 women will have a repeat infection, and 1 in 4 will suffer from chronic pelvic pain, infertility, or an ectopic pregnancy because of the infection.

Treatment

Acutely ill women should be admitted to hospital. Women managed at home should rest and avoid intercourse and their condition should be closely monitored. Initial therapy should be aimed at the likely pathogens but there is no consensus as to the optimal regimen. For the less severely ill woman, a single high dose of oral amoxycillin (3 g) followed by 10–14 days of a tetracycline (except in pregnancy), with or without metronidazole is suitable. With the use of such therapy, the complications of salpingitis, such as infertility, ectopic pregnancy, and pelvic adhesions can be reduced.

As many of these infections are sexually transmitted the GP must give the woman the opportunity to discuss her lifestyle and should also ensure that current sexual partners are free from asymptomatic infection. Guilt and blame may underpin subsequent depression, sometimes many years later, particularly if infertility results. The GP should seek to create an open climate within the consultation which allows these issues to be aired should the patient wish it.

Genital infections in men

This section of the chapter will deal principally with sexually transmitted infections (STD). Male anatomy does not lead to such a convenient separation between the urinary and genital tracts, hence the reader will find infections such as prostatitis and epididymo-orchitis principally described in Chapter 10 on the urinary tract. HIV infection and AIDS are addressed in Chapter 16 but provide an ever-present context to any discussion of STD.

Urethritis

Heterosexual men with sexually transmitted infections present most frequently to their GP complaining of a urethral discharge accompanied by burning on passing urine and itching around the meatus. Many men prefer to use the STD clinic and as a result these symptoms are seen in general practice much less commonly than vaginal discharge. In addition, many men with urethritis are asymptomatic and represent an important reservoir of infection which may only come to light when their partner develops symptoms.

Homosexual men rarely present sexually transmitted infections to their GP as they frequently feel that they will not be received with knowledge and understanding. However, it is important to remember that many sexually transmitted infections cause anal symptoms in men and women who have had anoreceptive intercourse, and rectal swabs should be cultured routinely when these patients are investigated for urethritis.

The syndrome is caused by infection with either *N. gonorrhoeae* or other organisms, principally *C. trachomatis* or *U. urealyticum* and occasionally *T. vaginalis.*[43]

Non-gonococcal urethritis (NGU) is the commonest sexually transmitted disease in men in the UK and Europe[44] and the role of *C. trachomatis*, found in up to half of cases, mirrors the incidence of the infection in women.

It is not possible to distinguish, on clinical grounds, which organism is responsible and these men must be investigated. The tests are much better done in the GU clinic. It is unwise to treat the infection 'blind' and if the patient absolutely declines referral the tests to be taken should be discussed with the local GU physician. At the very least, they should include a slide for a Gram-stain of the urethral discharge to identify the intracellular Gram-negative diplococci which are highly specific for gonorrhoea, urethral cultures for *N. gonorrhoea*, and the locally available test for *Chlamydia*. Testing the first 5 ml of urine voided has been shown to be as sensitive as examining the urethral discharge for *Chlamydia* and is useful in the general practice setting.[45] If treatment is undertaken in general practice it is important to establish the local regime and follow it. The possibility of other infections, including HIV, should be entertained and prevention of future infections discussed. The local complications of untreated infections with *N. gonorrhoea* and *C. trachomatis* include epididymitis, and more rarely prostatitis (see Chapter 10).

Sexually acquired reactive arthritis

Approximately 1% of men presenting with non-gonococcal urethritis develop sexually acquired reactive arthritis of whom one-third have Reiter's syndrome comprising urethritis, iritis, and arthritis.[46]

Sexually transmitted lesions of the external genitalia

Herpetic balanitis

Primary herpes infection of the penis results in clusters of painful vesicles or ulcers on the skin or mucous membranes of the penis. The clinical course and treatment is as described for women, men also become asymptomatic shedders of the virus. Studies have shown that susceptible female partners have a three times greater risk of acquiring the infection from infected men than vice versa.[47] It is important that men use condoms if they know that they have genital herpes although the problem of what to do if the couple wish to conceive remains. Sometimes, GPs are approached by couples in this situation, but this is a problem best addressed after discussion with the GU physician who will often see the couple together for a discussion.

Anogenital warts

Many studies have demonstrated that the majority of current partners of people with genital HPV infection have also been infected.[36] In men, the lesions are usually on the penis with the initial site of occurrence being the frenulum, coronal sulcus, or inner surface of the prepuce. Typical condylomata acuminata caused by HPV types 6 and 11 with a low oncogenic potential are less common than lesions not visible to the naked eye, unless 3–5% acetic acid is applied to them. Some of these lesions are caused by HPV types 16, 18, 31, and 33 which carry a high risk for the development of severe dysplasia.

Most studies of these penile acetowhite lesions have concentrated on the potential role of the man as a reservoir for infection of female partners. However, while most are asymptomatic, some do experience itching, burning, and dyspareunia.[48]

Treatment

Sometimes women with the finding of HPV infection in a cervical smear inquire about treatment for their current partner. If lesions cannot be seen by the naked eye it is acceptable to reassure the couple and ask the man to present with any lesions that do develop. Treatment should be reserved for those lesions which cause physical illness or psychosexual distress.[49] Obvious lesions may be treated with podophyllin with care, podophyllotoxin 0.5% in an alcoholic base is suitable, or patients referred to the GU clinic. The possibility of other sexually transmitted infections should be considered, anal warts are particularly common in homosexual men who should be referred for treatment and counselling about other infections including HIV disease.

Sexually transmitted infections: the GP perspective

The diagnosis and management of STD in general practice is controversial as it is widely held that these patients should all be referred to the GU clinic. There is no doubt that clinics provide an excellent and confidential service but there is also no doubt that some patients absolutely decline to attend them and request treatment in the practice setting.[45] *Chlamydia*, *Trichomonas*, herpes simplex, genital warts, and gonorrhoea are all infections presented by men and women to their GP. Frequently, the knowledge of family relationships and the confidential information given to the doctor raises difficult ethical issues about confidentiality, informed consent, and truth-telling.[50] Recording of the information in the medical records has implications for future insurance reports and in some instances there is a temptation to compromise the standard of clinical care and treat an infection 'blind' in order to resolve an emotionally charged situation.

Case history

A man of 35 had received treatment for chlamydial urethritis from a GU clinic in another city. He had been working there for several months, returning home at weekends. He had two children and his wife was 30-weeks pregnant. The infection had been the result of a brief relationship with a colleague at work, now over, but he could not be certain he had not infected his wife. He consulted in great distress to ask the GP to examine his wife at her next antenatal appointment and take a test for *Chlamydia* without her knowledge as he had read that the infection could harm her and lead to complications for the baby. The GP explained that she could not agree to this course of action as it would involve deceiving the wife. Eventually, he agreed to discuss the relationship with his wife and the couple were seen together by the local GU physician. The marriage went through a great deal of turmoil and the wife suffered postnatal depression.

This case history was subsequently used as a basis for role-playing for undergraduate teaching. Many of the participants were tempted to investigate and/or treat the wife without her knowledge and consent on the basis that the consequences overall for the family would be better.

Whatever the level of clinical responsibility that a GP decides to take in managing sexually transmitted infections it is imperative that there is a close working relationship with the local genitourinary medicine specialist and his/her team. Proper attention to prevention and contact tracing should be part of the care of all patients.

References

1. O'Dowd T. Clinical prediction of *Gardnerella vaginalis* in general practice. *J Roy Coll Gen Pract* (1987) **37**: 59–61

2. Mardh P-A. The vaginal ecosystem *Am J Obstet Gynecol* (1991) **165**: 1163–7

3. Westrom L. Wolner-Hanssen P. Pathogenesis of pelvic inflammatory disease *Genitourin Med* (1993) **69**: 9–17

4. Jonsson M, Karlsson R, Rylander E *et al*. The silent suffering women—a population based study on the association between reported symptoms and past and present infections of the lower genital tract. *Genitourin Med* (1995); **71**: 158–62

5. UK Family Planning Research Network. Patterns of sexual behaviour among sexually experienced women attending family planning clinics in England, Scotland and Wales. *Brit J Fam Plan* (1988) **14**: 74–82

6. Dekker J *et al*. Vaginal symptoms of unknown aetiology: a study in Dutch general practice. *Brit J Gen Pract* (1993) **43**: 239–44

7. Stewart D *et al.* Psychosocial aspects of chronic, clinically unconfirmed vulvovaginitis. *Obstet Gynecol* (1990) **75**: 852–6

8. Schmidt H, Hansen J, Korsager B. Microbiology of vaginal discharge in general practice. *Scand J Prim Health Care* (1986) **4**: 75–80

9. Westrom L, Mardh P-A. Acute pelvic inflammatory disease (PID). In: Holmes KK, Mardh P-A, Sparling PF *et al.* ed. *Sexually Transmitted Diseases.* 2nd edn. New York: McGraw Hill (1990) 593–613

10. DOH, BMA, Conference of Medical Royal Colleges. *Child protection: medical responsibilities.* Addendum to 'Working together Under the Children Act (1989)'

11. Van Oppen C, Feldman R (editorial) Antibiotic prophylaxis of neonatal group B streptococcal infections. *BMJ* (1993) **306**: 411–12

12. Odds F C. *Candida and candidosis.* 2nd edn. London: Balliere Tindall (1992)

13. Guillebaud J. *Contraception: hormonal and barrier methods.* London: Martin Dunitz (1992)

14. Mitchell S, Bradbeer C (editorial). Over the counter treatment for candidiasis. An opportunity to educate. *BMJ* (1992) **304**: 1648

15. Fong I, McCleary P, Read S. Cellular immunity of patients with recurrent or refractory vulvovaginal moniliasis. *Am J Obstet Gynecol* (1992) **166**: 887–90

16. Böhler K *et al.* Zinc levels of serum and cervicovaginal secretions in recurrent vulvovaginitis. *Genitourin Med* (1994) **70**: 308–10

17. Witkin S, Hirsch J, Ledger W. A macrophage defect in women with candida vaginitis and its reversal *in vitro* by prostaglandin inhibitors. *Am J Obstet Gynecol* (1986) **155**: 790–5

18. Spiegel CA. Bacterial vaginosis. *Clinical Microbiological Reviews* (1991) 485–502.

19. Eschenbach D, Hillier S, Critchlow C *et al.* Diagnosis and clinical manifestations of bacterial vaginosis. *Am J Obstet Gynecol* (1988) **158**:819–27

20. Southgate L., Treharne J., Forsey T. *Chlamydia trachomatis* and *Neisseria gonorrhoea* infections in women attending inner city general practices. *BMJ* (1983) **287**: 879–81

21. Oakeshott P *et al.* Testing for cervical *Chlamydial trachomatis* infection in an inner city practice. *Family Practice* (1992) **94**: 421–4

22. Taylor-Robinson D (editorial). *Chlamydia trachomatis* and sexually transmitted disease. What do we know and what shall we do? *BMJ* (1994) **308**: 150–1

23. Thejls H *et al.* Expanded gold standard in the diagnosis of *Chlamydia trachomatis* in a low prevalence population: diagnostic efficacy of tissue culture, direct immunofluorescence, enzyme immunoassay, PCR and serology. *Genitourin Med* (1994) **70**: 300–3

24. Frost E, Deslandes S, Bourgaux-Ramoisy D. Sensitive detection and typing of

Chlamydia trachomatis using nested polymerase chain reaction. *Genitourin Med* (1993) **69**: 290–4

25. Martin D *et al.* A controlled trial of a single dose of azithromycin for the treatment of chlamydial urethritis and cervicitis. *N. Engl J Med* (1992) **327**: 921–5

26. Southgate L, Williams R, Treharne J Detection, treatment and follow-up of women with *Chlamydia trachomatis* infections seeking abortion in inner city general practices *BMJ* (1989) **299**: 1136–7

27. Peeling R. *Chlamydia trachomatis* and *Neisseria gonorrhoea*: pathogens in retreat? *Cur Op Infect Dis* (1995) **8**: 26–34

28. Nicoll A, Moisley C. Antenatal screening for syphilis. *BMJ* (1994) **308**: 1253–4

29. Wolley PD, Kudesia G. Incidence of herpes simplex virus type 1 and 2 from patients with primary (first attack) genital herpes in Sheffield. *Int J STD and AIDS* (1990) **1**: 184–6

30. Koelle D M, Benedetti J, Langenberg A, Corey L. Asymptomatic reactivation of herpes simplex virus in women after the first episode of genital herpes. *Ann Intern Med* (1992) **116**: 433–7

31. Catotti D N, Clarke P, Catoe K. Herpes revisited. Still a cause for concern. *Sex Transm Dis* (1993) **20**: 77–80

32. Carney O *et al.* A prospective study of the psychological impact on patients with a first episode of genital herpes. *Genitourin Med* (1994) **70**: 40–5

33. Cassidy L *et al.* Are doctors in genitourinary medicine perceiving the psychological impact of recurrent genital herpes? *Genitourin Med* (1993) **70**: 357–8

34. Nagaswaran A, Kinghorn G. Sexually transmitted diseases in children: herpes simplex infection, cytomegalovirus infection, hepatitis B virus infection and molluscum contagiosum. *Genitourin Med* (1993) **69**: 303–11

35. Prober C G *et al.* The management of pregnancies complicated by genital infections with herpes simplex virus. *Clin Infect Dis* (1992) **15**: 1031–8

36. Koutsky L, Wolner P. Genital papillomavirus infections: Current knowledge and future prospects. *Obstet and Gynec Clin N Amer* (1989) **3**: 541–64

37. Koutsky L, Holmes K, Critchlow C *et al.* A cohort study of the risk of cervical intraepithelial neoplasia grade 2 or 3 in relation to human papillomavirus infection. *N Engl J Med.* (1992) **327**: 1272–8

38. Zur Hausen H. Human papillomaviruses in the pathogenisis of anogential cancer. *Virology* (1991) **184**: 9–13

39. Lorincz A *et al.* Human papilloma virus infection of the cervix: relative risk associations with 15 common anogenital types. *Obstet Gynecol* (1992) **79**: 328

40. Paavonen J. Pathophysiologic aspects of human papillomavirus infection *Curr Op Infect Dis* (1993) **6**: 21–6

41. Sheppard S, White M, Walzman M. Genital warts: just a nuisance? *Genitourin Med* (1995) **71**: 194

42. Higgins S, Stedman Y, Chandiok P. Severe genital ulceration in two females following self-treatment with podophyllin solutions. *Genitourin Med* (1994) **70**: 146

43. Kreiger J. *et al.* Risk assessment and laboratory diagnosis of trichomoniasis in men. *J Infect Dis* (1992) **166**: 1362–6

44. Oriel J. Male genital *Chlamydia trachomatis* infections. *J Infect* (1992) **25**: 35–7

45. Dryden M *et al.* Detection of *Chlamydia trachomatis* in general practice urine samples. *Brit J Gen Pract* (1994) **44**: 114–17

46. Keat A. Extra-genital *Chlamydia trachomatis* infection as sexually-acquired reactive arthritis. *J Infect* (1992) **25**: 47–9

47. Mertz G *et al.* Risk factors for the sexual transmission of genital herpes. *Ann Intern Med* (1992) **116**: 433–7

48. Wikström A *et al.* Papillomavirus-associated balanoposthisis. *Genitourin Med* (1994) **70**: 175–81

49. von Krogh *et al.* Self treatment using 0.25%–0.5% podophyllotoxin-ethanol solutions against penile condylomata acuminata: a placebo-controlled comparative study. *Genitourin Med* (1994) **70**: 105–9

50. Johnson A, Wadsworth J, Wellings K. Who goes to sexually transmitted disease clinics? Results from a national population survey. *Genitourin Med* (1996) **72**: 197–202

CHAPTER TWELVE

Infections of the bones and joints

There are two major conditions of the musculoskeletal system, septic arthritis and osteomyelitis, which may present in general practice. They may be difficult to diagnose and treat and are caused by a range of pathogens which differ depending on the clinical circumstances. Their presentation differs in children and adults.

There is very little written about the incidence of these infections in general practice: concerning acute bacterial infections, one of the GP authors of this chapter, during 25 years of practice, recalls about five cases of acute osteomyelitis in children, two adult cases of tuberculous spinal infection, and one acute and severe infection in a knee joint following an insect bite. Conversations with colleagues with equivalent experience also revealed answers of a similar order of magnitude; the reader may like to make comparable inquiries! Morbidity statistics from general practice confirm our clinical impression and report incidence rates for all bone and joint infections of 1 per 10 000 years at risk.[1] Despite their rarity the responsibility for early diagnosis and referral usually rests in primary care.

Septic arthritis

Aetiology

Some of the most important bacterial and fungal agents associated with septic arthritis in adults are shown in Table 12.1. Overall, *Staphylococcus aureus* infection is responsible for more than 70% of septic arthritis in adults. In young adults (20–30 years) the gonococcus is a major cause of joint infection and can occur either with a polyarthritis in which the organism is rarely cultured from joint fluid but is frequently grown from blood cultures, or as septic arthritis in a single joint from which the organism can usually be recovered. Amongst the streptococcal infections, it is commonly group A beta-haemolytic *Streptococcus* which is the infecting agent. When Gram-negative septic arthritis in adults occurs it is often in the context of an elderly debilitated patient with an underlying Gram-negative septicaemia, frequently related to an intercurrent urinary tract infection. Drug addicts are also at risk from Gram-negative septic arthritis, most commonly with *Pseudomonas aeruginosa*. Anaerobic organisms account for less than 1% of joint infections.

Table 12.1 *Bacterial and fungal agents that cause septic arthritis in adults*

Acute disease	Chronic infection
Staphylococcus aureus	*Brucella* spp.
Streptococcus spp.	*Mycobacterium tuberculosis*
Neisseria spp.	Atypical *Mycobacterium*
Gram-negative organisms	*Nocardia asteroides*
	Borrelia burgdorferi
	Fungi
	Candida albicans
	Sporothrix schenckii

In children under the age of 5 years, *Haemophilus influenzae* type b accounts for nearly one-third of cases, followed by *Staphylococcus aureus* and *Streptococcus* spp. Although group A beta-haemolytic streptococcus is an important agent in the over 2-year-old age group, in neonates, group B beta-haemolytic streptococcus and Gram-negative organisms, such as *Escherichia coli*, should not be forgotten. Infection with group A beta-haemolytic streptococcus can also result in a post-infectious polyarthropathy which may be part of the rheumatic fever syndrome or complicate a Henoch–Schönlein illness. *Salmonella* spp. may cause septic arthritis in children, but the well-known association of this organism with paediatric sickle-cell disease and osteomyelitis does not occur with septic arthritis.

A post-infectious arthritis as part of Reiter's syndrome (conjunctivitis or iritis and polyarthritis) may recur for many years as a chronic complication of infection with *Salmonella, Campylobacter, Shigella*, or *Yersinia*, as well as a sequel to non-specific urethritis. Patients with the HLA-B27 antigen show a predisposition to develop the syndrome.

Mycobacterial agents may be responsible for chronic joint infections. *Mycobacterium tuberculosis* or some of the atypical mycobacteria such as *M. fortuitum* or *M. marinum* can cause a monoarticular, slowly progressive arthritis, which will have granuloma formation demonstrated by histological examination. Mycobacteria can be grown from the joint specimens that are obtained, but only if the diagnosis is thought of and if appropriate cultures are made.

The fungus, *Sporothrix schenckii* is the second commonest cause after atypical mycobacteria, of a chronic monoarticular joint infection especially if there is an associated tenosynovitis. *Borrelia burgdorferi*, the aetiological agent of Lyme disease (see p. 000) can cause either an acute arthritis lasting for months in association with the acute manifestations of the disease, or a chronic arthritis which is less common, especially of the knee joint.[2]

A number of viruses are associated with a polyarticular syndrome affecting the joints usually as part of the systemic manifestation of the disease (Table 12.2). The association of hepatitis B with arthritis, and often urticaria, has

Table 12.2 *Viral diseases that have an associated arthritis*

Commonly associated	Rarely associated
Rubella	Varicella
Parvovirus	Echovirus
Mumps	Adenovirus
Hepatitis B	Influenza
	Epstein–Barr

been well documented. The arthritis usually occurs along with a rash several days or weeks before jaundice appears and tends to resolve with the onset of the jaundice. The joints of the hands are primarily involved but occasionally joint effusions in which hepatitis B antigen can be detected have been reported.

Whilst the arthritis associated with rubella occurs mainly in women, men are the predominant sufferers of arthritis in association with mumps. The arthritis is usually polyarticular and may continue for as long as three months. The rubella associated arthritis seen primarily in women occurs with the onset of the rash or shortly after. Whilst about 3% of children may suffer from arthritis in conjunction with receipt of rubella vaccine, nearly 40% of postpubertal females who receive the vaccine have an associated arthralgia.[3] Both the arthritis associated with the natural disease and that associated with the vaccine are self-limiting and resolution can be expected within 3–4 weeks.

Finally, human parvovirus B19 is now well documented as a cause of a symmetrical polyarthritis, especially in women.[4] This virus, now known to be the cause of Fifth disease or epidemic erythema infectiousum, is also associated with early spontaneous miscarriage. Early investigation of arthralgia or polyarthritis in young women which does not include a search for parvovirus will miss the infection and hence an opportunity to advise the woman to avoid pregnancy until the infection is over.[5]

Clinical features

A red, hot, swollen joint with limitation of movement is a *septic joint* until it can be demonstrated that it is not. It is a medical emergency and requires urgent referral to hospital for investigation and treatment. An audit at a teaching hospital with a large local catchment area showed that the presentation of an acute hot joint was relatively common, 84% occurred in the community of which one-third were first assessed in general practice and the remainder in the hospital casualty department. The most frequent diagnosis was acute pseudo-gout with only 20% having a proven septic arthritis.[6] Bacterial infection usually results from haematogenous spread from a distant focus, but can follow a penetrating wound, insect bite, or an intra-articular injection with corticosteroids. Rheumatoid or osteoarthritic joints are more susceptible. Children and adults who present with bacterial infection of a single joint complain of pain and tenderness over the area. The knee, followed by the hip, are the commonest joints involved in both groups of patients. The elbow and ankle joints are then the next most common joints affected in children, whilst in adults the shoulder and sacro-iliac joints are more commonly involved.

Examination of the febrile patient will reveal a tender, swollen joint with limited, painful movement: 90% of accessible joints will have a demonstrable effusion. In very young infants there will also be non-specific signs, including irritability, especially when the affected joint is moved. In patients who suffer from rheumatoid disease, individual joints can become infected as well as being involved in the systemic disease. In these patients, especially if steroids or immunosuppressive agents are being taken, it may be impossible to distinguish between an exacerbation of rheumatoid arthritis and a septic joint. It is therefore imperative that the joint fluid is urgently examined and cultured in case sepsis and not the underlying disease accounts for the new clinical presentation.

Young adults may present with multiple involvement of joints and a rash. If there is an appropriate history or a urethral discharge then a clinical diagnosis of gonococcal infection may be made, whilst chronic meningococcal infection may present similarly, but without the genital involvement. In addition, an associated inflammation of the tendon sheaths (tenosynovitis) often occurs with the disseminated gonococcal syndrome and in infections with viral and atypical mycobacterial infections.

Diagnosis and investigations

A variety of non-specific tests may be helpful in making the diagnosis of acute septic arthritis. The ESR will be elevated in both bacterial and viral disease, although it is likely to be higher in the former. In chronic infections there may be an associated anaemia. The white cell count is usually elevated, with a neutrophil leucocytosis.

Most joints, with the important exceptions of the hip and sacroiliac joints, will be accessible so that the joint effusion can be tapped for Gram-stain and culturing. This procedure is often done after urgent hospital referral, however, joint aspiration in practice may unexpectedly produce purulent material which should always be sent to the laboratory for culture. The patient requires hospital referral. The white cell count in the joint fluid is commonly elevated, but this does not necessarily indicate infection since other inflammatory conditions such as rheumatoid arthritis and crystal diseases of the joints can also provoke this response.

Although the glucose level in infected joint fluid is reduced in comparison to blood glucose, this is a fairly non-specific finding in a number of inflammatory conditions and does not really help in confirming the diagnosis. Fluid obtained from a rheumatoid joint should, as a matter of routine, be cultured, but the importance of referring such a patient to hospital urgently cannot be overemphasized if sepsis cannot be excluded.

Once effusion fluid is obtained the critical acute investigation is its Gram-stain. It will be positive in approximately 50% of cases and in 90% of cases with a bacterial aetiology the organism will be grown on culture.[7] A strong presumptive diagnosis can be obtained within one hour of obtaining the sample if the Gram-film is positive. Blood cultures are also essential since many cases of septic arthritis are haematogenously derived. This is an especially important investigation if the joint effusion cannot be sampled easily, as in septic arthritis of the sacro-iliac joint. Reports of the positivity rate of blood cultures varies from 10%–40%. In suspected gonococcal arthritis, rectal, urethral, and pharyngeal cultures may confirm the diagnosis.

Radiology of the joints may be of some diagnostic help since swelling of the joint capsule and the associated soft tissues may be seen. Radiological evidence of joint destruction is rare except with late presentations or in association with rheumatoid disease.

Prosthetic joint infections

A special note needs to be added concerning prosthetic joints, especially as hip replacements and now, increasingly, replacement of other joints such as elbow and knee joints, have become part of routine orthopaedic practice. Usually, these procedures are straightforward and uncomplicated, but between 1% and 5% of implanted joints may become infected with potentially dire consequences for the patient.

The aetiology of prosthetic joint infection is either by haematogenous spread or by direct infection either at the time of operation or subsequently from a contiguous focus. The vast majority of patients present with an indolent course, often several years after the operation, in which pain in the joint is the major feature. More acute symptoms such as fever or purulent discharge are less common.[8] Joint pain does not always indicate infection in this setting, however, since dislocation of the joint or loosening of the cement may also produce similar symptoms. Careful clinical evaluation and radiology are likely to help in the clinical differential diagnosis.

More than half of the infections which occur in prosthetic joints are caused by staphylococci, with coagulase negative staphylococci being implicated more frequently than *Staph. aureus*. Gram-negative bacilli and beta-haemolytic streptococci each cause about 20% of infections and the rest are caused by a variety of other organisms, including streptococci and anaerobes.

Prevention is by far and away the most important factor in avoiding infections postoperatively and a combination of perioperative prophylactic antibiotics, usually a beta-lactam, combined with a meticulous surgical technique involving good haemostasis has been shown to reduce infection rates.[9] If a prosthetic joint does become infected then a combination of strategies are usually employed but removal of the infected prosthesis is always involved. Many clinicians recommend a long course (6 weeks) of bactericidal antibiotics specifically directed at the infecting organism after removal of the prosthesis with later re-insertion of a new joint, often using antibiotic-containing cement.

Prophylactic antibiotics for patients with prosthetic joints

The question of prophylactic antibiotics for procedures such as dental work may be raised with the GP by patients with prosthetic joints. Since the consequences of prosthetic joint infections are so devastating some clinicians conceptually see this problem rather like endocarditis and some have recommended prophylaxis under the same circumstances. However, neither the incidence of prosthetic joint infections following presumed episodes of bacteraemia nor the efficacy of prophylactic antibiotics have been studied in this clinical setting. General practitioners should discuss this issue with the microbiologist or orthopaedic surgeon to determine the local view while research evidence is awaited.

Septic bursitis

Patients may sometimes develop an infection of the prepatellar or olecranon bursa, usually as a result of trauma or sustained pressure during such work as gardening, carpet laying, or plumbing. There may be pain, reddening, tenderness, and swelling of the bursa and the condition may resemble a septic arthritis. In bursitis, however, movement of the joint is painless. The infection is almost always due to *Staph. aureus* or *Strep. pyogenes* but diagnosis is made by Gram-stain and culture of the bursa fluid. The bursa must be aspirated or drained and parenteral antibiotics may be necessary. Early referral to a specialist is recommended.

Osteomyelitis

Case history

A 14-year-old girl presented with a 10-day history of fever, myalgia, and pain in her left knee. Her GP requested her admission to hospital because she was unwell with a pyrexia of 40 °C, and a tachycardia. The peripheral white cell count was 10×10^9/l. A urine specimen showed numerous white blood cells and grew a *Staph. aureus* in pure culture at $>10^5$ organisms/ml. An initial diagnosis of urinary tract infection was made. Subsequent blood cultures also grew *Staph. aureus*. The left knee joint was aspirated but culture of the fluid was sterile. A venogram initially reported a deep venous thrombosis but ultrasound of the lower end of the femur demonstrated a soft tissue swelling. The site was surgically explored and 300 ml of pus was drained. On further exploration, two sinuses at the lower end of the femur were noted. A subperiosteal collection was drained. Necrotic infected bone was excised from around the area of the metaphysis. Pus and bone obtained at operation *Staph. aureus*. Eight weeks after completing antibiotic therapy (IV flucloxacillin and oral fucidin for 4 weeks, followed by 2 weeks of oral therapy) the patient was re-admitted to hospital with a pathological fracture at the site of the previous infection.

Aetiology

Haematogenous osteomyelitis is almost invariably caused by a single organism. The most important aetiological agent in both children and adults is *Staph. aureus*. Gram-negative bacilli are the next most commonly encountered organisms, with *Haemophilus influenzae* and *Salmonella* being of special concern. Salmonellas are implicated in more than 80% of cases of osteomyelitis associated with sickle-cell disease. *Pseudomonas aeruginosa* can cause osteomyelitis especially against a background of predisposing illnesses, such as malignancy or connective tissue diseases, or in association with intravenous drug abuse.[11]

Polymicrobial osteomyelitis is more commonly seen in association with infection derived from a local source of infection. It tends to occur in elderly patients and may be related to recent surgery (often open hip surgery) with a subsequent wound infection or to a related, non-responding pressure sore.[12] These infections may involve a single organism such as *Staph. aureus* especially if they are associated with postoperative wound sepsis, but Gram-negative bacilli and anaerobes as well as mixed infections including *Staph. aureus* have also been implicated.

Mycobacterium tuberculosis is well described as a cause of chronic osteomyelitis. Although the spine is commonly the major site of infection, other bones including the hip and knee can also be involved. The presentation of spinal disease may be slow and insidious with chronic back pain and general debility; signs of cord compression develop later. This infection should be remembered, particularly in practices with a high proportion of patients who have previously lived in the Indian subcontinent.

Clinical features

Infection of the bone occurs by three routes: (1) haematogenous spread; (2) spread from an adjacent focus of infection (contiguous infection); or (3) occasionally by direct inoculation. The case history presents many of the salient features—and consequences—of acute, haematogenous osteomyelitis. Whilst in neonates, as with many infections, signs of osteomyelitis may be extremely soft and non-specific, in children its presentation is often dramatic with high fever, systemic toxicity, and severe pain with limited movement of the affected bone in a previously well patient. There may be obvious swelling of associated soft tissues with surrounding erythema. In adults the presentation may be less acute with pain and limitation of movement in the bone as the primary symptoms. Males are more than twice as commonly affected as females. In any of these situations the rule for the GP is that if the diagnosis occurs to you, you must positively rule it out, and this usually means immediate referral.

Approximately three-quarters of cases involve the long bones of the lower limb, especially in childhood and young adolescence. In young people, the metaphysis of growing bone is characteristically affected because of the vasculature of this area. Subperiosteal collections can occur because the periosteum becomes more adherent only in adulthood. In elderly patients with peripheral vascular disease or diabetes mellitus the small bones of the feet may become infected. Patients with sickle-cell disease, in whom osteomyelitis can mimic sickle-cell thrombotic crisis, those on haemodialysis, or intravenous drug abusers are all predisposed to bone infections and hence doctors working in inner city practices should be particularly aware of the possibility.

Diagnosis and investigations

The diagnosis of osteomyelitis can be confirmed using radiographic and laboratory tests. The ESR is likely to be raised but the white cell count may be unimpressive. If infection is due to *Staph. aureus* there may be a normal total white cell count but the differential may reflect a marked neutrophilia. The measurement of anti-staphylococcal and anti-streptococcal antibodies may help to confirm the diagnosis of deep sepsis. Bony X-ray changes of acute osteomyelitis will not become apparent for 10 days or more after the infection is established. There may, however, be changes in the appearance of soft tissues planes which suggest the diagnosis, especially in the appropriate clinical setting, which appear earlier than the bony changes. Radionucleotide scanning techniques especially with technetium are more sensitive.

It is both desirable and essential to establish the aetiological agent responsible for the infection. The duration of antibiotics and the potential for long-term disability make it mandatory that every effort is made to culture the infecting organism and to obtain its antibiotic sensitivities. Appropriate specimens include blood cultures, needle aspiration of the bone, joint fluid, specimens of pus or tissue obtained at operation or fluid from overlying wounds. Up to 85% of cases may be expected to have a bacteriological diagnosis established by culture of such in specimens.[10]

In acute haematogenous infections it is common to obtain a single organism, whereas in more chronic forms, or in infections resulting from secondary spread from an infected focus, mixed infections may be found. In chronic osteomyelitis where there may be associated sinus formation, the predictive value of sinus culture for organisms other than *Staph. aureus* is less than 50% when compared with culture of specimens obtained at operation.

Treatment of septic arthritis and osteomyelitis

Joint aspiration should be performed in patients with suspected septic arthritis since it has not only diagnostic but also therapeutic value. Many orthopaedic surgeons irrigate accessible joints as well. Antibiotic therapy, accompanied by repeated joint aspiration if the effusion accumulates, should provide adequate treatment but if after one week the effusion persists, formal surgical drainage may be required.

The antibiotic regime that is chosen will reflect either the specific clinical situation or, ideally, the antibiotic sensitivity of the organism responsible for

Table 12.3 *Empirical antibiotics in septic arthritis*

Age	Likely organisms	Suggested therapy
<1 month	Group B streptococci Gram-negative bacilli *Staph. aureus*	Gentamicin and flucloxacillin. Change to penicillin and gentamicin if group B streptococci confirmed
1 mth–5 yrs	*Haemophilus influenzae* Staph. aureus Gram-negative bacilli Group streptococci	Cephalosporin (*e.g.* cefuroxime) in addition to gentamicin and flucloxacillin
>5 yrs–adult	*Staph. aureus* Streptococci *Neisseria* spp. Gram-negative bacilli	Flucloxacillin and fucidin (orally) or a cephalosporin (e.g. cefuroxime)

the infection. If at presentation joint fluid is not available or if the Gram-stain is negative, then empirical antibiotics will be necessary. Table 12.3 shows the antibiotics used, but these are only empirical guidelines and any GP who has to start treatment for a patient awaiting admission or transfer to a specialist unit should discuss the patient with a microbiologist. If the Gram-film of the joint aspirate is positive then more specific treatment may be commenced. Thus for example, in a neonate with Gram-positive cocci in chains on a Gram-film from a joint aspirate, it would be sensible to start with penicillin and gentamicin as initial therapy rather than flucloxacillin and gentamicin. Similarly, a young adult with Gram-negative diplococci from the Gram-stain of a monoarticular joint effusion should be commenced on penicillin (in the USA, a cephalosporin such as ceftriaxone is currently first-line therapy because of concerns of beta-lactamase production in *Neisseria gonorrhoeae*). If Lyme disease has been diagnosed high dose intravenous penicillin would be appropriate.

The treatment of acute osteomyelitis is more difficult and is still somewhat contentious. Although most practitioners still advocate surgical drainage where this is possible there is dispute over which antibiotic regimes to use, the best route, and the duration of therapy. Staphylococcal sepsis should probably be treated with combination therapy since there is some suggestion that a more successful outcome can be achieved, especially in chronic osteomyelitis. In the UK a commonly used regime includes intravenous flucloxacillin with oral fucidin. In the USA, for staphylococcal infection, a penicillin-resistant beta-lactam such as naficillin is often used as a single agent in high doses. Long-standing recommendations from the USA for treatment of the condition in children, which are probably also applicable to adults, emphasizes the requirement for needle aspiration of the affected bone if subperiosteal pus is not obtained, with subsequent surgical drainage of the pus if any is aspirated. Appropriate intravenous antibiotics are recommended by this protocol for a total of four weeks, with monitoring of serum cidal levels. No oral therapy need subsequently be given. It should be noted that there are an increasing number of studies evaluating the role of oral antibiotics in the treatment of osteomyelitis. In selected patients where the organism and its antibiotic sensitivities are known, where there has been adequate surgical debridement, and where there is both patient compliance and appropriate monitoring (including serum cidal levels) oral therapy following a short course of intravenous therapy may be appropriate.[13] Cases of late relapses of acute osteomyelitis or of chronic osteomyelitis will require surgical referral for debridement and definitive surgical treatment, as well as long-term antibiotic therapy.

Implications for general practice

The overriding concern for the GP is to consider the possibility of a septic joint, especially in patients who may have other underlying joint problems such as rheumatoid arthritis. In the fit, young adult with a monoarticular swollen joint, septic arthritis will be the initial diagnosis but in the infant who is 'not quite right' it may be one of a number of diagnoses to be excluded. In more than 90% of adult patients with bacterial arthritis some predisposing factor may be found, including steroid therapy, pre-existing diabetes mellitus or trauma, but nearly a quarter of patients will have pre-existing arthritis.[14] The diagnostic difficulty then occurs of deciding whether a joint has flared up as part of the underlying process or as result of superseding infection.

Although most cases of bacterial arthritis resolve fully after treatment poor outcome of therapy is more likely in patients over 60 years with pre-existing rheumatoid arthritis, infections of the hips and shoulders, symptomatic for over 7 days before treatment, the involvement of four or more joints, and positive cultures after 7 days appropriate therapy.[15] It may fall to the GP to deal with the subsequent problems. For example, one study followed 60 paediatric cases of bone and joint infection. Four patients developed serious sequaelae (7%) involving limb shortening, joint destruction, and pathological fracture. In general, over a quarter of children may be affected by sequaelae such as shortening of a limb or reduced movement in the affected joint.[16,17]

Cases of osteomyelitis may present equally difficult diagnostic difficulties. In the very young child, the systemic signs of serious sepsis may overwhelm the presentation of the local source of infection and it is therefore a diagnosis which must be considered and for which careful examination should be performed. Most patients make a full recovery after an adequate treatment period but there can be subsequent sequaelae.

Case history

A 69-year-old woman was referred to the orthopaedic clinic with a one-week history of pain and swelling in her left knee. Six months earlier she had been commenced on steroids for polymyalgia rheumatica, with pain in her shoulders and an ESR of 116. She gave a past history of acute osteomyelitis at the age of 16 years (in 1939) which had been treated with surgical drainage and extended bed rest. Indeed, she recalls being forced to remain behind in her local London hospital when all the other children were being evacuated at the outset of war so that her treatment could continue! A small sinus had developed on the medial aspect of her knee but had been dry and healed for at least the preceding 20 years. The new effusion was tapped and a penicillin-sensitive *Staph. aureus* was isolated. When the patient had been admitted earlier in the year for investigation of her raised ESR and shoulder pain, a blood culture taken at that time had also grown a penicillin-sensitive *Staph. aureus* from one out of two blood culture bottles at 7 days incubation. The patient had been discharged home well and the blood culture isolate was thought to have been a skin contaminant. Retrospectively, it is likely that the blood culture isolate was relevant to her underlying diagnosis. Bone scan of the infected leg revealed the presence of a sequestrian, but the patient was unwilling to undergo surgery. She was weaned off her steroids, treated with 4 weeks of appropriate intravenous antibiotics, and was mobilized before discharge home on life-long, low dose penicillin V in the hope of preventing reactivation of her infection. When seen in the out-patient clinic 3 months following her discharge, the ESR was 5, the knee was dry with no effusion, and the patient was systemically well.

Late complications of osteomyelitis can include late relapses or the development of chronic osteomyelitis with the potential for amyloid disease and even a possible carcinoma. With the institution of antibiotics early in the disease process and with adequate antibiotic therapy, chronic forms of the infection are increasingly rare and these complications are now infrequently seen.

Cases of chronic osteomyelitis should be referred to an orthopaedic surgeon since the need for definitive surgery and appropriate type and duration of antibiotic therapy will require consideration. As demonstrated by the following case study, chronic osteomyelitis may present many years after the acute event.

References

1. McCormick A, Fleming D, Charlton J. *Morbidity statistics from general practice. Fourth National Study.* OPCS: London: HMSO (1995)

2. Goldings E, Jericho J. Lyme Disease. *J Clin Rheum Dis* (1986) **12**: 343–67

3. Benjamin C, Chew G, Silman A. Joint and limb symptoms in children after immunisation with measles, mumps and rubella vaccine. *BMJ* (1992) **304**: 1075–8

4. White D *et al.* Human parvovirus arthropathy. *Lancet* (1985) **1**: 419–21

5. Jobanputra P *et al.* High frequency of parvovirus B19 in patients tested for rheumatoid factor. *BMJ* (1995) **311**: 1542

6. Department of Rheumatology. *Audit of the management of the acute hot joint.* Royal Hospitals NHS Trust. November (1994)

7. Ward J, Atecheson S. Infectious arthritis. *Med Clinics N Am* (1977) **61**:313–29

8. Inman J, Gallegos K, Brause B. Clinical and Microbiological features of prosthetic joint infection. *American J Med* (1984) **77**:47–53

9. Norden C. A critical review of antibiotic prophylaxis in orthopaedic surgery. *Rev Infect Dis* (1983) **5**:928–32

10. Dich V, Nelson J, Haltalin K. Osteomyelitis in infants and in children. *Am J Dis Child* (1975) **129**: 1273–82

11. Meyers B, Berson B, Gilbert M. Clinical patterns of osteomyelitis due to gram-negative bacteria. *Arch Intern Med* (1973) **131**:228–33

12. Sugarman B, Hawes S, Musher D. Osteomyelitis beneath pressure sores. *Arch Intern Med* (1983) **143**:683–8

13. Morrissy R, Shore S. Bone and joint sepsis. *Ped Clinics N Am* (1986) **33**:1551–64

14. Kelly P, Martin W, Coventry M. Bacterial (suppurative) arthritis in the adult. *Am J Bone Joint Surg* (1970)**52**: 1595–602

15. Smith J, Piercy E. Infectious arthritis. *Clin Infect Dis* (1995) **20**:225–31

16. Howard J, Highgenboten C, Nelson J. Residual effects of septic arthritis in infancy and childhood. *JAMA* (1976) **236**:932–5

17. Strong M, Lejman T, Michno P. Sequelae from septic arthritis of the knee during the first two years of life. *J Ped Orthopaed* (1994) **14**:745–51

CHAPTER THIRTEEN

Skin and soft tissue infections

Skin and soft tissue infections are caused by a variety of bacteria, viruses, and fungi and are commonly seen in general practice. The average GP will see about 30 new cases per 1000 patients in any year. Patients also present with infestations some of which are secondarily infected. Many patients present directly to, or are followed up, by the practice nurse. The diagnosis and management of these conditions should form part of multidisciplinary continuing education and a practice clinical meeting on the subject would present an ideal opportunity to invite the local microbiologist and infection control nurse.

Bacterial infections

Most of the bacterial skin infections which are seen in general practice are caused by *Staphylococcus aureus* or *Streptococcus pyogenes*. While there are recognizable syndromes, which are discussed below, it is often necessary to start treatment on the basis of an ill-defined early clinical picture and before the results of microbiological culture are known. Streptococci are always susceptible to penicillin (or erythromycin in people with a penicillin allergy) but staphylococcal infection must be treated with a penicillinase-resistant antibiotic such as flucloxacillin. Some staphylococci are now resistant to erythromycin and the use of clarithromycin and azithromycin as alternatives for patients allergic to penicillin is not an ideal solution. This is a situation that might profitably be discussed with the local microbiologist.

The use of topical agents for minor skin infections is controversial.[1] They can cause skin sensitization, although many GPs have found topical fusidic acid a useful treatment for localized impetigo in children. This formulation is not used in hospital practice because of the production of bacterial resistance. Topical mupiricin should not be used except for methicillin-resistant staphylococci. Its casual use in general practice is to be avoided.

While several of the minor infections described below are sufficiently characteristic to allow empirical therapy, it is good practice to culture collections of pus to identify the responsible organism. Swabs from oozing surfaces may also be useful in directing the choice of an antibiotic.

Infections of hair follicles

Occasionally, patients present with an infection of the hair follicles that leads to small erythematous or pustular lesions. A severe form may occur in the beard area where it is known as sycosis barbae. The responsible organism is usually *Staph. aureus* and the infection responds to flucloxacillin and warm compresses. If the patient can stop shaving the situation is improved; if not, meticulous attention to hygiene and the use of disposable razors are good advice. Women may suffer from the condition in the axilla; frequent washing and avoiding the use of deodorants and shaving helps to prevent severe or recurrent infections.

If *Staph. aureus* infects an obstructed hair follicle then a boil results. These are extremely common infections and patients usually consult only if they are severe or recurrent. They start as a tender inflammatory nodule on the face, neck, or other hairy area and become fluctuant over several days. Eventually, they discharge pus and the pain is relieved. Signs of generalized infection are uncommon and although the patient is in great discomfort, drainage or warm soaks are generally adequate therapy with antibiotics reserved for severe lesions. The patient may welcome treatment and supervision by the practice nurse, especially if the boil is in an inaccessible place.

Some patients suffer from recurrent boils and need different management. Occasionally, undiagnosed diabetes may be present and this should always be excluded. Known diabetics, those who sweat profusely, and patients with poor hygiene are prone to recurrent infection. Often, the problem is due to nasal staphylococcal carriage in the patient or a family member and in persistent cases it is worth swabbing all the family members and treating carriers with antibiotic cream to the nostrils. Referral to a dermatologist may be necessary. Very occasionally, systemic rifampicin may be recommended to eradicate the organism in carriers.

If a staphylococcal infection spreads beyond an infected follicle into the subcutaneous fat a carbuncle results. This is a severe condition, often occurring on the back of the neck or back and is characterized by multiple drainage points and generalized signs of infection. As bacteraemia and metastatic spread may follow, the condition should be taken very seriously. Early referral to a surgeon is recommended as surgical drainage is usually necessary in conjunction with antistaphylococcal antibiotics.

Impetigo

Impetigo, an infection most commonly seen in young children, presents with a perioral crusting rash with spread to the nostrils and the hands; in a minority of cases there may be formation of bullae. The infection is still relatively common but is usually localized. While *Staph. aureus* is the usual causative organism, *Strep. pyogenes* may be responsible and it is not possible to distinguish clinically between them. Frequently, both organisms are isolated. In children with widespread impetiginized lesions on the trunk and limbs, underlying scabies must be considered and if present treated (see below). Similarly, impetigo of the scalp must not be diagnosed without excluding infestation with head lice; the secondary bacterial infection follows repeated scratching.

Treatment

Management of impetigo is with antibiotics active against *Staph. aureus* and *Strep. pyogenes*. Children with impetigo are contagious and time should be spent explaining to the parent about the use of separate towels, not sharing a bed, and encouraging the child not to touch the lesions. Families living in poor accommodation without facilities for frequent bathing or domestic washing machines will need particular understanding and support from the GP and health visitor. Children should be kept home from nursery or school until 48 hours after antibiotic treatment has started or until the lesions are dry and healing.

Erysipelas and cellulitis

In contrast, erysipelas is a disease of older patients, often female, and whilst involvement of the lower limbs is common, it can also present as a facial rash with a butterfly distribution. It is a superficial form of cellulitis with prominent lymphatic involvement. The patient is often extremely toxic and unwell and the rash characteristically has a palpable well-defined edge marking the outline of the oedematous tissues. The responsible organism is *Strep. pyogenes*, and the patient may need urgent admission for intravenous antibiotics.

Cellulitis is a spreading infection involving the subcutaneous tissues. The affected area is red, hot, swollen, painful, and ascending lymphangitis and regional lymph node involvement are common. The usual organism is *Strep. pyogenes* and less frequently *Staph. aureus* which enter through minor abrasions or long-standing ulcerating conditions such as venous ulcers. Prompt therapy with an oral antibiotic, such as flucloxacillin, usually produces a rapid response but these patients may become ill with fever and rigors and require hospital admission for investigation and intravenous antibiotics. This condition may be recurrent and patients come to recognize the early warning signs. It is reasonable for them to keep a course of antibiotics at home to start at once with the advice that should they do so they should also contact the practice.

Leg ulcers

The commonest cause of leg ulcers in UK general practice is disease of the arteries and veins. The medical and surgical management is beyond the scope of this section. However, in general, all practices need a team policy which includes a unified approach, assessment of the home environment, and inspection of the ulcer by doctor and nurse together at defined intervals. The mainstay of treatment for 'venous' ulcers remains elevation and exercise with expert bandaging by the nurse.[2] All ulcers are colonized by a wide range of organisms; this is not an indication for antibiotic therapy or the use of antiseptics. In particular, the use of topical antibiotics should be avoided with the ulcer kept clean by irrigation with saline. Occasionally, infection spreads beyond the margins of the ulcer and should then be dealt with as any other cellulitis (see above). Some of these patients may be admitted to primary care beds and it is important to involve the microbiologist in discussions about the use of antibiotics in the hospital setting.

Diabetic foot ulcers[3]

Diabetes leads to vulnerability to ulcers of the feet and infection plays an important role in their initiation. The use of systemic antibiotics is controversial unless there is cellulitis, constitutional upset, or a foul-smelling lesion. However, the nurse and doctor treating these patients should be vigilant for underlying osteitis which can be very difficult to diagnose. It is important to seek specialist advice if there are any doubts about the patient's progress as deterioration can occur quite rapidly, ultimately leading to avoidable amputation of the foot.

Necrotizing fasciitis

Streptococcus pyogenes (GAS) is a common primary pathogen of throat and skin and in Chapter 6 some discussion was made in debating whether it is necessary to confirm and interpret its presence in patients with sore throats. It is a frequent cause of the infections described above, many of which are minor and easy to treat. However, the organism is also responsible for rapidly fatal infections and the past decade has seen a resurgence of severe illness caused by GAS.[4] Intense media interest in necrotizing fasciitis in mid 1994 was accompanied by sensational headlines of 'flesh-eating bacteria' and many GPs were consulted by worried patients with minor skin infections as a result.

The increase is associated with changes in the virulence of some streptococci which produce pyrogenic exotoxin-A (scarlet fever toxin) and bear surface M-protein which enables the bacterium to resist phagocytosis.[5] These organisms are similar to those that caused the scarlet fever that was so feared at the beginning of the century.

GAS infections can be divided into the three major categories shown in Table 13.1. Severe invasive disease is rare but may present in general practice in children and adults. It is preceded by pharyngitis or infection through a break in the skin, both extremely common events highlighting one of the perennial difficulties for the generalist, namely the identification of the situation that is just a bit different from all of the others and which heralds the onset of a catastrophic infection. The organism then localizes in an area of tissue damage such as a bruise or a varicella lesion; in children the disease occurs most commonly in the later stages of chickenpox. For the

Table 13.1 *Different types of infections caused by beta-haemolytic group A streptococcus (GAS)*

Uncomplicated
- Pharyngitis
- Impetigo

Severe invasive disease
- Septicaemia
- Streptococcal toxic shock syndrome
- Necrotizing fasciitis
- Myositis

Delayed sequaelae
- Erythema nodosum
- Acute glomerulonephritis
- Rheumatic fever

---

first 3 days there is a flu-like illness getting worse with the onset of high fever, sore throat, lymphadenitis, vomiting, diarrhoea, and a scarlet fever rash. Any child recovering from chickenpox who develops these symptoms should be admitted to hospital immediately. During this time penicillin is effective but by the fourth day the infection cannot be controlled by antibiotics. There is multiorgan failure, disseminated intravascular coagulation, and intractable pain at the site of the infection which has developed into a fasciitis or myositis. The only effective treatment is radical surgery; the case fatality rate is 30–50% and over half the survivors have limbs amputated.[6]

Staphylococcal toxic shock syndrome

This disease is characterized by fever, mucous membrane hyperaemia, subcutaneous oedema, desquamating erythroderma, and rapid progression to hypotension and multiorgan failure. The syndrome has been reported in young women and has been related to the presence of vaginal staphylococci, menstruation, and the use of tampons. Health education for women about menstruation should emphasize the need to change tampons regularly, especially if super-tampons are used. The syndrome is not confined to this group, however, and is also associated with focal staphylococcal infections, often in children.[7]

Viral infections

A variety of viruses cause skin lesions which may be presented to the GP. The majority are due to the herpes simplex virus (types 1 and 2), the varicella zoster virus, and the human papilloma virus. *Molluscum contagiosum* and orf are also viral skin infections which are seen occasionally and may present diagnostic difficulty for the GP. Many generalized viral infections are accompanied by characteristic rashes or skin lesions; they are described in Chapter 14.

Herpes simplex

Skin infections with herpes simplex virus (HSV) occur as a result of direct inoculation on to the skin or mucous membrane. Genital herpes, usually caused by HSV-2 is described in Chapter 11 where a section on the characteristics and epidemiology of the herpes simplex virus is included. Herpes simplex is also an important cause of viral keratitis.

Clinical features

Primary infection with herpes simplex leads to vesicles on the lips, face, buccal mucosa, and throat in the majority of cases. The vesicles rupture, leaving painful ulcers or erosions which persist for about two weeks. The lesions then heal forming crusts on non-mucosal surfaces. The end of viral shedding coincides with the formation of dry crusts. Most of these infections are in children under 5; the incubation period is from 2 to 21 days. Although the primary infection may be mild or subclinical, it may be accompanied by systemic symptoms such as fever, malaise, headaches, and lymphadenopathy. During the primary infection the virus establishes latency in the dorsal root ganglion.

Reactivation of herpes simplex virus

Clinical triggers which are associated with the reactivation of the disease are well known to patients and doctors alike; they include sunlight, fever, menstruation, and stress. About 50% of patients experience a recurrence at a median time of one year. The commonest presentation in general practice is that of patients who have recurrent 'cold sores'.

Treatment of recurrent herpes labialis (cold sores)

Patients get to know their own triggers for recurrence of cold sores but it does no harm to reinforce the use of high factor sun block cream and that application of acyclovir cream, now available direct to patients from the pharmacy, has a beneficial effect if applied as soon as prodromal itching is noticed. However, it is not universally successful and oral prophylactic therapy may be recommended for patients with particularly frequent recurrences. Acyclovir 400 mg, twice daily has been shown to reduce the number of recurrences by 71% in culture-confirmed lesions compared with placebo in patients subject to six or more episodes a year of herpes labialis.[8] Acyclovir prophylaxis is less successful for herpes labialis than for genital herpes where up to 90% of lesions may be avoided.[9] General practitioners must weigh up the cost–benefit ratio in taking this decision, remembering to include the full weight of patient misery in the equation.[10]

Varicella zoster virus: herpes zoster

The varicella zoster virus infects and establishes latency in 90–95% of children by the age of 15.[11] Reactivation of the virus leads to shingles (zoster) usually much later in life.

Epidemiology and spread

Herpes zoster occurs at some time in the life of 10–20% of the population; usually in later life although it can present at any age. The age-related risk is believed to be due to waning of the immune containment of the virus. Although humoral immunity is not thought to be of major relevance in reactivation, cell-mediated immune mechanisms play a crucial role in controlling the virus. The lymphocyte response to varicella zoster virus antigens declines with advancing age, during immunosuppressive therapy, and with the development of lymphoproliferative malignancies. Patients with HIV infection are at high risk for developing zoster and this should be borne in mind within general practice when patients present.

Although patients with malignancy are at higher risk for herpes zoster, studies have shown that the converse is not true. General practitioners need not investigate otherwise healthy patients with shingles for silent cancers.

Clinical features

The onset of herpes zoster is marked by a prodromal phase lasting 1–4 days. During this time the patient complains of fever, malaise, headache, and localized parasthesiae. Other causes of severe localized pain such as appendicitis or migraine may be considered at first but the appearance of the skin eruption, usually involving one dermatome, but occasionally up to three, determines the diagnosis.

The skin eruption consists of groups of vesicles on an erythematous base. They become pustular (rarely haemorrhagic) by days 3–4 and form crusts by days 7–10 by which time they no longer contain viable virus. In otherwise healthy patients the lesions usually resolve within three weeks although scarring is common.

Complications and prognosis

The neurological and ocular complications of zoster are shown in Table 13.2. The principal cause of acute and chronic morbidity associated with the condition is pain. Post-herpetic neuralgia is commoner and lasts longer in older people and can cause unbearable distress to sufferers. It complicates about 9–14% of cases of herpes zoster and resolves within 2 months in 50% of cases and within 12 months in 80%.

The other neurological complications are much less common with motor neuropathies occurring overall in 5% of cases and in up to 12% of

Table 13.2 *Neurological and ocular complications of herpes zoster*

Neurological
- Post-herpetic neuralgia
- Motor neuropathies: (cranial nerves)
  - Ophthalmoplegia (3,4,6)
  - Ramsay–Hunt syndrome (7,8)
  - Also (9,10,12)
- Motor neuropathies: peripheral nerves
  - diaphragmatic paralysis
  - neurogenic bladder
- Guillain–Barré syndrome
- Encephalitis
- Myelitis

Ocular
- Lid ulceration and retraction
- Conjunctivitis, scleritis
- Anterior uveitis
- Keratitis
- Optic neuritis
- Thrombosis, haemorrhage
- Panophthalmitis

---

patients with cranial nerve involvement. About half of these manifest as the Ramsay–Hunt syndrome. This consists of lesions in the external auditory canal and ipsilateral facial and auditory nerve involvement. The patient also complains of vertigo and hearing loss. Most of the post-herpetic neuropathies are temporary with up to 75% of patients making a full recovery. Zoster in the ophthalmic distribution is followed by complications in over a third of cases. They result from sensory or motor neuropathies, direct viral invasion, and vasculopathy. They may lead to serious loss of vision and the GP must review these patients very frequently and refer immediately if ocular complications arise. An early discussion with the ophthalmologist is in any case a sensible course of action.

Investigations

The diagnosis of zoster is clinical and investigations are rarely relevant in general practice. However, studies have shown that some patients presumed to have zoster were in fact suffering from herpes simplex virus infections. Patients with maxillary or sacral nerve root involvement, or who have had previous vesicular lesions in the same distribution should be considered for further definitive diagnosis so that management can take into account the prevention of recurrences in the case of herpes simplex virus infections.

Treatment

Although oral acyclovir, famciclovir, and valaciclovir are all approved for the therapy of herpes zoster, clinical benefits have not been shown to be outstanding and the effect on post-herpetic neuralgia is equivocal. While definitive research evidence is awaited therapy should be reserved for the elderly, the immunocompromised and those with ophthalmic zoster and decided on a case-by-case basis.[12,13] Patients should be informed that although the lesions are vesicular they are potentially infectious to people who are not immune to chickenpox. The lesions should be covered if possible and family visits to susceptible adults should be postponed accordingly.

Post-herpetic neuralgia should be treated with analgesics and amitriptyline has been shown to be useful if the symptoms persist. All elderly patients with zoster should be followed up, reviewed, and if necessary, referred, until a satisfactory resolution of persisting pain is achieved.

Case history

A previously healthy man of 65, a retired owner of a shoe shop, appeared to make an uneventful recovery from thoracic herpes zoster (T12). Two weeks later he developed a feverish illness with generalized aches and pains. The GP visited and and thought he looked unwell but found no localizing signs to aid diagnosis. The next day the patient experienced weakness in his legs and difficulty in walking to the lavatory. The following day he was worse with the weakness also affecting his hands. He was admitted to the the local hospital and subsequently transferred to the regional neurology unit where the diagnosis of Guillain–Barré syndrome secondary to herpes zoster was made. His recovery was slow, but after several months he was able to walk and resume a normal life.

Human papilloma virus

Human papilloma viruses (HPV) are associated with benign papillomas, usually of the hands, feet, and genitals, and the potential for malignant transformation.

A great deal is still to be discovered about HPV and the factors which allow the presence of chronic infection in some patients. While immunocompromised patients with depressed cell-mediated immunity are subject to severe wart infections, immunocompetent patients in whom infections resolve are not certain to avoid the development of new warts at some future date.

Most warts will resolve within months if left alone; certainly, they are gone within two years. However, children are commonly seen with warts on their hands and feet and parents request that they be treated, sometimes as a result of ill-informed pressure from school.

Treatment of warts including plantar warts (verrucas)[14]

Plantar warts are very common, and few people escape infection although many are subclinical and hence go undetected. General practitioners and practice nurses seeing children with plantar warts should spend time explaining the natural history to the parents particularly that they will get better by themselves. If a decision to treat the wart is made then about 80% will be cured within 12 weeks using a topical salicylic acid preparation carefully applied to the wart only. The child and parent must be prepared to apply the paint daily having first pared the wart with an emery board or pumice stone. The wart may then be covered with a plaster unless a preparation in a collodian gel is used. Some practitioners prefer preparations containing podophyllin applied less frequently. Mosaic plantar warts are particularly difficult to treat and 3% formaldehyde soaks poured into a shallow dish and the wart area soaked for 15–20 minutes may prove effective. All of these treatments may cause pain and irritation and patients should be asked to return if they are worried; in any case it does no harm for the practice nurse to check progress at least once.

Some practices prefer to use an ablative treatment, liquid nitrogen cryotherapy being the commonest. The technique involves freezing the wart and 1 mm of surrounding skin for a maximum of 10–25 seconds. The procedure should be repeated at about three-week intervals until the warts have cleared. This can be very painful and is not suitable for younger children. The local dermatologist, or other experienced GPs should be approached for training before embarking on this approach. Overall, the results from cryotherapy are no better than those from properly applied wart paint.

The most important thing to emphasize to parents is that this is a universal infection, it gets better by itself (slowly) and that there is no need to exclude the child from swimming or gym. Warts that are being treated may conveniently be covered by a plaster. If the practice has a range of strategies and a practice policy for treating this common complaint, referral to the dermatologist should be unusual.

DNA pox viruses

Molluscum contagiosum: Epidemiology and clinical features

Molluscum contagiosum is a benign cutaneous lesion caused by a large DNA pox virus. It is relatively uncommon:[15] a study in Dutch general practice reported an incidence of 2.4 per 1000 person years with a peak incidence between the ages of 6 and 10 years. There was a higher incidence in the first half of the year with the sexes affected equally. Overall, one in six Dutch children aged 15 years had visited their GP at least once in their lifetime for molluscum contagiosum. There were few adult cases.[16] Occasionally, the infection may be sexually transmitted (3% of all cases) and it may also occur in a severe form in immunocompromised individuals.

Table 13.3 *The clinical stages of orf*

Maculopapular	Erythematous macule or papule
Target	A red centre, middle pale ring, outer red halo
Acute	Erythematous weeping nodule
Regenerative	Dry with black dots on the surface
Papillomatous	Papillomas appear on the surface of the lesion
Regressive	Dry crust

The lesions commonly occur on the face, neck, axillae, and groins; each one forms a small dome-shaped pearly papule with a central umbilication which may be crusted. The lesions tend to occur in groups, sometimes along scratch marks, and although they enlarge at first they tend to regress within 7 to 9 months.

Treatment

Once a lesion becomes inflamed it may be squeezed with blunt forceps thereby expressing the cheesy material it contains. This is often enough to effect a cure but as the lesions respond well to cryotherapy with liquid nitrogen some GPs adopt this approach. Others curette solitary lesions as a minor surgical procedure.

Orf

Orf is an infection of sheep and goats caused by a DNA pox virus which is transmitted to humans by inoculation from infected lesions, exudate, or contaminated objects such as fences, hedges, and barn doors. It is therefore most commonly seen in country practice but holiday-makers can present in town settings on return where the diagnosis may easily be missed! In humans, the disease usually presents as a solitary lesion on the fingers or hands after an incubation period of less than 4 weeks. It often gets better within another 6 weeks having gone through several characteristic stages. Complications are unusual but include secondary bacterial infection which provides the only indication for antibiotic therapy.

Fungal infections

Superficial fungal infections seen in general practice are due to dermatophytes or yeasts. Until relatively recently the treatment of some of these infections was unsatisfactory with both patients and doctors daunted by the need for lengthy courses of drugs with potentially toxic side-effects. However, new and effective treatments have become available making the need for precise diagnosis more important. In addition, the increasing incidence of fungal infections in immunocompromised patients has led to the use of unusual drug regimes many of which will be prescribed in general practice under specialist supervision.

Epidemiology

There are few reports from general practice with accurate figures about the incidence of these infections. Poyner[17] reported the annual incidence of dermatophyte infections in 1992 in his group practice of 25 000 patients as 8.6/1000: 215 patients presented of whom 50% had infections on the feet, 22% on the trunk, 20% in the groin, and 4% in the nails. The prevalence of fungal foot infections is estimated to be between 10% and 15% of the population with up to a third of these involving the toe-nails. Many patients do not seek advice for these problems or if they do they prefer to see a chiropodist.

Dermatophyte infections

Dermatophytes are fungi that invade the superficial layers (stratum corneum) of the epidermis, hair, and nails. Infection is acquired from other humans, animals, and soil and is spread as a result of contact with keratin debris carrying fungal hyphae. The dermatophyte fungi responsible for skin disease in humans are classified into three genera; *Microsporum*, *Trichophyton*, and *Epidermophyton*. There are several species within each genus and, overall, about 10 species cause the infections known as 'ringworm'. This lay term is misleading and upsetting to patients but it is still widely used. Although certain species tend to occur in particular sites, the clinical term 'tinea' is used irrespective of the organism and is followed by the Latin word describing the body site. (e.g. tinea pedis, tinea capitis). *Trichophyton rubrum* causes most of the skin and nail infections and *Microsporum canis* is the principal cause of scalp ringworm.

Diagnosis

The clinical features and differential diagnosis of dermatophyte infections at different sites is shown in Table 13.4. These infections are sometimes difficult to diagnose; the important thing is to consider the possibility when first examining the lesions. The diagnosis should be confirmed, preferably before starting treatment and in any case steroid cream should not be applied if there is any doubt as it leads to the loss of the defined margin, extension of the infection, and pustule formation (tinea incognito). It is rarely so urgent to begin treatment that investigations cannot be done and most patients will be happy to wait once they understand why there is a delay.

Investigations

Using a scalpel held at right angles, skin scrapings can be taken from the advancing margin of the lesion, they should be collected on to black paper if possible. Infected nails should be clipped or scraped from the diseased nail surface and the clippings sent to the laboratory; in the case of tinea capitis, skin scrapings and hairs from the affected area should be sent.[18]

Table 13.4 *The clinical features and differential diagnosis of dermatophyte infections*

Site	Clinical features	Differential diagnosis
Feet (Tinea pedis)	Itchy, scaling between 3rd and 4th toes Dorsum of feet, sole of foot, defined	Erythrasma *Candida albicans* *Staph. aureus* Eczema Psoriasis
Groin (Tinea cruris)	Itchy, symmetrical scaly, erythematous, usually men, look for other sites of infection	Intertrigo Flexural psoriasis Seborrhoeic dermatitis *Candida albicans*
Body (Tinea corporis)	Itchy, erythematous scaly plaques, defined, elevated margins, central clearing	Discoid eczema Psoriasis
Scalp (Tinea capitis)	Children, usually from kittens, scaling, broken hairs; if severe, pustular, scarring alopecia	Alopecia areata Psoriasis Eczema
Nails (Onychomycosis)	Asymmetrical, thickening, discoloration	Psoriasis Lichen planus Onychogryphosis *Candida*

Treatment

The majority of superficial infections will respond to topical therapy; if systemic therapy is contemplated it should be based on proven infection as prolonged therapy may be required to effect a cure. The antifungals have been described in Chapter 5. It is well to remember that the older and cheaper preparation, Whitfield's ointment (benzoic acid 6% and salicylic acid 3% in an emulsifying agent), is also quite effective for localized tinea.

Trunk and groin. Localized infections can be treated topically with an imidazole or terbinafine cream. Extensive disease in adults should be treated systemically with either terbinafine 250 mg daily for 2–4 weeks or itraconazole 100 mg daily for 4 weeks. Other members of the household should be examined and treated if necessary. Both of these regimes lead to 80–90% cure rates.[19] Extensive infections in pregnancy should be referred for a specialist opinion as griseofulvin is contraindicated and the newer drugs are not licensed for use in this situation.

Scalp infection. This infection affects children and should be treated systemically with griseofulvin in a dose of 10 mg/kg of body weight or 1 g daily in adults until there is no further evidence of infection. Up to 3 months of therapy may be necessary.[20] If the lesions are boggy and pustular (kerion) then a systemic antistaphyloccocal antibiotic should be prescribed. Selenium sulphide shampoo is a useful adjunct therapy as it lessens the spread of infective spores and allows an infected child to remain at school.

Foot infection. Topical treatment is best for infections confined to the toe cleft. The patients may well have tried remedies from the pharmacist already. All the imidazole creams are suitable, and terbinafine cream is also highly effective. If the disease affects the dorsum of the foot or the thickened horny layer of the sole, terbinafine 250 mg daily for 2–6 weeks is indicated. Itraconazole 100 mg daily is an alternative and is more effective than griseofulvin. Ideally, patients with this infection should avoid swimming pools and communal changing facilities unless their feet are covered. They should keep their feet dry, wear clean preferably cotton socks daily, and avoid closed synthetic footwear.

Nail infection.[21] This is the most difficult dermatophyte infection to treat and toe-nails are particularly difficult due to their slower rate of growth. In people aged over 50 it is very difficult to get a satisfactory result even after two years of therapy with griseofulvin. Patients on this drug should have their liver function tests monitored and many feel it is not worth taking prolonged, possibly toxic oral therapy for this problem. However, terbinafine 250 mg daily for three months has a cure rate of over 80%,[22,23] and amorolfine lacquer gives good results for distal nail infection although it is very expensive.[24]

Case history

A woman of 72 had seen her GP regularly to monitor severe hypertension. On each occasion she commented on her finger nails which still showed signs of the chronic fungal infection which had been confirmed over two years previously. She did not wish to take oral treatment, keeping her hands dry had no effect, and she seemed resigned to living with the unsightly appearance. One day she mentioned that she had read of a 'nail varnish' that worked wonders and asked if she could try it. The GP looked up the cost of amorolfine lacquer and gulped! Six months later after twice weekly application, the patient's nails were better and she remarked on how wonderful it was to overcome a chronic health problem and have her hands looking nice again.

Yeast infections

Candidosis

It is unusual for *Candida albicans* to be a primary cause of skin disease, it is usually secondary to another problem, such as napkin dermatitis, flexural psoriasis or an immunocompromised patient. It can however cause a chronic paronychia, usually in the finger nails, where there may be a shiny red bolstered nail fold with pus exuding from underneath. *Candida* vulvo-vaginitis is described in Chapter 11, where a detailed description of the yeast can also be found.

All of the topical azole agents and nystatin are effective and sometimes better results are achieved using a combined preparation with hydrocortisone. Candidosis infection should be suspected in babies with nappy rash if the flexures are primarily involved and there are satellite lesions near the spreading margin of the rash. Mothers should be encouraged to leave the child exposed when circumstances allow and to change nappies frequently.

Elderly people who wear dentures are prone to oral candidosis and may also develop an angular cheilitis. The oral lesions form white plaques with an underlying red base which can bleed on touching and the angular cheilitis presents with fissues and erythema. These patients should remove dentures at night, put them in an antifungal solution, see the dentist to check the fit, and use topical oral treatment with a combined preparation to the corners of the mouth.

Case history

An elderly man of 87 had seen his GP regularly for five years. He had always been reserved, with few friends and declined to see the practice nurse. As a vegan, his diet was a source of concern and when he developed an angular cheilitis he was investigated for anaemia. In fact, the situation only resolved when the GP discovered he could now only open his mouth wide enough to remove his dentures with great difficulty and so slept with them in. The local dentist was very encouraging and made him a new set which he now wears. The GP recommended oral miconazole gel and the patient made a complete recovery.

Pityriasis versicolor and seborrhoeic dermatitis

Pityriasis versicolor is characterized by spreading, discrete, brown, scaly patches on the trunk. If the skin is exposed to sun then hypopigmentation occurs. The infection is caused by a hyphal form of *Pityrosporum* yeast called *Malassezia furfur*. It is now also recognized that the infection is important in the aetiology of various forms of seborrhoeic dermatitis. Treatment with a selenium shampoo to the scalp and body is effective in both conditions. Itraconazole 200 mg daily for 5 days results in a 90% cure rate for pityriasis versicolor, and ketoconazole shampoo is the most effective, but also the most expensive treatment for the severe dandruff which is the commonest manifestation of seborrhoea. Systemic therapy for seborrhoea must be reserved for patients with AIDs who may suffer from widespread, poorly controlled disease.

Infestation

Scabies

This cutaneous infestation is caused by the mite *Sarcoptes scabiei*, a common problem in modern general practice, has been with mankind for 3000 years—it has been described in ancient China, India, and the Middle East.[25] The severe itching associated with the infestation has a depressing and debilitating effect which led to it being particularly troublesome during some military campaigns. It was notorious during the Napoleonic Wars and the American Civil War from which the terms 'seven year itch' and 'camp itch' originated.[26]

The life cycle of Sarcoptes scabiei

The mite, *S. scabiei*, is white, has four pairs of legs, the male measures about 0.22 mm × 0.18 mm and the fully grown female about 0.4 mm × 0.3 mm. The gravid female creates burrows at the base of the stratum corneum of the epidermis in which she lays 2–3 eggs a day. Within 72 hours, larvae emerge and make new burrows although less than 10% become adults. The larvae moult, producing nymphs, and moult twice more before reaching maturity when they mate. The whole process takes about 10–17 days and the mites live for 30–60 days. The males spend most time on the surface but enter shallow burrows to feed or mate. The process of burrowing is initiated by the secretion of a solution which produces a minute depression in the skin of the host; penetration takes 1–10 minutes and burrowing a further 30 minutes. Transmission of the mite to a new host is dependent on its ability to survive away from the body. Survival times are longest in cool damp environments and the estimated time of survival at room temperatures is about 2 days.

Epidemiology

The incidence of scabies in UK general practice, based on the Royal College of General Practitioners' weekly returns data, has risen from 1.8/1000 in 1987 to 3.6/1000 in 1993. The global morbidity from scabies since 1900 appears to have encompassed three pandemics with roughly 30-year cycles.

The risk factors for acquiring the infestation relate to close personal contact with an infected person, in particular sharing clothes or sharing a bed. In so far as these risk factors are associated with sexual behaviour or poverty and overcrowding, then these factors are also relevant. Live mites have been recovered from dust samples in 64% of homes of sufferers, but in environments where temperatures were higher, bedlinen was changed frequently, and regular vacuuming occurred, contamination of fomites was lower.[27] Scabies can and does infect all kinds of people, excellent personal

Table 13.5 *Common sites of adult mites in scabies*

- Interdigital spaces of the hands
- Flexor surfaces of the wrists
- Extensor surfaces of the elbows
- Anterior axillary folds
- Female breasts (skin of nipples)
- Periumbilical area
- Penis and scrotum
- Buttocks

hygiene is not protective and the 1990s are a time of high incidence in the pandemic cycle.

Clinical features

Infected people harbour surprisingly few mites with 50% of cases having five or less. The itch is due to sensitization to mite antigens and does not start until a month or more after infestation. This is important in determining the source of infestation and also in the spread of the disease as this can occur during the early stages when the patient is unaware of the infestation. Patients experiencing a re-infestation develop symptoms and signs within 24–48 hours due to previous sensitization.

The cutaneous reaction to the mite consists of a widespread eruption of erythematous, papular, and vesicular lesions. The adult mites are confined to burrows in relatively few sites (Table 13.5), and some have proposed that the rash may be related to shallow burrowing by the numerous immature mites which do not reach maturity. The rash is extremely irritant, especially at night, and frequent scratching leads to excoriation, and eczematization with secondary infestation with *Strep. pyogenes* or *Staph. aureus* occurring in some cases. Untreated, the lesions progress to scaly skin and eventually heavy crusting from hyperkeratosis. This state is known as Norwegian scabies and if the crusts are removed, mite density on the undersurface may exceed 1400 mites/cm^2. This condition is principally seen in patients with AIDS.

Diagnosis

The diagnosis is confirmed by finding evidence of the mite or its debris. This may not be easy but it is important to try (Table 13.6).

Treatment

Although the oldest and cheapest treatment for scabies is benzyl benzoate it requires three applications and is irritant. The modern treatment of scabies revolves around the use of three scabicides: lindane, malathion, and permethrin. Lindane is a toxic substance and should not be used for children under 10 years, during pregnancy, and breast-feeding; for people of low body weight and in epilepsy.[28] Malathion is suitable for children but is

Table 13.6 *Skin scrapings for the diagnosis of scabies*

1. Examine the common sites for adult mite burrows and search for papular and vesicular eruptions
2. If a burrow is obvious it is sometimes possible to remove the mite from its position just in front of the papule at the head of the burrow. Use a sterile needle to try
3. Find an area of papules that have not been scratched. Put a few drops of liquid paraffin on the skin and scrape the skin surface with a no. 15 scalpel blade to remove top of papules and burrow
4. Remove oil and contents and place on to a glass slide and view under the microscope. Faecal pellets are the most likely material, but eggs and mites may be seen.

not as effective as permethrin in children for whom the treatment of choice is permethrin 5% cream.[29] The importance of careful prescribing and rotation of scabicides during a time of high incidence cannot be overemphasized, particularly in view of the higher proportion of the population who are immunocompromised and who suffer from very severe infestations if they are unlucky enough to encounter the mite.

Once a scabicide has been chosen then the patients should be prescribed enough for one treatment. All members of the household and others in close physical contact should be treated. This is crucial to success but can sometimes lead to difficult and sensitive negotiations within the consultation for which time should be set aside. It is often helpful to provide the patient with literature to explain the need for family treatment and to be ready to discuss the matter with absent family members should they appear or telephone later. It is important to synchronize the treatment for everybody who needs it or it may be ineffective.

The treatment should be applied just before bedtime, and it is better not to bathe first as it may increase systemic absorption. The treatment should be applied all over the body, paying particular attention to the webs of the fingers and toes and under the finger nails. Children are more likely to have an infestation on the face and behind the ears and these sites should be treated. When the hands are washed during the next day a new application to them is ideal. A bath should be taken after 24 hours and treatment with calamine and antihistamines given for a few days as the itching may intensify immediately after treatment. Families may need support in dealing with scabies and the offer of follow-up by the practice nurse will be welcome to some.

Lice

There are three cutaneous infestations with lice: on the scalp (pediculosis capitis), the body (pediculosis corporis), and lice of coarse body hair (pediculosis pubis, crabs).

Pediculosis capitis

This infestation is commonest in childhood where the lice and recently laid eggs amy be found on the hair close to the scalp. Dead eggs (nits) further up the hair shaft indicate old infection and do not require treatment.

Treatment of pediculosis capitis

Head lice are best treated by lotions rather than shampoos and they should be applied to the dry hair and scalp according to the manufacturer's instructions, allowed to stay for 12 hours, and then washed off. Lotions in an aqueous base are to be preferred. Malathion and permethrin are both suitable but the GP should confer with the health visitor or school nurse to discover the current local recommendations. A systematic review of clinical efficacy of topical treatments concluded that only for permethrin has sufficient evidence been published to show efficacy.[30] All family members should be treated and, ideally, all class members to ensure success. Head lice can be cleared over a 2 week period by regular 'wet combing'.

Treatment of pediculosis corporis

This infestation is relatively uncommon but may be seen in homeless people sleeping out. The infestation makes the sufferer feel unwell and there may be associated lymphadenopathy. On examination there are widespread papules and excoriation often with associated impetigo. Treatment is with carbaryl, malathion, or permethrin but the most important aspect is to provide clean clothing and bathing facilities.

Treatment of pediculosis pubis

This condition is caused by crab lice (*Pthirus pubis*) which infest coarse body hair, principally pubic, axillary, and eyelashes. The mode of transmission is by direct body contact and is often during intercourse in the case of pubic lice. Patients who have this infestation should be given the opportunity to discuss the possibility of sexually transmitted infections and should be investigated or referred as appropriate. The lice are about 2 mm in length and difficult to see; the nits appear as small whitish dots glued to the hair shaft. The treatment is with non-alcohol based preparations of malathion and carbaryl which are extremely effective as a single application.

Imported skin and soft tissue infections

The speed and frequency of air travel has lead to some unusual skin and soft tissue infections presenting in general practice.

Leprosy

Although leprosy is still one of the most important infectious diseases, affecting many millions of persons world-wide,[31] the disease is of virtually no risk to the traveller. Transmission of the organism responsible, *Mycobacterium leprae*, is not by casual contact but by nasal secretions of patients with untreated, early forms of the disease. The GP is very unlikely to see cases in the UK, unless there is a large immigrant population within the practice area.

Case history

A man of 60 who had lived all of his adult life in the UK returned to visit his relatives in Pakistan in November 1991. After his return he presented to his Hertfordshire GP with pain in and around his left eye. The pain lessened but recurred in March 1992, associated with tiredness and watering of both eyes. The GP entertained a working diagnosis of sinusitis and awaited events. In late April the patient developed a rosacea-like rash on his face with facial oedema. Subsequent swelling of the hands and feet were followed by an urgent referral to hospital where an allergic reaction was diagnosed. Worsening of the facial oedema and rash, arthralgia, and the development of anaesthetic skin lesions developed during May and June 1992 with several urgent admissions arranged by the increasingly alarmed GP. Eventually, a skin biopsy in June 1992 confirmed the diagnosis of leprosy. The patient also had a complete left foot drop, weakness of the intrinsic small muscles of the left hand, and an inability to close both eyes completely.

Clinical features

The organism invades skin and peripheral nerves and the clinical presentation essentially depends on the host's immune response to infection. Two major forms of the disease (lepromatous and tuberculoid leprosy) are recognized, although intermediate forms also occur. Lepromatous leprosy occurs when an individual is lacking a cellular immune response to the bacteria. It is characterized by widespread erythematous or brown, papular or nodular, non-anaesthetic skin lesions. Later, the skin of the face, especially the nose and ear lobes becomes thickened, and rhinitis, testicular atrophy, and ocular damage are common. There are large numbers of organisms demonstrable in nasal smears or in skin biopsy specimens. Patients with tuberculoid leprosy mount an effective cellular immune response to *M. leprae* and have fewer skin lesions but damage to peripheral nerves mediated by delayed-type hypersensitivity reactions. There are a limited number of erythematous or hypopigmented, macular, anaesthetic skin lesions which may have a raised edge. The nerves near the skin lesions are thickened. The neuropathy of leprosy leads to palsies and the anaesthesia to ulceration and loss of tissue.

Cutaneous leishmaniasis

Leishmaniasis is caused by protozoa of the genus *Leishmania* which are transmitted to man by sandflies. The Leishmania that are capable of causing infection in man are divided into four groups: *L. tropica* in the Old World and *L. mexicana* in the New World produce localized forms of cutaneous disease; *L. braziliensis* is the cause of an aggressive form of cutaneous disease termed espundia, and *L. donovani* is the aetiological agent of visceral leishmaniasis or kala-azar.

In Mediterranean countries, the Middle East through to India and in Central Asia and China, the characteristic lesion caused by *L. tropica* is a slowly-growing ulcerating skin lesion with a granulating base (oriental sore or Delhi boil) at the site of the bite. This eventually heals spontaneously leaving an atrophic scar.

A similar disease occurs in South America and is caused by *L. mexicana*. Sometimes, the sandfly bite is on the ear and, if the infection involves the cartilage of the pinna, then a chronic destructive lesion occurs (chiclero's ulcer). Infection with *L. braziliensis* is also found in areas of South America. The initial lesions are similar to those described above but sometimes, several weeks or years later, destructive secondary or metastatic lesions develop at mucocutaneous junctions of the nose and mouth. Diagnosis of cutaneous leishmaniasis is established by demonstrating the parasite (Leishman–Donovan bodies) in histological samples.

Onchocerciasis

Onchocerciasis or river blindness is a chronic disease caused by the filaria *Onchocerca volvulus* in tropical Africa and in some areas of Latin America. It characteristically affects the skin and eyes. The infection is transmitted to humans by the bites of blackflies and is uncommon in travellers but common in those who have spent several years in endemic areas. The adult worms lie in subcutaneous nodules, 2–3 cm in diameter, situated particularly on the trunk and legs in those contracting infection in Africa. The microfilariae are in the skin and eyes. In the skin they produce intensely itchy papules, sometimes with joint pains. After some time, lichenification and atrophy of the skin occurs, resulting in spotty depigmentation of the shins and lower abdomen (leopard skin). In the eye there is keratitis, iritis, and chorioretinitis ultimately causing blindness. The diagnosis can be confirmed by finding microfilariae in small snips of skin. Treatment is with diethylcarbamazine (DEC) or ivermectin, either of which have to be given repeatedly as neither kills the adult worms.

Loaisis

Infections with the filarial nematode *Loa* only occur in West Africa. The adult worms migrate continuously in the subcutaneous tissues at about 1 cm per hour and so-called 'Calabar swellings' are egg-sized lesions that occur on the skin as worms are passing. The worm can also occasionally be seen crossing the conjunctiva. The microfilariae are found in the blood during the day and their discovery confirms the diagnosis. There is an eosinophilia. Treatment is with ivermectin or DEC.

Cutaneous larva migrans

This disorder, also known as creeping eruption, is a migratory, intensely itchy, skin eruption caused by larval nematodes of various species, usually dog or cat hookworms. Hookworm eggs are shed in the animal's faeces, often on beaches or other sandy areas. The larvae hatch and penetrate human skin: the track marks the route of the parasite as it wanders aimlessly in the skin. Without treatment, the lesions gradually disappear, but resolution can be speeded by application of liquid nitrogen, ethyl chloride, or topical thiabendazole (crushed tablets in petroleum jelly is a suitable preparation) to the advancing edge of the track.

References

1. Corbett R. Topical antibiotics. *Practitioner* (1990) **234**: 494–6

2. Simon D, Freak L, Kinsella A *et al.* Community leg ulcer clinics: a comparative study in two health authorities *BMJ*; **312**: 1648–51

3. Johnston C. Diabetic skin and soft tissue infections. *Curr Op Infect Dis* (1994) **7**: 214–18

4. Stevens D, Tanner M, Winship J *et al.* Severe group A streptococcal infections associated with a toxic shock-like syndrome and scarlet fever toxin A. *N Engl J med* (1989) **321**: 1–7

5. Cleary P, Kaplan E, Handley J *et al.* Clonal basis for resurgence of serious *Streptococcus pyogenes* disease in the (1980)s. *Lancet* (1992) **339**: 518–521

6. Burge T. Watson J (editorial). Necrotising fasciitis. *BMJ* (1994) **308**: 145–54

7. Resnik S. Staphylococcal toxin-mediated syndromes in childhood. *Semin Dermatol* (1992) **11**: 11–18

8. Rooney J, Straus S, Mannix M *et al.* Oral acyclovir to suppress frequently recurrent herpes labialis: A double blind placebo controlled trial. *Ann Intern Med* (1993) **118**: 268–72

9. Kaplowitz L, Baker D, Gelb L *et al.* Prolonged continuous acyclovir treatment of normal adults with frequently recurring genital herpes simplex virus infection. *JAMA* (1991) **265**: 747–51

10. Worrall G. Acyclovir in recurrent herpes labialis: justified as oral prophylaxis only in severely affected people. *BMJ* (1996) **312**: 6

11. Whitley R. Therapeutic approaches to varicella-zoster virus infections. *J Infect Dis* (1992) **166**: 51–7

12. Lancaster T, Silagy C, Gray S. Primary care managment of acute herpes zoster: systematic review of evidence from randomized controlled trials. *Br J Gen Pract* (1995) **45**: 39–45

13. Whitley R, Straus S. Therapy for varicella-zoster virus infections: Where do we stand? *Infect Dis Clin Pract* (1993) **2**: 100–8

14. Sterling J. Treating the troublesome wart. *Practitioner* (1995) **239**: 44–7

15. Steele K. Primary dermatological care in general practice. *J Roy Coll Gen Pract* (1984) **34**: 22–3

16. Konig S, Bruijnzeels M *et al.* Molluscum contagiosum in Dutch general practice. *Brit J Gen Pract* (1994) **44**: 417–19

17. Poyner T. The GP's approach to fungal skin infections. *Prescriber* (1993) **4**: 3 68–71

18. Kock C, Sampers G, Knottnerus J. Diagnosis and management of cases of suspected dermatomycosis in the Netherlands: influence of general practice based potassium hydroxide testing. *Brit J Gen Pract* (1995) **45**: 349–51

19. Roberts D, Evans G. Management of superficial fungal infections. *Practitioner* (1993) **237**: 153–7

20. Management of scalp ringworm. *Drugs Therap Bull* (1996) **34**: 5–6

21. Denning D, Evans E, Kibbler C *et al.* Fungal nail disease: a guide to good practice (report of a Working Group of the British Society for Medical Mycology). *BMJ* (1995) **311**: 1277–81

22. Goodfield M, Andrew L, Evans E. Short term treatment of dermatophyte onychomycosis with terbenafine. *BMJ* (1992) **304**: 1151–4

23. Hay R, Stratigos J. Therapeutic potential of terbinafine in dermatomycoses. proceedings of a symposium. *Brit J Dermatol* (1992) **126**: 2–69

24. Reinel D. Topical treatment of onychomycosis with amorolfine 5% nail lacquer: comparative efficacy and tolerability of once and twice weekly use. *Dermatol* (1992) **184**: 21–4

25. Parish L. History of scabies. In: Orkin M, Maibach H, Parish L *et al.* ed. *Scabies and pediculosis.* Philadelphia: Lippincott (1977) 1–7

26. Trice F, Manson R. Camp itch: a retrospective study 100 years later. *South Med J* (1966) **59**: 10–14

27. Arlian L. Biology, host relations, and epidemiology of Scarcoptes scabei. *Ann Rev Entomol* (1989) **34**: 139–61

28. Wilkinson C. Is the treatment of scabies hazardous? *J Roy Coll Gen Pract* (1988) **38**: 468–9

29. Molinari F. Update on the treatment of pediculosis and scabies. *Ped Nurs* (1992) **8**: 600–2

30. Vander Stichele, Dezure E, Bogaert M. Systematic review of clinical efficacy of topical treatments for headlice. *BMJ* (1995) **311**: 604–8

31. Lienhardt C, Fine P (editorial). Controlling leprosy: multidrug treatment is not enough. *BMJ* (1992) **305**: 206–7

CHAPTER FOURTEEN

Generalized infections

This chapter includes infections that affect several or most of the body systems and which do not therefore fit naturally into other Chapters of this book.

Viral

The immunization of children has substantially modified the pattern of childhood viral illnesses. Nevertheless, these infections, which also may occur infrequently in adults, still comprise an important part of general practice and they will be discussed in some detail here.

Chickenpox (varicella)

The varicella zoster virus was first described by Ruska in 1943 following electron microscopy of fluid from chickenpox vesicles. In 1953, Weller reported that the fluids from vesicles from patients with chickenpox and shingles induced similar cytopathic changes in cultured cells. Subsequent work has established that the two conditions are caused by the same virus. The virus is a herpesvirus and the organization of the viral genome shows similarities to that of other herpesviruses.

Epidemiology

Primary infection usually results in chickenpox. In the USA there are about 3 million cases each year, principally in children aged 1–14 years. World-wide there are estimated to be about 60 million cases each year: few (5%) individuals reach adulthood without catching the disease. The infection is easily communicated and the attack rate among non-immune household contacts is greater than 90%. Chickenpox is acquired by direct contact with either varicella or zoster lesions or by the inhalation of infectious respiratory secretions. The incubation period varies between 9 and 21 days (median 14 days) although it may be shorter in the immunocompromised individual. The patient begins to shed virus for two days before the rash appears until all the lesions are crusted over. The infection is not spread on fomites, and immune individuals in contact with a patient with chickenpox do not become colonized with the virus and therefore do not transmit the infection. Chickenpox occurs throughout the year but the incidence in temperate countries peaks sharply in the spring.

Clinical features

The onset of chickenpox may be marked by fever and fleeting pains in the muscles and joints. These systemic symptoms precede the rash which is intensely itchy, vesicular, and first appears on the face, scalp, or trunk. The lesions typically appear in three crops and involve the entire body with up to 500 vesicles present in the course of the infection. The rash begins with macules which become papules and then vesicles on erythematous bases. Initially, the fluid in the vesicles is clear, but it then becomes cloudy. Finally, the vesicles rupture leaving a shallow ulcer which crusts over. New lesions rarely appear after the first 4 days and most are crusted by day 6; permanent scarring occurs if the lesions are scratched. Lesions at all stages may be present on the same body area. The diagnosis is usually straightforward when other factors, such as the age group, season, exposure, and appearance of the rash, are considered although the differential diagnosis includes disseminated zoster, disseminated herpes simplex, and hand, foot, and mouth disease. The vast majority of patients with chickenpox acquire lifelong immunity to further attacks, although these have been reported.

Prognosis

Chickenpox is usually a benign infection in healthy children, although various complications can occur in the new-born, the immunocompromised, and occasionally in healthy adults. The infection may run a particularly mild course in infants under one year because of the presence of maternal antibodies. The risk of a fatal outcome for chickenpox is directly related to age and immune competence. The risk of dying from the infection for healthy adults is 30 per 100 000 cases, more than 15 times greater than that for normal children aged 1–14 years. Although less than 2% of varicella infections occur in adults (>20) nearly 25% of all varicella-related deaths occur in this group.

Dermatological complications

The commonest complication in healthy under-fives is secondary bacterial infection of the skin lesions by group A beta-haemolytic streptococci or *Staphylococcus aureus*.

Patients with skin conditions such as eczema, burns, or cutaneous lymphoma and patients who are immunocompromised may develop serious cutaneous complications during chickenpox. These include haemorrhagic or bullous lesions, fulminating purpura due to disseminated intravascular coagulation, and necrotizing fasciitis.

Neurological complications

The commonest neurological complications associated with chickenpox is varicella encephalitis which occurs most frequently in children aged 5–14 years. Encephalitis, which occurs in 1/1000 cases of varicella, takes two forms: (1) the cerebellar form most commonly seen in children; and (2) the focal form usually seen in adults. Children with encephalitis develop nausea, vomiting, nystagmus, ataxia, and neck rigidity: fortunately the syndrome usually follows a self-limiting course with full recovery. Adults with encephalitis have a much graver prognosis as the focal form carries a 35% mortality and is characterized by focal neurological signs and fits. Reye syndrome, which is an acute encephalopathy associated with fatty change in the liver or hepatitis, carries a case fatality rate of about 20%. The syndrome is preceded by an acute viral illness which is reported to be varicella 20–30% of the time. The use of aspirin during the viral illness appears to predispose the patient to develop Reye's syndrome and is therefore contraindicated in the treatment of fevers in childhood. Now that salicylates are no longer used in children under the age 12 years, Reye's syndrome has become a rarity.

Respiratory complications

The onset of cough, dyspnoea, and fever, 1–6 days after the rash has appeared indicates varicella pneumonia which has recently been reported in 3% of previously healthy adults with chickenpox.[1] This is the commonest serious complication in adults and although the presentation may also include pleuritic chest pain and haemoptysis there are often few signs on examination of the chest. A chest X-ray will show a patchy or diffuse bilateral infiltrate with a peribronchial distribution; pulmonary function tests may show diffusion abnormalities for several months. Varicella pneumonia does not occur when the rash is mild. Adults with chickenpox managed at home require regular monitoring and a chest X-ray if they are unwell. Local arrangements for achieving this investigation while avoiding unnecessary admission to hospital will challenge relationships between primary and secondary care: the patient is contagious and will not be welcome in an ambulance or X-ray department without proper prior arrangements!

HIV and chickenpox

Chickenpox in patients infected with the HIV virus may be complicated and sometimes lethal. Although herpes zoster is a common event during HIV infection, varicella is seen less frequently and may present in its classic form thereby indicating a primary infection. These patients are more likely to develop complicated varicella, even if they are asymptomatic in relation to their HIV infection.

Chickenpox in pregnancy

This has implications for the unborn child, 10% of whom experience an intrauterine infection. Varicella during the first trimester may be associated with the congenital varicella syndrome which is characterized by atrophy of the brain cortex, chorioretinitis, limb hypoplasia, and cicatricial scarring. Studies of the incidence of this rare syndrome are few and contain small numbers: 2 infants of those born to 27 women with first trimester varicella were affected and in another series 4 babies born to 140 women with varicella

Table 14.1 *Period of maximum risk in perinatal varicella infections[24]*

Day of maternal onset*	−8 to −5	−5 to 2	2–8
Transfer of maternal antibody	Yes	No	No
Period of maximum risk	No	Yes	No
Antibody response of baby	No	No	Yes

*Delivery is day 0.

in pregnancy were affected. Infants whose mothers have had varicella at any stage of pregnancy have an increased risk of herpes zoster early in life.

Maternal infection in the perinatal period (5 days before to 2 days after delivery) may lead to neonatal varicella which in some reports is particularly associated with viral pneumonia and which itself has a case fatality rate of up to 30%. These figures, however, are based on cases seen in hospital and give a biased view of the overall outlook for these babies. A prospective study of 240 infants born to women with perinatal varicella, in 118 of whom the maternal onset of infection was between 5 days before to 2 days after delivery, failed to reveal a single death due to the infection (Table 14.1).

General practitioners frequently see children with chickenpox. However, managing the infection in relation to pregnancy is an uncommon situation because most adults are immune. It is important that clear guidelines for good practice are available to all practices, including indications for the use of varicella zoster-immune globulin. The particular circumstances of these women must be discussed with the virologist so that the GP is in a position to advise on the best management.

If another member of the household develops chickenpox it is important to be certain of the maternal antibody status before recommending she return home with a new-born infant. If the mother is not immune and exposure cannot be avoided the possibility of giving the infant varicella-immune globulin should be discussed with the virologist or paediatrician.

Investigations

Although the clinical diagnosis of varicella infection is usually straight-forward, confirmation may be necessary in atypical cases, in pregnancy, or immunosuppressed patients. The virus may be cultured from the vesicular fluid with positive results obtained in 4–10 days. A smear prepared from the base of a lesion may also be examined for the presence of multinucleate giant cells typical of either a Varicella-zoster virus (VZV) or a herpes simplex infection. The two infections may then usually be distinguished clinically. Antibodies to VZV infection develop from day 3 to day 5 of the varicella rash and persist, although the levels fall with time. Antibody tests for varicella are available, and patients in whom an accurate diagnosis is important should be discussed with the local virology laboratory who will advise on the tests currently available and the correct procedure for using them.

Treatment

Antiviral management should be considered in all immunocompromised patients who develop varicella because of the risk of serious complications. Reports of severe chickenpox associated with steroid treatment have led to suggestions that all patients on steroids should be warned to seek medical attention should they be in contact with chickenpox or shingles and if they are uncertain of their own immunity.[23] Patients with pneumonia should also be treated. Intravenous acyclovir is the drug of choice and patients likely to benefit from this therapy require early admission to hospital.

Attacks in healthy children are managed symptomatically[4] with paracetamol (not aspirin), and calamine lotion if the parent wishes to use it. Some GPs find antihistamines useful in combating pruritis and the patient should wear light loose cotton clothing which covers the majority of the lesions and helps to prevent scarring from scratching. Parents should pay particular attention to hygiene to avoid secondary infection. Perineal lesions in children still wearing nappies may be a particular problem.

Three recent placebo-controlled trials, designed to evaluate oral acyclovir therapy for varicella, demonstrated an effect on disease progression in healthy children aged 2–12 years, adolescents, and young adults. In one study adolescents aged 13–18 received 800 mg four times daily for 5 days. They experienced a significant reduction in the duration of the fever and new lesion formation. Treated patients had fewer lesions in the acute phase and less scarring at 28 days.[5] Taken together, these studies show acyclovir to be a safe and effective treatment for varicella provided that it is commenced within 24 hours of the appearance of the rash.[6] General practitioners managing adolescents and adults with varicella should discuss the relevance of oral acyclovir with the local microbiologist despite the costs. The current view is that resistance of VZV to acyclovir is unlikely to occur in healthy hosts when the drug is given for a short effective course.[7]

Prevention

The isolation of individuals infected with VZV from those still susceptible to infection remains the most effective means of prevention. People without a history of varicella are likely to become infectious about 10–14 days after exposure to the infection and remain so until all the lesions are crusted (about 8 days in all). Significant exposures are:

• Continuous household contact

• More than 1 hour of indoor play

- Adjacent beds in hospital
- Prolonged face to face contact with infectious health worker
- New-born of mother with onset −2 to +5 days of delivery

When managing a patient with varicella the GP should consider whether the household includes susceptible individuals who might be at high risk of complications from chickenpox. These include patients on immunosuppressive treatment including steroids, or with leukaemia or lymphoma, neonates and premature babies, susceptible pregnant women, and HIV positive individuals. Efforts must be made to establish their immunity to varicella and advice from the virologist sought on the advisability of administering varicella zoster-immune globulin. Live attenuated varicella vaccine was developed in Japan in the 1970s and has been licensed in a number of countries. Major questions still to be resolved are the duration of immunity and the incidence of zoster following immunization.[8]

Case history

A 24-year-old woman, the daughter of a GP, was surprised to develop chickenpox after contact with a colleague in the office, as she thought she had had it as a child. She was moderately unwell but the infection ran a normal course and was beneficial in that it was the occasion of her giving up smoking! Her husband developed the infection 2 weeks later and felt extremely unwell during the first 24 hours after the appearance of the rash. A request for a home visit was deflected by a receptionist who said 'we never visit for chickenpox'. The couple and their 3-year-old daughter drove to her parents home and following a rigor that night, and on the advice of the microbiologist, the husband was started on a course of oral acyclovir by the local GP. He had a severe infection complicated by conjunctivitis but made a complete recovery. The child developed the illness a full month after the mother first became ill. Although the rash was widespread there was remarkably little constitutional upset and she made a rapid recovery. In all the family were affected by the infection for six weeks during which time the adults were away from work either ill or caring for the others.

Herpes zoster

Reactivation of the varicella virus leads to the development of herpes zoster which is discussed in Chapters 6 and 13.

Measles

This is a distinct exanthematous viral infection characterized by fever and involvement of the respiratory tract. Although the primary site of infection is the respiratory epithelium of the nasopharynx, measles is a systemic infection with characteristic multinucleated giant cells found in the reticuloendothelium and in the respiratory epithelium.

The infection is caused by the measles virus which is a single-stranded RNA virus of the paramyxovirus group. The virus is closely related to the canine distemper virus and both are classified within the *Moribillivirus* genus. The natural host for the measles virus is man and one infection confers lifelong immunity.

The measles virus is transmitted by droplets spread by coughing or sneezing. It is highly communicable for about a week with infectivity at its highest between the late prodromal phase of the illness until about 4 days after the onset of the rash. About 95% of people who are infected become ill, although a very mild form without the rash is recognized.

Epidemiology

In the early 1980s, estimates of death from measles among children were estimated to be 2.5 million world-wide. By 1989, the figure was reported to be nearer 1.5 million: measles is still the commonest vaccine-preventable cause of death in children in the world.

Measles occurs world-wide with a peak incidence in temperate climates between February and April with epidemics every two to four years. Before the introduction of vaccines the infection was essentially universal in the UK with 95% of people living in cities infected by the age of 15 years. Each year, 100 000–800 000 children were affected. The introduction of the measles, mumps, and rubella (MMR) vaccine has given a renewed opportunity to eradicate measles.

Clinical features

Children with measles have coryza, conjunctivitis, cough, fever, malaise, and a maculopapular rash. They are unwell and feel very miserable. The incubation period is 9–11 days before the prodromal symptoms and signs appear. The child appears to have a bad cold with infection of the conjunctiva and increasing fever. Examination of the buccal mucosa opposite the upper molars may reveal Koplik's spots which are clusters of bluish-white papules on an erythematous base. These lesions are present in about 80% of measles cases and are considered diagnostic. It is worth looking for them when examining any unimmunized child who is ill with a cold as an early diagnosis can improve management and allow the possibility of immunization of other unprotected children in the family.

The rash usually starts on the neck and spreads to include the face, body, and extremities over a 2–3 day period. Initially the lesions are erythematous and maculopapular but later they become confluent, the rash fades after 5–7 days, sometimes with transient brown staining of the skin and a fine desquamation. The second phase of fever is at its peak at 48–72 hours after the onset of the rash and then subsides. Usually the last symptom to resolve is the non-productive cough.

The commonest complications of measles are otitis media and pneumonitis which occur in about 5–9% and 1–6% of cases, respectively. Other complications are rare but may be very serious; encephalitis is seen in about 0.5–1 cases/1000 and subacute sclerosing panencephalitis in about 5/million cases.

The onset of immediate complications is marked by a third phase of increasing fever which should alert both parents and GPs that the disease is not running an uncomplicated course. Death from measles usually follows the onset of complications in children with poor nutrition or other health problems.

Neurological complications

Post-measles encephalitis is thought to be an autoimmune disease, and manifests some 4–7 days after the onset of the rash. The patient experiences fever, headache, irritability, lethargy, and sometimes fits. The condition is fatal in about 15% of patients and another 30% have permanent neurological damage. Subacute sclerosing panencephalitis is a rare, late complication which is characterized by a progressive impairment of the intellectual and motor capabilities of the patient, and is invariably fatal. Research has shown the condition to be linked to the presence of a measles-like virus in the brain tissue. In the USA, the epidemiology of measles has been altered by mass immunization. The condition now occurs most frequently in young adults due to vaccine failure or postponement of exposure. The trend may follow in the UK with increased immunization; adults with measles usually have a severe illness and need close monitoring for complications.

Respiratory complications

Pneumonia may be caused by the measles virus itself or by secondary bacterial or viral infection. Measles pneumonia is particularly severe in immunocompromised patients.

Investigations

Most cases of measles are diagnosed clinically, although as more children are immunized younger GPs will see few cases and may not be alert to the typical clinical picture. The differential diagnosis of measles includes all illnesses with a maculopapular exanthema (Table 14.2).

The diagnosis can be confirmed by serology if necessary; diagnosis from saliva collected by wiping a specially designed sponge swab around the gum margin for about a minute is available in the UK.[9] Use of this method has demonstrated that the clinical diagnosis of measles is often inaccurate and it has been proposed as a simple test to improve the accuracy of case reporting

Table 14.2 *Differential diagnosis of measles*

- Rubella
- Enterovirus infection
- Erythema infectiosum
- Drug eruption
- Meningococcal infection

on which to base measles control programmes, such as the immunization of all British schoolchildren undertaken in 1994.[10]

Treatment

Measles runs a benign course in the great majority of British children. Some healthy children experience complications and hence all children should be carefully monitored once the diagnosis has been made. The initial examination should include inspection of the eardrums and a careful examination of the chest, as well as noting the overall condition of the child. The natural history of the infection should be explained to the parents and the child should be reviewed after the appearance of the rash at the time of maximum fever and later if the temperature spikes again indicating the onset of complications. The role of telephone follow-up and of a nurse working to a protocol to follow up milder infections might be debated within the practice.

The circumstances under which referral to hospital should be considered are shown in Table 14.3. No specific treatment is available, but fluids and antibiotics may be used as necessary. Croup may be managed at home using steam but the situation must be carefully monitored. Antibiotics are indicated for chest infections and otitis media.

Prevention

Measles is prevented by immunization. If a case of measles occurs within the practice there has been a failure of this approach and it would be worthwhile arranging to meet all concerned to discuss the possible reasons. The effectiveness of the arrangements for inviting patients for immunization, the relationship between the practice team and the family, and the practice policy for dealing with groups who frequently remain unimmunized should all be reviewed.

When a child presents with measles the GP should think of preventing the

Table 14.3 *Indications for hospital referral in children with measles*

Urgent
- Increasing respiratory distress
- Unresponsive croup
- Persisting tachypnoea
- Convulsions

Consider
- Unexplained drowsiness
- Marked toxicity
- Persisting high fever
- Recurrence of high fever
- Difficult social circumstances

illness in other children in the family. Unprotected individuals over 6 months of age who are within 72 hours of direct contact should receive measles vaccine. Those who were in direct contact more than 72 hours previously, are aged less than 6–12 months or in whom the vaccine is contraindicated, should receive human normal immunoglobulin. The concerned GP should discuss any problems with the local community paediatrician.

The infection is spread by coughing and sneezing and the child is infectious for about a week, particularly during the late prodromal phase and for the first four days of the rash. Parents must understand these facts and the child should be kept away from other susceptible children during this time.

Rubella

This is a mild viral illness with a rash caused by a spherical RNA virus with a pleomorphic envelope. However, the disease has another, devastating, effect; if a woman in the very early weeks of pregnancy is infected, major damage occurs to the unborn child.

Epidemiology

The infection is spread by droplets and infected individuals are infectious from 10 days before the rash appears to 14 days afterwards.

In the past, epidemics of rubella occurred about every 6–9 years. The rates varied between 2–10 cases/100 000 in the four weekly returns from the Royal College of General Practitioners, until 1989 when the MMR immunization was introduced.

Clinical features

The diagnosis of rubella is difficult, as other infections produce similar features (Table 14.4). The infection usually runs a benign course, children are usually relatively well although adults have more pronounced prodromal symptoms and are more susceptible to the arthralgia and viral septic arthritis which is the only occasional complication.

Table 14.4 *Clinical features of rubella*

- Coryza
- Sore throat
- Transient fever
- Tender post-auricular and cervical lymphadenopathy
- Splenomegaly
- Petechiae of the soft palate
- Discrete, non-confluent, macular rash

Table 14.5 *Manifestations of congenital rubella*

- Meningoencephalitis
- Nerve deafness
- Cataract
- Chorioretinitis
- Microcephaly
- Learning disabilities
- Disorders of behaviour and language

Congenital rubella syndrome

Primary infection with rubella in the first four months of pregnancy is associated with a major risk of fetal damage. The effects of the infection are more severe the younger the fetus is (Table 14.5). The syndrome is diagnosed by the demonstration of the rubella virus or antigen with a monoclonal antibody test or the detection of persistent or rising titre of IgG or presence of IgM antibody.

Diagnosis of rubella in pregnancy

Although the infection is usually obvious it may be subclinical with an equal risk of fetal damage. Rubella is as difficult to diagnose in adults as children and hence all women with rubella-like illnesses and exposure to rubella in pregnancy should be investigated. The relevance of previous assays which may have been done some years earlier, and the problems of false positive results with the rubella HAI test which is now no longer used, means that definitive diagnosis is necessary despite a previous history of immunization or immunity. Re-infection has been documented, usually among women with close and prolonged exposure to rubella, but large series have not been reported and the risk to the fetus is not well documented.

In addition, the possibility of vaccine failure always exists; it occurs after about 2–5% of vaccinations, no antibodies are produced and subsequent infection is accompanied by a typical primary antibody response.[11] For all these reasons care must be taken to establish immunity in every pregnancy and to diagnose women at risk. If the GP is initiating or supervising these investigations it is important to provide full details of symptoms, date and type of contact, previous rubella immunization, and dates and results of previous tests for rubella antibody. As the question of abortion may arise is is vital to discuss the issue with the woman and her partner. Women opposed to abortion may decline investigation, but it is important to ensure that they understand the risks if they continue the pregnancy after a rubella infection. Management of pregnant women with suspected rubella requires excellent administrative and communication skills. Results must be obtained promptly and appropriate action must follow. Close liaison with the virologist and the obstetrician is mandatory if distress is to be kept to a minimum.

Any mismanagement of the situation is likely to lead to a complaint or legal action.

Mumps

Mumps is a generalized illness which normally presents with a parotitis or meningitis or more rarely with pancreatitis, orchitis, or oophoritis. Occasionally, it leads to deafness. The illness is caused by a single-stranded virus of the paramyxovirus family.

The infection is distributed world-wide and is usually seen in school-age children and adolescents. The introduction of MMR vaccination and the immunization of all British schoolchildren from 1994 will have a profound effect on the incidence of the disease in the UK.

Clinical features

The usual presentation is with painful parotid swelling which fills in the angle of the jaw, extends forward on to the cheek, and may raise the ear lobe. It is uncomfortable rather than tender and while there may initially be an accompanying fever there is relatively minor constitutional upset. The openings of the salivary ducts into the mouth may be red and oedematous. Clinical meningitis occurs in 1–10% of individuals with parotitis and about 50% of those with mumps meningitis also have parotitis. Mumps meningitis is a short self-limiting disorder presenting with headache, neck stiffness, and a positive Kernig's sign. These patients are best discussed with the specialist and admitted for investigation if there is any doubt about the cause of the symptoms.

Mumps orchitis, even when bilateral, rarely causes sterility.

Human parvovirus (B19)[12]

Aetiology and epidemiology

Human parvovirus B19 is a small DNA virus which was discovered in the UK in 1975. The infection occurs world-wide and appears throughout the year in all age groups, either as sporadic cases or during outbreaks of erythema infectiosum (slapped cheek disease). The range of seroprevalence is 2–15% in children of 5 years and under, 15–60% in 5–19-year-olds, and 30–60% in adults.[13]

Clinical features

Although asymptomatic infection has been reported in about 20% of children, the commonest presentation of the infection is with a childhood illness which starts about one week after infection with a viraemia and mild systemic symptoms. This is followed 1–4 days later by a facial rash (the slapped cheek appearance) with a generalized lace-like rash over the trunk and extremities which may become confluent. The rash may reappear for some weeks with exertion, emotion, or temperature.[14]

Parvovirus infection and polyarthritis

In some outbreaks of erythema infectiosum, arthralgia and a symmetrical peripheral polyarthritis is a prominent feature. The hands are most frequently affected, followed by the knees and wrists. The symptoms may persist for several months but are eventually self-limiting. Occasionally, the arthritis may be the only presentation of the infection, particularly in adults.

Transient aplastic crisis and severe anaemia

Parvovirus B19 causes suppression of red cell production by infection and lysis of red cell precursor cells. While individuals with normal haemopoiesis can cope with the insult, those with conditions leading to increased red cell destruction or loss may develop a transient aplastic crisis. General practitioners who work in areas with a higher incidence of sickle-cell disease and beta-thalassaemia should be aware of this possibility, as these patients may become very ill and need admission and transfusion.

Parvovirus infection in pregnancy

This may result in fetal death from anaemia or hydrops foetalis in less than 10% of cases. There is no evidence that fetal survival is associated with increased congenital abnormality and so abortion is not indicated if infection is not followed by miscarriage or intrauterine death and still-birth. A prospective study of women with confirmed infection found that the number of spontaneous abortions in the first trimester was not increased but the mid trimester rate of spontaneous abortions was ten times that expected.[15,16] The infection may be confused with rubella and it is imperative to establish a diagnosis which is achieved by detecting parvovirus IgG and IgM. This situation is best managed in consultation with the virologist and obstetrician.

Hand, foot and mouth disease

Clinical features

This infection is caused by a Coxsackie virus, usually A16. It commonly occurs in children under 10 years and is characterized by a sore throat, fever, and malaise followed by the appearance of a few small, lax vesicles with an erythematous margin on the palms of the hands and the soles of the feet, and painful vesicles in the mouth.

Treatment

This is symptomatic and directed at pain relief and the reduction of fever if the child is at risk of febrile convulsions.

Roseola infantum

Clinical features

This infection is seen in babies aged 6 months to 3 years and is caused by human herpesvirus type 6. The first symptoms are a high fever with lymphadenopathy during which the child is relatively well. After a few days the fever subsides and is followed by a centrally distributed maculopapular rash which fades after one or two days. The infection is often confused with rubella or measles.[17] Complications are very unusual although susceptible children may experience a febrile convulsion.

Bacterial infections

Human spirochaetal diseases

Spirochaetes are bacteria which are widely distributed in nature. Of the order Spirochaetales, there are six genera of which three contain organisms which are pathogenic for humans. While syphilis and yaws have been discussed elsewhere, Lyme disease and leptospirosis are important generalized infections which are occasionally seen in general practice and which can be difficult to diagnose. Both of these infections are zoonotic and infection is acquired by direct or indirect contact with the animal reservoir.

All infections due to spirochaetes show similar features; skin or mucous membrane as the portal of entry, bacteraemia early in the infection with clinical manifestations, and widespread dissemination throughout the tissues and body fluids, and then one or more further stages of the disease usually with periods of latency in between.

Lyme disease

This multisystem disease was first described in 1977 from the study of a cluster of children in Lyme, Connecticut who were thought to have juvenile rheumatoid arthritis. The association of the illness with erythema migrans and the rural setting lead to the hypothesis that this was an arthropod borne infection linked to other syndromes described earlier in Europe.[18]

The disease is carried by a tick-borne spirochaete, *Borrelia burgdorferi*. In Europe, the responsible tick is *Ixodes ricinus* which occurs in many parts of the UK with a peak activity in late spring, early summer, and autumn. The hosts are small mammals such as field mice and voles and large mammals such as deer, sheep, and horses. The ticks are inactive at temperatures of less than 5 °C and do not withstand drying out. The tick has three forms in its life cycle, larvae, nymphs, and adults and all three may bite humans.[19] The risk of acquiring the infection from a single bite is unknown, although it seems higher the longer the tick is attached. Prevalence studies in the UK indicate that serious disease is uncommon; healthy blood donors in the New Forest, UK, where the disease is endemic have an overall seroprevalence of 4% and

Table 14.6 *The clinical features of Lyme disease*

Early localized disease: a few days to a month after the tick bite
- Erythema migrans
- Fatigue/malaise/lethargy
- Myalgia
- Arthralgia
- Regional/generalized lympadenopathy

Early disseminated disease: weeks to months after the tick bite
- *Central nervous system*: meningitis, encephalitis, cranial nerve palsies especially facial nerve, peripheral neuropathy, myelitis
- *Heart*: conduction defects, mild cardiomyopathy (rare in the UK)
- *Musculoskeletal system*: migratory arthritis of one or more large joints
- *Skin*: multiple areas of erythema migrans
- *Eye*: anterior and posterior uveitis, panophthalmitis

Chronic or persistent disease: months to years after the tick bite
- *Central nervous system*: chronic encephalopathy, chronic peripheral neuropathy, ataxia, dementia, sleep disorder
- *Musculosketal system*: migratory polyarthritis, chronic monoarthritis (usually the knee joint)
- *Skin*: acrodermatitis chronica atrophicans, localized scleroderma-like lesions

---

forestry workers in the same area had a seroprevalence of 25%. Most of these workers could not recall an illness suggestive of Lyme disease supporting the hypothesis that many infections are asymptomatic.[20]

Clinical features

Lyme disease is a multisystem disease which can be described in three broad categories based on the clinical features and the time since acquisition. While some patients experience all three, some present initially with the later features of Lyme disease (Table 14.6). The striking lesion in early localized disease is that of erythema migrans. It starts as an erythematous macule or papule at the site of the tick bite which is usually painless although it may itch or burn. The rash spreads out from the site with a reddened leading edge and the central skin returning to near normal appearance sometimes attaining a diameter of up to 70 cm. Spirochaetes are present in the leading edge and may be cultured from skin biopsies but the lesion eventually resolves spontaneously.

Many organs may be involved in the early disseminated stage of Lyme disease as shown in Table 14.6, and it is important for the GP to be aware of the possibility of the infection in endemic areas or those at risk. The diagnosis of late Lyme disease is likely to be made by specialists but it may occasionally be the lot of a GP to have an inspired hunch, but only if he/she is aware of the possibility in the first place!

Investigation and treatment

The diagnosis is established from the clinical picture, a possible exposure to tick bites, and the detection of antibodies. ELISA tests may give false positives and it is important to establish the diagnosis by further testing using other techniques. This stage of the investigation is best conducted in discussion with the microbiologist.

The infection is treated with antibiotics; erythema migrans responds to amoxycillin 500 mg, 3 times a day, or doxycycline 100 mg, twice daily for 10–21 days. Other manifestations of the infection should be referred or discussed to ensure that correct antibiotic regimes are followed.

Prevention

The risk of infection is minimized if tick bites are avoided or discovered early. Those at risk should keep covered, use an insect repellent, and inspect exposed skin and clothes for ticks every few hours, remembering the larvae and nymphs are very small. Pets should wear tick collars

Leptospirosis

Leptospira are finely coiled thread-like spirochaetes, 6–20 mm long, and have a distribution world-wide. Human disease is due to a single species of spirochaete, *L. interrogans*, which has 19 serogroups and ten times that number of serotypes. Pathological serogroups include: *icterohaemorrhagiae, hebdomanis, hardjo, canicola, pomona,* and *gryppotyphosa.*

Leptospirosis is a zoonosis. Man is an incidental host who becomes infected through direct or indirect contact with the reservoir animal which excretes leptospiras in the urine for a long time without any evidence of disease. Different serotypes tend to have different animal reservoirs: *canicola* preferentially infects dogs; *hardjo* infects cattle; *gryppotyphosa* infects voles; and classical *icterohaemorrhagiae* infects rats.

Transmission results from direct contact with the body fluids of reservoir animals or indirect contact with contaminated water or soil, and the infection is endemic in the UK. Of 299 cases confirmed in England and Wales between 1985 and 1989, disease from cattle caused 157 cases, with 87 from rats. The absence of infection from dogs is attributed to canine immunization and is another reason for advising pet owners to have their animals fully immunized. There were 15 deaths during the period and a further 92 cases were acquired abroad.[21] The leptospiras gain access through abrasions of the skin or through mucous membranes. A primary bacteraemia results in multiplication in all body tissues until the development of an immune response after 7–14 days. Thus, the disease has initial features relating to bacterial multiplication in many organs and a second phase resulting from the interaction between the spirochaete and the immune response. (See Table 14.7 for precautions against leptospirosis.)

Table 14.7 *Precautions against leptospirosis*

- Avoid swimming in lakes and rivers
- Wear protective clothing and footwear
- Cover cuts with waterproof plasters
- Shower after watersports in freshwater areas
- Do not touch rats without wearing gloves
- Remember the possibility of leptospirosis in at-risk groups

Clinical features

The incubation period is usually 1–2 weeks. Subclinical infection is common in those exposed to infected animals and of those who are ill, only about 10% have an icteric illness. The symptoms are often biphasic. The initial clinical features are non-specific with high fevers, intense frontal headache, severe myalgia, and conjunctival suffusion. This initial phase of the illness lasts for 5–7 days and complete or partial resolution then occurs. In many individuals the second phase never occurs but, in some, a day or two later the immune phase of the illness develops with aseptic meningitis as the principal feature. Hepatomegaly, abdominal pain, pulmonary, or cardiac involvement with cough and breathlessness may also occur. In severe forms of the disease (Weil's syndrome) the immune phase is complicated by jaundice, renal failure, haemorrhage, and vascular collapse. This is fatal in about 10–20% of patients.

The initial phase, if mild, is difficult to distinguish from influenza, atypical pneumonia, viral meningitis, or viral hepatitis. Where there is a history of recent travel, brucellosis, rickettsial infections, malaria, and dengue may also need exclusion. Laboratory findings are helpful in the differential diagnosis: icteric leptospirosis is associated with a neutrophilia (which is uncommon in typhoid or scrub typhus) and mild thrombocytopenia. The elevated bilirubin is not associated with markedly elevated transaminase levels (unlike hepatitis).

Leptospirosis is usually diagnosed by serological means although they are not usually available in time to influence the clinical management. Agglutinating antibodies appear after about one week of illness and reach a maximum only after about three weeks: convalescent specimens are needed to confirm the diagnosis.

Treatment

In severe infections hospitalization and full supportive care is the mainstay of treatment. Antibiotics should be given to all cases, since they shorten the duration of early disease and limit the renal damage in more severely unwell individuals. Seven days of either intravenous penicillin or oral doxycycline, or amoxycillin should be given. Vaccines are not available for human use but do exist for animals.

Case history

The teenage son of one of the authors was shocked to find that his teacher, who had been off sick with the 'flu', had died from Weil's disease. He had been fishing in the local river and had got a fish hook stuck in his hand. The significance of this event was not appreciated when he developed a fever two weeks later.

Enteric fever (typhoid and paratyphoid)

Enteric fever is an acute systemic illness caused by infection with a small number of *Salmonella* strains. The organisms responsible (*S. typhi* and *S. paratyphi A, B,* and *C*) are Gram-negative bacilli that are by and large exclusively human pathogens (only *S. paratyphi C* can infect other animals). Infection is usually acquired from water or food contaminated by another human with acute infection or chronic carriage of the organisms. The pathogen may be concentrated in molluscs such as mussels. Typhoid is endemic in many parts of the world where water supply, hygiene, and food preparation are poor. In the UK, it is generally seen in immigrants from endemic areas or in people returning from holidays abroad, particularly Asia. Typhoid may occur in epidemics which can usually be traced to common source exposure. Sources of outbreaks in Europe included canned beef (which caused 507 cases in Aberdeen in 1964), and contaminated water supplies in Zermatt, 1963.

Clinical features and investigations

The infective dose of *Salmonella* is large (ID_{50} is 10^7 organisms). After ingestion, the organisms invade the intestinal epithelium and enter the lymphatic tissues of the small intestine.

The incubation period of typhoid is 10–14 days and there is then fever, headache, and general malaise. The temperature classically rises in a stepwise manner during the first week. Confusion and lethargy, cough, diarrhoea or constipation, nausea, and a variety of other symptoms may occur, and approximately 25% of patients have a relative bradycardia. The patient looks unwell by the end of the first week and careful examination may reveal small erythematous macules that blanch on pressure, so-called rose spots, particularly on the abdomen and chest. The spleen and liver may also be palpable. During the second week of the illness the high fever is maintained and abdominal pain and diarrhoea may become more prominent. The temperature tends to resolve by lysis during the third week but at this stage gastrointestinal haemorrhage and/or bowel perforation occasionally occur.

Patients with typhoid are often anaemic, with a slight leucopenia (5–6000 × 10^9/l), and relative lymphocytosis. Biochemical tests of liver function are elevated to about twice normal. Confirmation of typhoid or paratyphoid is made by culture of the organism from the blood: septicaemia occurs about 5–10 days after onset. Positive stool cultures are less relevant since asymptomatic carriage of *S. typhi* can persist for many years after an acute infection. The Widal reaction, which measures agglutinating antibodies to *Salmonella*, is often requested but difficult to interpret since the background levels vary in different populations and the antibodies remain elevated for a long time following typhoid immunization. The diagnostic value is questionable and many microbiologists no longer recommend its use.

Treatment

Without therapy, the disease lasts for 3–4 weeks but appropriate antibiotics lead to improvement in symptoms within a day or two and defervescence usually within 5 days. Suitable antibiotics are ampicillin, trimethoprim or co-trimoxazole, chloramphenicol, and quinolones, such as ciprofloxacin or ofloxacin, given for 2 weeks, always providing that the organism is sensitive *in vitro*.

Approximately 20% of patients with typhoid continue to asymptomatically excrete the organism in the stool for 2 months after the onset of the illness and about 5% go on to develop prolonged (more than one year) carriage of organisms. It is particularly likely to occur in those with biliary tract disease. Eradication of organisms from a chronic carrier is sometimes attempted. Ampicillin in high dosage (sometimes with probenecid), co-trimoxazole with rifampicin, and ciprofloxacin alone have all been used with some success for the treatment of chronic *S.typhi* carriage.

The diagnosis of enteric fever is notifiable to the Public health Authorities which have the responsibility for deciding when an individual may return to school or employment.

Brucellosis

This is a zoonosis caused by three species of *Brucella* that are pathogenic for man: *Br. melitensis*, *Br. suis*, or *Br. abortus*. They are intracellular pathogens and in man may result in either acute or chronic infection. The organisms are excreted in the milk of infected animals and humans may become infected by either:

- Eating fresh soft cheeses or drinking milk from infected cattle
- Handling carcasses or meat of infected animals (veterinarians, farmers, abattoir workers, etc., are at particular risk)
- Tending or milking infected animals.

Brucella melitensis is the most likely species to infect man. It is found mainly in goats, sheep and camels in the Mediterranean region, the Middle East, South Africa, South America, India, and China. *Brucella suis* occurs mainly in pigs but also occasionally in cattle and rabbits. It is found in both North and South America and South East Asia. The animal host of *Br. abortus* is usually cattle or buffalo and is found most commonly in cattle-rearing areas world-wide, such as South America.

The short-stay traveller is not usually at great risk of *Brucella* infection, but imported cases usually occur in travellers to the Middle East, and immigrants and returned expatriots from this region. Following entry to the body, brucellae are phagocytosed but are capable of remaining viable within cells (particularly *Br. melitensis*). The organisms then localize in mononuclear cells of the reticuloendothelial system and giant cell granulomata develop in the bone marrow, spleen, liver, and lymph nodes.

Clinical features and diagnosis

The clinical features of brucellosis are very variable and depend somewhat on the individual host's immunity and the species involved: *Br. melitensis* and *Br. suis* cause more serious disease than *Br. abortus*. There is an incubation period of 3–4 weeks and then the illness may be acute or subacute in onset. In the acute form there is a high fever, sweats, generalized aches and pains, anorexia, and lethargy. The liver, spleen, and lymph nodes may be enlarged. In a minority of patients, acute brucellosis is complicated by problems affecting almost any organ system. Skeletal involvement is particularly common with arthritis of the large joints and spine, often causing disabling back or hip pains. The clinical features of complicating endocarditis, hepatitis, haemolytic anaemia, epididymo-orchitis, meningo-encephalitis, myelitis, or depression may also be present.

Re-exposure to *Brucella* in seropositive persons (particularly in veterinarians or laboratory workers) may cause hypersensitivity reactions which produce relapsing or chronic symptoms mimicking brucellosis.

The diagnosis of brucellosis is best confirmed by cultural isolation of *Brucella* from the blood and bone marrow. Sero-diagnosis also contributes to the diagnosis. By the time of diagnosis in the acute phase both IgM and IgG antibodies are usually present: with adequate treatment IgG disappears or decreases to very low levels. In the chronic phase or with exacerbation or re-infection IgG antibodies rise again. The serum agglutination test (SAT) measures both IgG and IgM; pretreatment with 2-mercapto-ethanol (2-ME) removes the IgM antibodies. The complement fixation test measures IgG. Thus, in acute brucellosis there will be a rise in both IgG and IgM agglutination titre. In more persistent active infections, the SAT titre remains elevated and does not fall, the 2-ME test is usually positive and the complement fixation titre is positive.

Prevention and treatment

Vaccinating cattle and goats to produce *Brucella*-free herds, has largely eliminated brucellosis is countries with organized agriculture. Human vaccines are not widely available or reliably protective and prevention of human disease largely depends on steps to prevent milk-borne transmission, for example:

• Heating milk to 60 °C for 10 minutes kills brucellae and, hence, pasteurized milk should if possible be drunk. If pasteurized milk is unavailable, milk should be boiled before drinking or use in milk dishes.

• Meat that is thoroughly cooked is unlikely to be infected.

A combination of rifampicin (600–900 mg/day) with doxycycline (200 mg/day) for 6 weeks is currently considered the treatment of choice for brucellosis. Tetracycline and intramuscular streptomycin is cheaper but more difficult to administer. Endocarditis requires prolonged combination treatment with additional co-trimoxazole; valve replacement may be required.

Typhus

Rickettsia are obligatory intracellular Gram-negative bacilli. Apart from louse-borne epidemic typhus the major human rickettsial diseases are zoonoses transmitted to humans by insects, either directly through bites or by faecal contamination of skin abrasions.

The predominant pathology of rickettsial diseases involves infection and damage to the vascular endothelial cells. This results in small vessel obstruction and micro-infarcts. All varieties of typhus cause fever, headache, and skin rashes.

Travellers are usually at risk of one or other of the non-epidemic forms of typhus, as a result of walking through tropical bush, and these illnesses are not a risk for the usual hotel tourist or business traveller.

Epidemic louse-borne typhus

Louse-borne typhus is not particularly a tropical disease: in the past it has been prominent in Europe and Asia during periods of war and social upheaval and is now limited to mountainous areas of Africa, Asia, and South America. Refugee workers may be at risk but it is not a disease of tourists. There is no zoonotic reservoir and the body louse (*Pediculus humanis*) is infected for its lifetime with the organism, *Rickettsia prowazeki*. It is the louse faeces that are infectious and these enter either through contaminated skin abrasions or are inhaled.

Clinical features

After an incubation period of 1–3 weeks there is abrupt fever, severe intractable headache, and myalgia. The fever remains high and unremitting, and the patient is often prostrate. A fine pink macular rash spreads from the axillae to the whole body and may become petechial or frankly haemorrhagic. Complications include delirium, organic confusion, meningitis, cranial nerve palsies, hepatitis, and vascular collapse. Secondary infections may occur. The fever settles in approximated two weeks but there is a considerable morbidity in the way of post-infectious fatigue, which can last for several months. Untreated, the mortality may be 25% or more.

Clinical differentiation must be from enteric fever, viral haemorrhagic fevers, and other forms of typhus. Diagnosis usually requires serological identification. This includes the non-specific Weil–Felix reaction and more specific rickettsial serology. The Weil–Felix reaction depends on the agglutination of various strains of *Proteus vulgaris* by the serum from patients with rickettsial infections. In epidemic typhus the reaction is to the OX-19 and, to a lesser extent, OX-2 strains. OX-K is negative.

Unfortunately, serology takes several weeks to become positive and therapy has to be started on clinical grounds. Treatment is with tetracycline or chloramphenicol until defervescence. Control involves delousing measures. There is a typhus vaccine used for those at particular risk.

Endemic murine typhus

Murine typhus is caused by *Rickettsia typhi* and is found world-wide. It is spread by the faeces of the rat flea (*Xenopsylla cheopis*). The clinical illness is similar to louse-borne typhus but somewhat less severe. The serological reactions and treatment are identical to those given above. The two diseases can only be distinguished by isolation of organisms or special procedures at reference laboratories.

Rocky Mountain spotted fever (RMSF)

This illness is caused by *Rickettsia rickettsii*, which is transmitted to humans by the bite of hard ticks, often the dog tick. It is not limited to the Rocky Mountain states of the USA but is found in both North and South America. Most cases occur in children. The incubation period is about one week and the onset is sudden with fever, chills, myalgia, and headache. The rash appears within 3–5 days of the fever: initial lesions are on the extremities and are maculopapular, later spreading to the trunk and becoming petechial and purpuric. Neurological, renal, and cardiovascular complications are common and death occurs in about 5% of cases, often within very few days of onset. Prompt therapy with a tetracycline or chloramphenicol results in rapid recovery.

Other tick-borne spotted fevers

There are a variety of other tick-borne rickettsial illnesses that may affect travellers exposed to ticks in the Eastern hemisphere. They are known by a variety of different names: Marseilles fever, South African tick typhus, Mediterranean fever (*fièvre boutonneuse*), Asian tick typhus, and Queensland tick typhus. In most respects these illnesses resemble RMSF. An important feature, however, is the presence of an eschar at the site of the tick bite. This is a small painless ulcer with a central black necrotic area resulting from the endothelial damage caused by the rickettsiae.

Scrub typhus

This is caused by *Rickettsia tsutsugamushi* transmitted by larval mites (chiggers) in the Far East and Pacific Islands. The mites usually feed on rodents in area of bush or scrub. Following infection there is local multiplication and formation of an eschar with local lymphadenopathy: 10–14 days later there is fever, headache, and myalgia, often ocular pain and apathy. A macular rash appears on the trunk a few days later still and the lymphadenopathy becomes generalized. Untreated, the mortality of 5–20% is usually due to cardiac failure. The serological response is to OX-K and treatment with tetracycline or chloramphenicol is rapidly effective.

Viral haemorrhagic fevers

A number of zoonotic viruses, some arthropod-borne and some spread by direct contact, have haemorrhagic manifestations as well as causing specific organ damage. They tend to engender great public and media anxiety.

Lassa fever

This zoonotic arenavirus is carried in otherwise healthy rodents in many bush areas of West Africa south of the Sahara: in some villages in the northern plains of Nigeria as many as 50% of the population have evidence of past infection with lassa virus. There are also foci of human disease described as far south as Mozambique. Human infection occurs when rodent urine contaminates household surfaces and foodstuffs. Presentation occurs 4–14 days after exposure (a history of appropriate travel or contact is important). The majority of indigenous human cases are mild but expatriates are particularly likely to progress to severe disease. Fever, back and retrosternal chest pains, and generalized myalgia is followed by an ulcerative pharyngitis, facial oedema, and hypotension. These symptoms are non-specific and differentiation must be from malaria, typhoid and other septicaemia, typhus, yellow fever, and infectious mononucleosis. In severe cases, a notable finding is elevated liver enzymes and the disease can be confirmed as Lassa fever by serology or by virus isolation in special facilities. In West Africa, normal barrier nursing procedures, the avoidance of needlestick injury, and other body fluid contamination are enough to prevent spread of infection to staff and other patients. However, the possibility of nosocomial spread and the severity of the disease have led to the use of much more stringent precautions for cases imported into Western nations. These include the use of isolation tents, chemical treatment of all body fluids, and special arrangements for laboratory investigations.

In the absence of a vaccine, control depends on reducing rodent exposure.

Other haemorrhagic fevers

There are a number of other haemorrhagic fevers that the average traveller may hear about but which are not a meaningful risk. *Congo-Crimean* haemorrhagic fever is spread by ticks from domestic animals to man in Asia and Africa. *Argentine* haemorrhagic fever and *Bolivian* haemorrhagic fever are, as their names suggest, endemic in South America. Those at risk tend to be farm workers and the clinical features resemble those of Lassa fever. Haemorrhagic fever with renal syndrome (HFRS) is caused by a number of different rodent-transmitted viruses distributed widely (including Scandinavia and Western Europe). Presentation occurs after 2–3 weeks incubation with a febrile illness followed by a hypotensive phase in which there may be haemorrhagic features and renal failure (hence the name!).

Yellow fever

Yellow fever is a severe haemorrhagic fever caused by a flavivirus transmitted by infected *Aedes aegypti* mosquitoes. The disease is endemic in tropical South America and Africa; the epidemiology of infection differs between urban and jungle areas and on each side of the Atlantic. The incubation period is short, in the order of 3–7 days and disease presents with fever and chills lasting for about 48 hours. In most patients, there is then uneventful recovery but in 10–20% of individuals, after a period of apparent improvement, the illness progresses rapidly with haemorrhagic manifestations, nephritis, hepatitis, and pneumonitis. Death occurs in up to 50% of cases within a week. Yellow fever has been largely controlled among travellers by the use of vaccine (see p. 000). Vaccination is almost 100% effective and gives protection for 10 years or longer. It is a mandatory procedure for some travel to endemic areas and all travel from endemic to receptive areas (areas without yellow fever but with mosquitoes capable of transmitting the disease). Despite this, deaths from yellow fever have occasionally been recorded in tourists travelling to endemic countries that have not insisted on certificates of vaccination.

Dengue

Dengue is an acute febrile illness caused by a flavivirus transmitted by *Aedes* mosquitoes in tropical Central America, the Caribbean, Asia, South East Asia, the Pacific and, to a lesser extent, Africa. Epidemics occur with high attack rates and it is by far the most commonly seen arbovirus infection in travellers. The disease has become very much more common in the past 50 years with perennial problems in Thailand and other parts of South-East Asia and epidemics in Cuba and the Caribbean in 1981.

Dengue fever

Classical dengue fever ('breakbone fever') has an incubation period of 3–7 days, following which there is a prominent fever, severe myalgia and arthralgia, headache, and retro-orbital pain. After 3–5 days, an erythematous blanching rash spreads from the trunk to the extremities. Hepatomegaly and lymphadenopathy may be present. After a few days, the fever settles but convalescence is often prolonged.

The diagnosis is suggested by exposure in an endemic or epidemic area, marked leucopenia (often less than $1500 \times 10^9/l$), and thrombocytopenia. Diagnosis can only be confirmed serologically. There is no specific treatment.

Dengue haemorrhagic fever

This is relative common in children in South East Asia and the Caribbean but rare in visitors. It probably results from re-infection with a different serotype of dengue virus and immune complex vascular damage, which leads to increased capillary permeability, hypovolaemia and disseminated intravascular coagulation (with haemorrhagic features). Haemorrhages into the skin, gums, and gastrointestinal tract and circulatory failure may follow. The mortality in untreated cases may be as high as 50%.

Plague

Yersinia pestis is a Gram-negative bacillus that is transmitted amongst various wild rodents by fleas. It is endemic in many parts of the world, countries reporting cases during the past decade include Vietnam, Peru, Brazil, Madagascar, Tanzania, Burma, and the USA. Transmission to humans is usually through fleas from urban rats.

Much of the pathology of plague is due to endotoxins and exotoxins which cause activation of the complement and coagulation pathways resulting in disseminated intravascular coagulation (DIC) and shock.

The most common form of human plague is bubonic plague. After an incubation period of less than a week, there is sudden onset of fever, rigors, and painful local suppurative lymphadenitis (buboes), usually in the groin, axilla, or neck. These buboes are very tender and are surrounded by oedema. The disease progresses to septicaemia with DIC. Occasionally, septicaemic plague occurs without the prior development of a bubo.

A further severe and often fatal form of plague is pneumonic infection with cough, dyspnoea, blood-flecked sputum, and respiratory failure. Untreated, plague has a mortality of almost 50%. Treatment may be with streptomycin, tetracycline, or chloramphenicol: tetracycline is the drug of choice. Prophylactic antibiotics can prevent the onset of infection with tetracycline again the drug of choice; children under 8 years of age can be given ciprofloxacin if absolutely necessary.

Media reporting of an outbreak of plague in India in 1994.[22] The outbreak of bubonic plague in Mararasta State and pneumonic plague in Gujarat State in India in 1994 with the subsequent world-wide media coverage and restrictions on travel highlight the relevance of infections once thought to be of historic importance only to the developed world. All UK general practitioners were expected to be on the watch for symptoms in travellers returning from India and to inform the general public, as they raised the subject during everyday consultations.

The media over-reaction also demonstrates the emotive sway and fear of this infection in the public mind. The greatest pandemic in history, the Black Death, centred on the year 1348 and is widely known. The plague reached a peak in London in 1665 with some 68 000 deaths in that year. Although isolated outbreaks in Europe continued, including one in England between 1906 and 1918, no major epidemics occurred subsequently. It is not widely known that the plague remains endemic in the USA with 11 case reports between 1993 and 1994.[23]

Trichinosis

This illness is caused by the nematode *Trichinella spiralis* and is acquired by eating encysted larvae in the undercooked flesh of pigs and other carnivores. The cysts develop into adults in the small bowel: severe infections cause diarrhoea and abdominal pain. Larvae are produced which penetrate the bowel wall, migrate in the circulation, and encyst in muscles. In severe infections of muscle there is fever, muscle weakness, and tenderness, and periorbital oedema lasting for a few weeks. Eosinophilia is usually a pronounced feature. Serology and muscle biopsy confirm the diagnosis, but the value of anthelminthic therapy with thiabendazole (which kills the adults) and mebendazole (which may be effective against larvae) is uncertain.

Trichinosis is prevented by adequate cooking of meat: the smoking and salting of meat is not reliable.

References

1. Wallace M *et al.* Treatment of adult varicella with oral acyclovir. A randomised, placebo-controlled trial. *Ann Intern Med* (1992) **117**: 358–9

2. Department of Health. *Corticosteroids and varicella zoster virus. CMOs update 2.* London: DoH (1994)

3. Rice R, Simmons K, Carr R. Near fatal chickenpox during prednisolone treatment. *BMJ* (1994) **309;** 1069–70

4. American Academy of Pediatrics Committee on Infectious Diseases: The use of oral acyclovir in otherwise healthy children with varicella. *Ped* (1993) **91**: 674–6

5. Balfour H H *et al.* Acyclovir treatment of varicella in otherwise healthy adolescents. The collaborative acyclovir varicella study group. *J Ped* (1992) **120**: 627–33

6. McKendrick M. Acyclovir for childhood chickenpox. Cost is unjustified. Balfour H. No reason not to treat. Controversies in management. *BMJ* (1995) **310;** 108–10

7. Arvin A. Progress in the treatment and prevention of varicella. *Curr Op Infect Dis* (1993) **6**: 553–7

8. Friedman Ross L, Lantos J. Immunisation against chickenpox: better to confine immunisation to those at high risk. *BMJ* (1995) **310**: 2–3

9. Brown D, Ramsay M, Richards A *et al*. Salivary diagnosis of measles: a study of notified cases in the United Kingdom, (1991–3). *BMJ* (1994) **308**: 1015–17

10. Letter from the CMO, Dr K Calman. Measles and rubella immunisation campaign. *PL CMO* **94**: 12

11. Miller E. Rubella infection in pregnancy: remaining problems. *Brit J Obs Gyn* (1989) **96**: 887–8

12. Cohen B. Parvovirus B19: an expanding spectrum of disease. *BMJ* (1995) **311;** 1549–52

13. Cohen B J, Buckley M M. The prevalence of antibody to human parvovirus B19 in England and Wales. *J Med Microbiol* (1988) **25**: 151–3

14. Mortality and morbidity weekly report. Risks associated with human parvo B19 infection. *JAMA* (1989) **261**: 1406–8; Part 2; **261**: 1555–63

15. Public Health Laboratory Service Working Party on 'Fifth Disease'. Prospective study of human parvovirus (B19) infection in pregnancy. *BMJ* (1990) **300**: 1166–70

16. Pattison J (editorial). Human parvovirus B19. *BMJ* (1994) **308**: 150–1

17. Tait D, Ward K, Brown D. Measles and rubella misdiagnosed in infants as exanthem subitum (roseola infantum). *BMJ* (1996) **312**: 101–2

18. Steere A. Lyme disease. *N Engl J Med* (1989) **321**: 586–96

19. Nathwani D, Hamlet N, Walker E. Lyme disease: a review. *Brit J Gen Pract* (1990) **40**: 72–4

20. O'Connell S. Lyme disease in the United Kingdom. *BMJ* (1995) **310**: 303–8

21. Ferguson I (editorial). Leptospirosis update. The risk is small and may be reduced by simple precautions. *BMJ* (1991) **302**: 128–9

22. Cook G. Plague in india: an inappropriate media response. *Curr Op Infect Dis* (1994) **7**: 639–643

23. Human plague–United states, (1993–1994) *MMWR* (1994) **43**: 242–6

24. Felsher J, Freifield A. (NIH conference) The epidemiology, natural history and complications of varicella-zoster virus. 223–6. In Strauss S E. Moderator. Varicella-zoster infections: biology, natural history, treatment and prevention. *Ann Intern Med* (1998) **108**: 221–37

CHAPTER FIFTEEN

The prevention of infection during travel abroad

In 1949 UK residents made 1.7 million visits abroad. In 1995 the figure was 41.5 million, of which 7.7 million were beyond Europe. An increasing number of these trips are made to countries in the Far East, Africa, and other subtropical and tropical areas and the speed of air travel ensures that many individuals are returning home within the incubation period of tropical diseases.[1] Therefore, general practitioners within the UK are likely to see many more patients with infections caused by exotic organisms.

These developments have had a substantial impact on UK general practice. Many people attend for immunization and advice before travel, others seek help on their return. In addition, doctors practising in areas with a high proportion of individuals from minority ethnic groups, including those who have fled repression and war in their own countries, may present with a different spectrum of disease. It is for these reasons that we have included a chapter on travel and infection.[2]

Omissions and inaccuracies in advice before travel are common[3] and may put the doctor at risk for legal action should harm befall the patient. With more and more travellers holidaying further afield each year potential problems are likely to increase. The Medical Defence Union's advice to doctors is:

There must be a very real possibility of a claim for negligence being made against a doctor who deliberately overrides a country's recommendations and the patient contracts one of the specified diseases. It is likely to prove extremely difficult to mount an adequate defence against this claim.

The guidelines in Table 15.1 should minimize errors.

Organization of a travel clinic

If a general practice undertakes to provide advice and immunization for travel abroad several matters should be discussed and decided before starting. Who will be involved, how much responsibility will the nurses take, and will the sessions be organized as clinics or integrated into the daily work of the practice

Table 15.1 *Essential background information for primary health care workers advising travellers*

- Doctors, nurses, and staff should make every effort to obtain current knowledge of the world-wide distribution of disease
- Accurate, up-to-date vaccination and malaria prophylaxis information must always be to hand
- Conditions of stay in countries to be visited must be addressed (i.e. travellers living rough or in good hotels will require different advice,
- General health advice must be available: additional advice concerning malaria prophylaxis (both physical protection against mosquito bites and chemoprophylaxis), water purification, food
- Current information concerning the prevalence of AIDS is now regarded as essential
- Records of vaccinations given or recommended, together with health advice, should be recorded

---

in a less formal way? The following issues should be explored before deciding that a clinic is to be the preferred option.

- Perform an audit of likely population requirements. Identify (from local knowledge) the usual travel pattern of practice population

- Locate the nearest yellow fever registration vaccination centre. Decide if yellow fever registration is sensible (see Appendix 1)

- Plan the integration of the travel clinic within the practice. The involvement, support and enthusiasm of all the staff is vital for success. Decide on the timing and consider evening or Saturday sessions. Clinics, while normally nurse-run, should be held at a time when a doctor is available to help with problems or emergencies

- Arrange staff training (doctors, nurses, and reception staff). Appropriate training usually has to be in-house and success will depend on the enthusiasm and motivation by one or two members of the practice. The basic training will in many respects be the same as for childhood immunization but there will be additional emphasis on how to give advice on the prevention of infection while abroad. Vaccination information is available from many sources (see Appendix 1).

Clinic efficiency

One member of staff should be primarily responsible for the clinic arrangements. Duties will include organizing the appointment system, ordering and maintaining supplies, submitting claims for reimbursement by the family health service authority or health board, and constant updating of information. The smooth running of a clinic is assisted by constructing a travellers' questionnaire, ideally to be completed by the patient before attending (see Appendix 2).

General practitioners and practice nurses are frequently asked for information and advice by patients intending to travel abroad both for business and holiday purposes. Travel agents sometimes provide information but this may be suspect and out of date. It is probably unreasonable to expect a travel agent to provide anything more than general vaccination advice. A busy travel agency is hardly the best venue for medical decisions and there is anecdotal evidence that wrong or even dangerous advice may sometimes be given. With the knowledge that our patients only retain about 20% of the content of a medical consultation, it is unlikely that, amidst the intensity of foreign booking, any greater proportion of holiday health advice will be retained. Nonetheless, basic advice concerning vaccination and healthy living abroad should be provided in written form by travel agents. The Department of Social Security pamphlet *The travellers' guide to health*', T1, which replaces SA 40/41, is useful for this purpose.

'Go and see your doctor' may not, however, be the most best advice in all circumstances. Travel medicine does not usually form part of the undergraduate curriculum although the subject, which is rapidly becoming a new specialty, is of considerable importance to the GP and practice nurse.

Some practices may look on travel immunization and advice as a strain (albeit income-producing) on practice time and resources. This attitude can result from lack of organization and poor basic knowledge. Others have found that travel medicine, properly timetabled within the working week, can be a stimulating extension of normal practice activities. Many patients consult their doctor in circumstances of doubt, anxiety, fear, or pain. A new and positive dimension is seen when the healthy patient attends, looking forward to a holiday and with few of the underlying worries that may prompt attendance for other preventative purposes. Doctors, reception staff, and nurses all gain much from such encounters, both in the satisfaction of providing sound medical advice and in dreaming about foreign travel!

For those practices unable to offer advice a satisfactory alternative is offered by specialized travel clinics. Each clinic provides a full range of immunizations, individual health briefings, specific malaria prevention advice, and a retail service. Several clinics are sited in general practice and are run by GPs and nurses. Clinics have direct computer link to the ever-changing world situation as the information is constantly updated from the London School of Hygiene and Tropical Medicine. These clinics offer a service which represents the ideal standard for general practice travel clinics. Much more than the mere availability of a vaccination service is required in advising international travellers and to emphasize that point the term 'travel clinic' is appropriate and will have the advantage of reminding travellers, doctors, and nurses that the implications of travel extend far beyond 'having the right injections'.

Vaccines administered before travel

Some of the vaccines administered before foreign travel in UK general practice are for diseases that are only contracted abroad, and are described in this section. It is important to remember, however, that diseases prevented in the UK by vaccination programmes are still prevalent in other countries. Travellers who have not been immunized, or who require boosters, may therefore be susceptible to polio, tetanus, diphtheria, hepatitis B, and tuberculosis and should be advised accordingly.

Typhoid

Typhoid vaccination should be considered for all persons travelling abroad except those travelling to Canada, the USA, Australia, New Zealand, and Northern Europe, although the efficacy of vaccination in preventing travellers from non-endemic countries from acquiring typhoid has not been unequivocally demonstrated. Three typhoid vaccines are available.

1. Whole cell vaccine

The former mainstay vaccine is a parenteral heat-killed *Salmonella typhi* whole organism vaccine, one injection of which will give around 70–80% protection which fades after 1 year. To provide protection for 3 years it is necessary to give two doses at an interval of 4 to 6 weeks. Thereafter, a single reinforcing dose will give protection for a further 3 years no matter what time interval has elapsed since the primary course (Table 15.2). Repeated injections increase the risk of hypersensitivity and reinforcing doses should, therefore, only be given when foreign travel is planned and the 3-year protection period has run out. During a 'crash' vaccination programme a primary course of one single dose is worth giving as it will provide a high degree of protection for 1 year.

2. Oral Ty 21a vaccine

An orally administered, live-attenuated strain of *S. typhi* Ty21a containing 10^9 organisms/dose is available. The vaccine is administered in a three-dose alternate day schedule but the efficacy of this vaccine has not been assessed in travellers from non-typhoid endemic countries and it has been suggested that

Table 15.2 *Vaccination schedule for whole cell typhoid vaccine*

Age (years)	1st dose	Interval	2nd dose	Booster
1–10	0.25 ml	4–6 weeks	0.25 ml	3 years
Over 10	0.5 ml	4–6 weeks	0.5 ml	3 years

The vaccine should be given by deep subcutaneous or intramuscular injection.
   Booster doses (0.1 ml) may also be given by the intradermal route and result in less adverse reactions.

individual doses need to contain a larger number of viable organisms.[4] As the vaccine contains live organisms it must not be given to HIV-positive people and should not be administered at the same time as oral polio vaccine.

3. Vi polysaccharide vaccine

A parenteral vaccine composed of purified Vi antigen was introduced to the UK in 1992. One injection is sufficient and the local and systemic reactions are much milder than those associated with the traditional parenteral vaccine. A single dose gives 70–80% protection for at least 3 years. Those at risk should be re-immunized every 3 years.

Contraindications for all types of typhoid vaccine

- Not advised for children under 1 year of age
- Should not be given in the presence of acute febrile illness
- Caution necessary in pregnancy. While there is no information suggesting that typhoid vaccine is unsafe in pregnancy, it must only be used if there is a definite indication

Cholera

There is no cholera vaccine currently available in the UK. Certificates of vaccination against cholera should not now be required by any country.

Hepatitis A

General practitioners frequently give active or passive immunization against hepatitis A without determining the susceptibility of the patient to the infection. While patients without risk factors are unlikely to be immune, those with a history of jaundice, or who have been born, lived, or travelled in areas where the infection is endemic are highly likely to be immune. It would seem sensible to immunize the first group without screening but to screen the high-risk group for antibody to hepatitis A and only immunize those who are negative. The immune group can be reassured they will never need testing or immunizing again.[6,7]

Passive protection

Travellers may be given passive protection using human normal immuno-globulin injection (HNIG), which is also available under the proprietary names of Gammabulin and Kabiglobulin. Passive immunization may prevent or modify the course of hepatitis A and is recommended for outside North America, Australia, New Zealand or Europe. Any (live) vaccine required prior to the journey should be administered in the first instance at least 3 weeks before Gammaglobulin.

All immunoglobulins are prepared from blood donations which are known to be HIV-negative and the processing of the plasma also renders passive immunization against hepatitis A, safe from HIV infection.

Hepatitis A vaccines

These vaccines are formaldehyde-inactivated virus.[8] They are available for all age groups over the age of 1 year. The initial dose is followed by a booster at 6–12 months and confers immunity for up to 10 years.

The vaccines are administered by intramuscular injection in the deltoid region. For adults over the age of 16 years, a combined hepatitis A plus B vaccine is now available.

Japanese B encephalitis

Japanese B encephalitis vaccine is strongly recommended for those travelling to endemic areas. It is particularly important for travellers in rural areas. The disease is seasonal. The vaccine is unlicensed and available on a named patient basis.

Several different vaccinations are available but can be difficult to obtain. Patients should be referred to their nearest specialist centre in these circumstances. The vaccine should be stored below 10 °C, and protected from sunlight. It must not be frozen.

Dosage

The primary vaccination is by two 1 ml subcutaneous doses given at an interval of 1–2 weeks. Additional protection may be afforded to those aged over 60 and those entering an epidemic area for the first time, by giving a further dose 1 month later. Immunity is maintained by a booster 1 ml dose given subcutaneously every one to four years. This is only necessary if re-entering an endemic area. The dosage for children under 3 years is 0.5 ml subcutaneously, spaced at the same time intervals as for an adult.

Contraindications

- Acute or severe infection
- Pregnancy
- Diabetes
- Immunocompromised traveller
- Heart, kidney, or liver disease

Tick-borne encephalitis

A killed vaccine is available on a named patient basis and is recommended for those where prolonged exposure is likely—camping, working, or walking in high-risk areas. The full primary course consists of three intramuscular injections of 0.5 ml. The time interval between the first and second injection should be 4–12 weeks, and between the second and third, 9–12 months. This regime will give protection for three years but may be reinforced within a period of 6 years by a single booster dose. A reduced primary course of two injections gives protection for 1 year. The interval between first and second doses may be reduced to 2 weeks. There is no lower age limit but it is usually given to children over the age of 1 year.

Contraindications. These include acute or severe illness and central nervous system disease.

Meningococcal meningitis

In some areas of the world the risk of contracting meningococcal meningitis is quite high and it is essential that up-to-date advice about meningococcal meningitis is obtained when constructing a vaccination programme for travel abroad. Since 1988, Saudi Arabia has required immunization of pilgrims on the Haj annual pilgrimage.

The current vaccine contains antigens of group A and C meningococcus only and is a dead vaccine. Once prepared, the vaccine should be used within the hour and must be stored at between 2 °C and 8 °C. Vaccine gives protection for 3 years or more and protective antibodies usually appear within 5 days of vaccination. Where there is high risk, re-vaccination should be offered after 2 years. The highest risk is to travellers under the age of 35, and particularly children. In endemic areas, vaccination may be offered from the age of 3 months, although its efficacy at this early age cannot be guaranteed. It is certainly known to be effective from the age of 2 years and onwards.

Dosage

In adults and children over the age of 2 years a single dose of reconstituted vaccine is recommended. Children from 3 months to 2 years of age should receive a single dose of reconstituted vaccine followed 1–3 months later by a second dose.

Contraindications. Immunization should be postponed during acute or severe infection. Children under 2 years of age and pregnant women should not be immunized unless visiting a highly endemic area.

Yellow fever

In order to obtain a valid certificate of yellow fever vaccination the procedure must be carried out at a recognized yellow fever vaccination centre. These centres are approved by the World Health Organization and are able to issue a valid international vaccination certificate. All centres in the UK are listed in *Immunisation against infectious disease* (HMSO 1996).

Yellow fever is a live vaccine and gives a high level of immunity that will continue for at least ten years and may be lifelong. The International Certificate becomes valid ten days after primary vaccination and is valid for ten years. Upon re-vaccination validity is immediate. Many countries require a certificate for all visitors, whilst some require only a certificate for those who have visited or travelled through an endemic area. An airplane stop in such an endemic area qualifies as a visit to that country.

Contraindications

- Acute febrile or acute illness
- Aged under 9 months.
- Immunosuppressed traveller
- Extreme hypersensitivity to neomycin, polymyxin, egg, or chicken protein
- Pregnant women, but if yellow fever risk is high, then dangers of vaccination less than danger from disease
- When another live vaccine has been given within 3 weeks
- HIV-positive individuals should not receive yellow fever vaccination without assessment of their CD4 count

Some countries may accept a medical certificate stating that vaccination is contraindicated on medical grounds

Reactions to yellow fever immunization are generally mild although myalgia, headache, or fever may occur in about 10% of vaccinees. Severe reactions, such as encephalitis, are very rare and usually confined to infants.

If possible yellow fever vaccination should not be given within 3 weeks of another live vaccine. If time does not allow such spacing, then the vaccines should be given at the same time using different sites. Local reactions at injection sites are common.

Dosage

Vaccination is with 0.5 ml by deep subcutaneous injection, the preferred site being middle third of deltoid in upper arm. The same dose is given regardless of age.

The vaccine should be stored at 2–8 °C. Protection from light is necessary. The vaccine must be used within one hour of reconstitution.

Health education and the prevention of infection while travelling

The general principles for the prevention of infection apply where ever an individual is living or travelling and the possible sources of infection (human, animal, and environment), and portals of entry into the body remain the same. However, differences in climate, food, sanitation, animal and insect species, and a lack of awareness of hazards make foreign travel potentially dangerous unless the individual is prepared and sensible.

In advising a traveller the GP should have some idea of the purpose of the trip and give general advice about infections caught from other people, animals, insects, and the environment, which may be acquired via water, food, sex, or tissue penetration (see Table 2.2). Some of the general advice which follows might be used to devise handouts for patients receiving immunization before travelling. Some authors have challenged the assumption that travel prophylaxis is worthwhile and have argued that the costs of hepatitis-A and typhoid immunization are not justified.[9] However, they underline the importance of advice about avoiding infection by adopting appropriate behaviour.

General precautions

Water

Generally, if water is clear, contains no sediment, and smells of chlorine, it is probably safe. Ideally, travellers should drink only bottled water, or be advised that other drinking water must be boiled. In many countries ice in drinks should be avoided.

Water may be disinfected by the addition of chlorine or certain proprietary purification tablets to drinking and cooking water. Preparing a tincture of Iodine 2% (4 drops of iodine per litre of water) is also effective although both of these procedures will leave the water tainted in taste but it can be improved by the addition of soluble vitamin C. However, a special combined iodine resin and charcoal filter is available; the Travel Well and the smaller Trekker Travel Well (and the very small pocket Travel Well). It has been developed by MASTA, at the London School of Hygiene and Tropical Medicine. This device produces drinking water that is safe from bacteria, viruses, and parasites that can cause gastroenteritis, typhoid, cholera, dysentery, giardiasis, polio, and hepatitis. Carbon filters are of very doubtful value as they can become easily contaminated.

Tissue penetration

Travellers may be put at risk in many countries of the world from infections which enter the body via small abrasions or penetrate intact skin. Those who participate in bathing, canoeing, water-skiing, and other water sports are particularly at risk. Travellers should wear waterproof footwear when walking in endemic areas, particularly in rivers. They should avoid the usual village river crossings and always cross upstream of villages and such crossings. They should avoid swimming in lakes and rivers and should not walk bare-footed in the rural tropics.

Food

Generally, foods that can be peeled are safe, if not they should be sterilized. Shellfish is best avoided in many countries. Vegetables and salads should be thoroughly washed in bottled or purified water to eliminate unwanted fertilizers and contamination from food-handlers. Meat must be well cooked and eaten hot. Desert trips with 'local banquets' may ruin the remainder of a holiday. Milk, soft cheeses, and pate may be the source of infection with *Brucella* or *Listeria*. Ice-cream and cream may be the source of *Salmonella*. Remember that cruise ship passengers are not immune, as sanitary requirements are not of a universally high standard. High class cruise ships sometimes fail to pass health inspection. Almost 2.4 million cruise ship passengers passed through the Port of Miami in 1986 alone. Of 55 cruise ships sailing regularly from US ports, 22 failed sanitary inspection. Many hotels do not adequately control refrigeration and refrigerator temperatures. Pregnant women should be particularly careful when eating food abroad (toxoplasma). Unpasteurized cow, sheep, or goat's milk should not be drunk. Food that has been unrefrigerated for more than two or three hours should not be eaten.

HIV and hepatitis

Homosexual and bisexual males should avoid anal intercourse abroad, particularly in an endemic area. If this advice is not followed then special toughened contraceptive sheaths must be used. Heterosexual intercourse, particularly with prostitutes, should also be avoided in endemic areas. There is considerable evidence that many travellers take risks despite the public health campaigns of recent years.[10,11] In some parts of Africa, over 90% of prostitutes are estimated to be HIV-positive. Patients must be warned that casual intercourse is dangerous and that condoms must always be used. Spermicidal jelly, particularly that containing Nonoxynol-9 may give some additional protection. The risks from other sexually transmitted infections should also be explained.

Intravenous drug users must never share needles or syringes. Intravenous transfusion with blood or blood products should be avoided in many countries outside Northern Europe, North America, Australia, New Zealand, Singapore, and Hong Kong. Packs of sterile medical equipment are available for travellers and individuals should be advised to take them when visiting endemic areas (see Appendix 1). Any procedure that involves penetration of the skin with needles should not be undertaken (e.g. tattooing, acupuncture). Visits to dentists or doctors practising in endemic areas may be risky, since the re-use of syringes or needles may be a common practice.

If while travelling in a group a transfusion is required, then attempts should be made to receive compatible donated blood from a fellow traveller. If this is not possible a British Embassy or Consular official should be contacted for advice concerning screened blood.

Infections acquired from animals

Travellers should be warned that the following animals may harbour rabies.

- Dogs
- Skunks, raccoons, foxes, and insectivorous bats in North America

- Foxes in the Arctic, vampire bats and mongooses in the Caribbean
- Vampire bats in Central and South America
- Foxes, wolves, raccoon dogs, and insectivorous bats in Europe
- Wolves, jackals, and small carnivores, such as mongooses and civets, throughout most of Africa and Asia

Man is usually infected with the bite of a rabid dog but a skunk bite in mid-western USA, or a jackal in Africa could involve a very serious risk of rabies. Rabies is endemic in most parts of the world and there is current concern that rabies could reach the UK from Europe through the Channel tunnel. Rabies occurs in North America, Greenland, Canada, the former USSR, China, New Territories of Hong Kong, and most tropical areas.

The prevention of rabies amongst travellers has a low priority but this situation needs reviewing. Pre-exposure vaccination against rabies must be considered for travellers who run particularly high risks, such as animal collectors, zoologists, botanists, hunters, cave explorers, and those who travel rough, overland in endemic areas. Even travellers visiting cities in endemic areas are at risk from rabid dogs. Unnecessary contact with animals (e.g. stroking stray dogs or exploring bat-occupied caves should be avoided).

Pre-exposure prophylaxis. This human diploid cell vaccine is given as 3 doses on days 0, 7, and 28. A booster is given after 2–3 years. It is available for all ages over 1 year. It is given into the deltoid by subcutaneous injection, the intradermal route may also be used, but is not yet licensed. When rapid immunization is necessary the intradermal route may be used in all four limbs. This procedure is not covered by the manufacturer's product licence.

Post-exposure prophylaxis. The aim of this procedure is to neutralize the inoculated virus before it enters the nervous system. All mammal bites should be carefully cleaned and medical attention sought. Prophylactic antibiotics are usually advised as is booster tetanus vaccination. The area of the bite should be scrubbed thoroughly with soap and water under a running tap for at least five minutes and then rinsed with plain water. Any foreign material must be removed. If possible, the area should be irrigated with a virucidal agent (e.g. 40–70% alcohol or 0.1% aqueous iodine). Wounds should not be sutured and occlusive dressings should be avoided. If possible, it should be ascertained if the dog responsible for the bite has been vaccinated against rabies. The information available may or may not allow an accurate assessment of the risk but if doubt exists in an endemic area, post-exposure prophylaxis must be given even if the bite is several months old.

The standard post-exposure course of human diploid cell strain vaccine

(HDCSV) is 1 ml, intramuscular (deltoid) injection on days 0, 3, 7, 14, 30, and 90. Injections must not be given into the buttock.

Insect-borne disease

Malaria is the most important insect-borne disease and is discussed below. While the mosquito is the common vector of many diseases, other vectors such as sandfly, tick, louse, and flea are also important (Table 15.4). Prophylaxis against insect-borne disease depends on prevention of bites and often advice in this sphere is poor, lacking, or not adhered to by the traveller.

Malaria

Work to develop a vaccine against malaria continues. Despite the fact that malaria confers natural immunity on its human host, the complicated life cycle of the four malaria parasites has led to profound difficulties in the process.[12] All travellers to malaria endemic areas are strongly advised to use an appropriate drug regime and personal protection measures to prevent malaria (Table 15.5). General practitioners must make sure that travellers to endemic areas understand the danger from malaria. One aspect of advice that is frequently overlooked concerns avoiding mosquito bites. The general approach is relevant to other insect vectors.

Phillips-Howard *et al.*[13] found that annual rates of reported infection amongst travellers to Oceana (Papua New Guinea, Solomon Islands, etc.) were 4100 per 100 000 travellers. In Africa, emigrants returning to visit friends and relatives were at greatest risk, particularly in Ghana and Nigeria (1303 and 952 per 100 000, respectively).

Business travellers to Kenya experienced the highest attack rates in East Africa (465 per 100 000). Visitors to west Africa who did not comply with their chemoprophylactic regimes were at a 2.5-fold higher risk of infection than fully compliant users. The authors called for the travelling public to be encouraged to take protective measures against malaria and comply with prescribed chemoprophylactic regimes.

Wiselka *et al.*[14] highlighted the problems for people born or normally resident in the UK visiting relatives abroad. The authors reviewed 114 episodes of malaria in 110 patients who were admitted to the Infectious Diseases Unit in Leicester during the five-year period from February 1983 to January 1988. Most patients presented in the summer months, 68% were under 40 years of age, 39% were born in the Indian subcontinent, 23% in East Africa, and 23% in Britain: 82% of patients with falciparum malaria had recently returned from Africa, whereas 82% with vivax malaria had visited Asia; 36% had been given antimalarial prophylaxis but only half took medication correctly. General practitioners who care for minority ethnic groups must ensure that they understand the risks: the practice should have leaflets available in the relevant languages, and opportunities to talk

Table 15.4 *Transmission of diseases by insects*

Vector	Disease
Mosquitoes	Malaria
	Filariasis
	Dengue
	Yellow fever
	Japanese B encephalitis
Sandflies	Leishmaniasis
	Sandfly fever
Ticks	Tick-borne encephalitis
	Lyme disease
	Typhus (tick, scrub, endemic, epidemic)
Mites	Typhus
	Scabies
Tsetse files	Sleeping sickness
Reduviid bugs	Chagas' disease
Lice	Typhus
Fleas	Bubonic plague

to community groups about prevention of malaria and other travel-related illnesses should be sought.

Chemoprophylactic regimes

This chapter contains no specific country or regional advice for chemoprophylaxis since to do so in such a dynamic field would be inappropriate and dangerous. Consultation with a source of current and expert knowledge is essential and if the GP is in doubt about advice he/she is giving it should be confirmed by a telephone call to the Malaria Reference Laboratory or other centres listed in the British National Formulary.

Malaria transmission occurs over large areas of the world, many of which are increasingly visited by holiday-makers. It is found in:

- The Middle East

- Central and South America

- Oceania

- The Indian Subcontinent

- South East Asia (Thailand) Indonesia, People's Republic of China, Philippines, Burma, Kampuchea, Vietnam, and Laos

Drug resistance of *Plasmodium falciparum* to chloroquine has been reported from many countries with a striking advance from East to West Africa with

Table 15.5 *Personal protection measures against mosquitoes*

- Sleep in a securely screened room
- Use a mosquito net, but check that it has no holes and is securely tucked in around base or mattress. The box net is much the best and is suspended from two parallel nylon lines fixed across the room using adhesive wall hooks.
- Mosquito net protection is enhanced if the net is soaked in permethrin. Repeat every 6 months
- Mosquito nets must be used to cover cots
- Air conditioning helps eliminate mosquitoes
- Synthetic pyrethroids vaporized when using 'plug-in electric mats' are effective against mosquitoes. Electronic buzzers are **not** effective
- Spray-type insect repellents should be used to kill any mosquitoes the in room before retiring
- After dusk and in the early morning long sleeves, skirts, or trousers should be worn
- In late afternoon, shady areas must be avoided as some mosquitoes are active during the day
- Special wrist and ankle bands impregnated with 'DEET' (diethyl toluamide) are highly effective as is deet aerosol spray
- Preparations made from eucalyptus oil

---

almost all of the countries of sub-Saharan Africa now reporting chloroquine-resistant malaria.

Resistance to other antimalarials is also commonly found. In addition, there are reports of rare but severe reactions to Fansidar (pyrimethamine 25 mg, sulfadoxine 500 mg), which may cause severe or fatal Stevens–Johnson syndrome, and Maloprim (pyrimethamine 12.5 mg, dapsone 100 mg) and amodiaquine, which may cause agranulocytosis. Both Fansidar and Maloprim may have a role, the former in emergency self treatment and the latter as a second-line drug where the benefits of use are judged to outweigh the risks.

The spread of drug-resistant strains of *P. falciparum*, the reduced risk in some areas, new information on adverse drug reactions and new chemoprophylactic agents lead to recommendations from the Malaria Reference Laboratory, London in 1993,[15] which were revised and extended in 1995[16] (see also Table 15.6). The situation is complex and careful assessment is required before advice can be offered. Travellers, even to low-risk areas, should be warned to avoid mosquito bites, to take prophylaxis, and follow the instructions *to the letter*, and to seek medical advice urgently should they develop a fever.

Risk of malaria World-wide: 1995[16]

North Africa and the Middle East. The risk is very low in most tourist areas. *Plasmodium vivax* malaria occurs in Far Eastern and Southern Turkey, Syria, and Iraq. Chloroquine-resistant falciparum malaria occurs in Oman, the Emirates, Yemen, Iran, and Afghanistan.

Sub-Saharan Africa. The risk is high throughout this area, except in the extreme south. Cloroquine-resistant falciparum malaria is common.

South Asia. The risk to travellers exists throughout except in high mountains. Although *P. vivax* is usual, falciparum malaria occurs and is commonly resistant to chloroquine.

South East and East Asia. The most difficult areas for advice are South East and East Asia. Malaria risk is high in some areas and multidrug resistance common. Specialist advice should always be sought because of increasing mefloquine-resistance, particularly on the Thai-Cambodian and Thai-Burmese borders.

Oceania. There is a high risk of chloroquine-resistant falciparum malaria and reports of chloroquine-resistant vivax malaria.

Latin America. There is a risk of malaria throughout South and Central America with some chloroquine-resistant falciparum malaria occurring. There is a high risk of chloroquine-resistant malaria in the Amazon basin and adjacent countries to the north and west.

Drug interactions and contraindications

The usual drugs for malaria prophylaxis are shown in Table 15.6 and includes chloroquine and proquanil which are both available over the counter in the UK. However, some preparations should be prescribed with caution (see below). Travellers who intend to go to high-risk areas should be acquainted with basic details of drug safety as well as efficacy for their own particular circumstances, so that they can evaluate local advice should they need and/or receive it.

Chloroquine and proquanil. Both drugs are relatively safe in healthy people and in pregnancy and have few serious side-effects. Chloroquine is unsuitable for individuals with epilepsy and care with both drugs should be exercised for people with impaired renal function.

Mefloquine. This should be prescribed with caution. When used for pro-phylaxis it may cause severe neuropsychiatric effects, including psychoses and seizures in 1 of every 10 000–15 000 users. It has not been associated with any fatalities. When used at therapeutic levels the prevalence of serious side-effects is some 10-fold greater. During prophylaxis, 40% of these events occur after the first dose and 75% by the third dose. Contraindications include any history of convulsions (or history of convulsions in close family member)

Table 15.6 *Regimes for malaria prophylaxis for individuals over 12 years old*

- *Prophylaxis in areas without drug resistance*
  - Chloroquine 300 mg (2 tablets) weekly (available without prescription)
  - Proquanil 200 mg (2 tablets) daily (available without prescription)
- *Prophylaxis in areas of chloroquine-resistant P. falciparum*
  - Mefloquine 250 mg (1 tablet) weekly

  - Chloroquine 300 mg (2 tablets) weekly
        Plus
  - Proquanil 200 mg (2 tablets) daily

  - Maloprim (pyrimethamine + dapsone) (1 tablet) weekly
        Plus
  - Chloroquine 300 mg (1 tablet) weekly
- *Prophylaxis of mefloquine-resistant P. falciparum*
  - Doxycycline 100 mg daily
- *Some areas of limited risk*

No chemoprophylaxis but **strict** attention to avoiding mosquito bites and seek urgent medical advice at the onset of a fever

and patients with a history of overt psychiatric problems (particularly mood swings).

Mefloquine should be avoided during the first trimester of pregnancy and lactation. If mefloquine has been prescribed then pregnancy should be avoided for three months after the last dose. Caution should be exercised in renal insufficiency or severe liver failure. It should not be given to airline pilots and should not be used for standby treatment.

There are possible drug interactions between mefloquine and:

- Beta blockers
- Digoxin
- Calcium channel blockers
- Metoclopramide
- Oral anticoagulants
- Oral hypoglycaemic agents

Fansidar. This drug is contraindicated in people with an allergy to sulphonamides.

Doxycycline. This antibiotic is unsuitable for children under 12 years, in pregnancy and lactation and causes gastrointestinal upsets, in particular oesophagitis.

Malaria prophylaxis in pregnancy

It is most important that pregnant women travelling to malaria endemic areas take adequate prophylaxis and take careful precautions to avoid mosquito bites. Pregnant women are at high risk of severe malaria and it is obviously sensible to avoid high-risk areas on a planned trip, particularly if chloroquine resistance is present. Expert advice regarding malaria prophylaxis should be obtained from a recognized reference source. The risk to the fetus from antimalarials is relatively small and certainly much less than the risk to the pregnancy should malaria be contracted.

Proquanil is the safest drug in pregnancy. Proquanil plus chloroquine may be used, but both regimes should be supplemented with folic acid. As neither regime gives complete protection in areas of drug resistance, the individual should be asked to reflect on whether her journey is really essential. Mefloquine may be given during the second and third trimester of pregnancy. If mefloquine has been prescribed then pregnancy should be avoided for three months after the last dose, although pregnancy during a course of the drug is not considered an indication for termination of pregnancy.[16] This advice should be stressed to women going on holiday to sub-Saharan Africa.

Asplenic patients

Individuals without spleens are at very high risk from malaria and should avoid travel to areas of risk if possible.

Emergency malaria self treatment

Standby treatment has developed in response to the need for travellers to take more responsibility for their own protection than previously. Uniform recommendations for prophylaxis can no longer be made. Emergency treatment (Table 15.7) is particularly important for the back-packer in remote and high-risk areas, although overprescription of these drugs is to be avoided as they are not an alternative to proper medical care.

Travellers who are prescribed self-therapy must be instructed to seek medical attention promptly should symptoms develop even though standby treatment has been taken. Written instructions must be carried indicating that if a fever of 38°C or more should develop after arriving in a malarious area, medical advice must be sought. Standby treatment should be taken only if medical advice is not immediately available that day, or the condition is deteriorating.

Antimalarials must always be commenced 1–3 weeks before entering a malaria endemic area and continued for 4 weeks after leaving. The precise timeframe depends on the choice of prophylaxis. Even after all recommended precautions have been taken, any fever must be reported and the doctor informed concerning recent travel.

No chemoprophylaxis is absolutely certain to prevent the occurrence of malaria.

Table 15.7 *Emergency malaria self treatment*

- *Quinine hydrochloride, dichloride, or sulphate* (**not** bisulphate)
  - 300 mg, 2 tablets 3 times per day for 7 days or for 3 days followed by 3 tablets of Fansidar once
  - Quinine is not a suitable standby if mefloquine is used as a prophylactic
  - Quinine is the only safe standby drug in pregnancy. Therapeutic levels do not cause abortion

- *Fansidar* (sulfadoxine pyrimethamine)—3 tablets taken together. This regime carries a small risk of Stevens–Johnson syndrome

- *Mefloquine*—15 mg/kg not exceeding 4 250 mg tablets in a split dose

- *Quinine + tetracycline*—Quinine 300 mg, 2 tablets times daily for 3 days with tetracycline 250 mg 4 times daily for 7 days

---

Planning a vaccination programme

Travellers should allow at least four weeks prior to departure for commencing a vaccination programme. This does not always occur in practice and the GP is sometimes put under duress to organize a crash course at limited notice. This is particularly difficult to organize when the traveller intends 'roughing it' through several, or distant countries. The plan for each individual must always include:

1. The number of injections for a primary course.
2. Ideal interval dates between injections.
3. Minimum interval between injections.
4. Frequency of booster dose.
5. Preferred injection route.

The GP must always check the current situation from an authoritative source. Tables 15.8 and 15.9 show programmes for visitors to the Gambia and India and illustrate the range of issues that must be addressed.

The section which follows demonstrates the programme of immunization and advice which is recommended for a traveller to rural India who is leaving shortly. If a practice is unable to arrange care at this standard then it is safer to refer the patient to a specialist centre.

Table 15.8 *A vaccination programme for a traveller intending to visit the Gambia*

Ascertain if the individual has had:
- *Polio* vaccination within the past 10 years
- *Tetanus* within the past 10 years
- *Typhoid* fever within the past 3 years (this is probably unnecessary if the traveller is over the age of 35 and has had five previous regular boosters)
- *Yellow fever.* Travellers are required to have an international vaccination certificate (or an exemption certificate) if entering from an infected country
- *Hepatitis A.* This is a significant risk if antibody-negative and particularly if travelling or living in rough or rural conditions.
- *Meningitis:* the vaccine is recommended for long-stay rural travellers

Optional, but to be considered:
- *Rabies*, unless vaccinated within the past 1 or 2 years (particularly important if living rough)
- *Tuberculosis.* Children should be immunized at any age. Adults should have skin test if there is any doubt about their immune status
- *Hepatitis B* transmission is through contaminated blood, blood products, or through sexual contact with an infected person. Vaccine is available

- *Malaria:* Risk is present throughout the year and prophylaxis is vital for the traveller. Details of current recommendation must be obtained from an authoritative body. Treatment must commence 1 week before travel and be continued for at least 4 weeks on return. In addition, the GP should discuss personal protection measures against the mosquito (Table 15.5 and 15.6)

- *AIDS:*
Advice concerning prevention of HIV should be given. The two most important factors are:
    – avoiding local sexual contact of any kind
    – avoiding transfusion with blood or blood products and injection or transfusion of fluid with contaminated medical equipment (pack of sterile medical equipment should be advised (see Appendix 1).

The principal infecting AIDS virus in Gambia seems to be HIV-2 rather than HIV-1. Screening of blood products for HIV-2 is most unlikely to have been carried out

---

Recommended immunizations

James, a 20-year-old fit healthy male student requires immunizations for a month-long trip (April/May). He intends to fly to India and then travel on to Nepal, spending approximately two weeks in each country. He is unsure of where he will be staying, intending to pack a rucksack and stay wherever and whenever he wishes.

The trip has been arranged rather hurriedly and he intends to leave England in 18 days' time. Due to the imminent departure date, the countries being visited, and the living conditions he can expect, it is important to obtain a detailed history of past vaccinations and start his immunization regime straightaway.

The recommended immunizations for the India and Nepal during April and May are that James should be 'in date' for:

Polio. He last had a booster at the age of 14 at school and therefore no booster dose is required.

Tetanus. He last had a booster dose at the age of 14 and is therefore in date.

Typhoid. He has never had typhoid immunization before. There are two options:

(1) Vi polysaccharide vaccine (Typhim Vi; this is not a live vaccine). A single dose by intramuscular or deep subcutaneous injection, re-immunization after 3 years if he remains at risk.
(2) Oral Ty 21a vaccine (Vivotif). This is a live vaccine which is unstable at room temperatures. Dose is one capsule on alternate days for three doses. He must be instructed to keep the vaccine in a refrigerator between doses. If he intends to be a regular traveller an annual booster of three doses would be advised.

Japanese B encephalitis. Due to the significant risk of this disease with outbreaks occurring March to May in the southern-most states of India, and being of particular risk to rural travellers, vaccination would be advised. The ideal regime is two doses with a minimum 10-day interval between.

Meningococcal meningitis A and C. This disease mainly occurs in the under-thirties, and due to meningitis outbreaks in New Delhi from November to May and throughout Nepal from November to May, James would be advised to be vaccinated. A single dose at least 10 days before travel to an 'at-risk' area is recommended.

Rabies. This vaccine would be recommended because of the countries being visited and rural travel where risk of rabies incidence is increased. The ideal regime is three doses at days 0,7 and 28. This time the gap cannot be shortened; James only has time for two doses rather than the ideal three. Therefore, two doses should be given, along with advice on what to do if bitten, licked, or scratched by possibly infected animal. He should complete his primary course on returning from his trip to ensure adequate primary immunization for any future travels.

Table 15.9 *Vaccination and advice programme for a student back-packing in rural india*

The following are advised but current requirements must always be checked:
- *Polio* within the past 10 years
- *Tetanus* within the past 10 years
- *Typhoid* within the past 3 years
- *Cholera* not normally recommended
- *Meningococcal meningitis* (if not vaccinated within past 3 years). Variable but significant risk present in many areas
- *Hepatitis A*. Significant risk if antibody-negative

- Malaria:
Prophylaxis essential in all areas throughout the year. Current recommendations must be obtained from an authoritative source. Antimalarials to be commenced 1 week before travel and to be continued for 4 weeks after return. The GP must give the traveller advice concerning personal protection measures against mosquitoes (Tables 15.5 and 15.6). Standby treatment should be provided (Table 15.7).

Optional, but to be considered:
- *Rabies* within the past 1–3 years, depending on the level of risk
- *Tuberculosis*. Children of any age must be immunized. Skin test for adults to determine immune status
- *Hepatitis B*. Certainly essential for health care worker or people living in a confined situation in an institution.
- *Japanese B encephalitis*, if no vaccination within the past 3 years. (Particularly required for visits to northern districts)

General advice:
- In times of typhoon or flood, the risk of water-borne diseases increases and advice concerning avoidance must be given
- Advice concerning prevention of AIDS and HIV must also be given

---

Tuberculosis. James was immunized at the age of 13 and is therefore in date.

Hepatitis B. As the risk of infection for people staying for short periods is dependent on sexual exposure and contact with blood, needles, and syringes, vaccination would not routinely be necessary, but advice on what to do in the event of accident or injury would be given. He would be advised to consider taking a travel pack with sterile needles with him.

Hepatitis A. Immunoglobulin is recommended for travel to India and Nepal and is given shortly before departure. It should ideally be given 21 days after a live vaccine, or if there is a shortage of time, it can be given at the same time. Alternatively (but bearing in mind the cost), hepatitis A vaccine (Havrix) may be given. The immunization consists of two doses spaced by 2 weeks to 1 month apart. The two doses will provide adequate antibody levels for 12 months and a booster dose at 6–12 months will provide cover for up to 10 years.

The schedule

Date of departure: *23 April*
5 April: Typhoid Vi polysaccharide vaccine (Typhim)
            1st Japanese B encephalitis
            Meningococcal A and C
            1st rabies

12 April: 2nd rabies

19 April: Hepatitis A vaccine
            2nd Japanese B encephalitis

Malaria
Prophylaxis and advice are **essential**.

Caring for the increasing proportion of our patients who undertake foreign travel is not complete without the ability to deal with the infections that they present on their return. Unfortunately even those who prepare carefully may fall ill, their problems are dealt with below.

See Appendix 1 for useful addresses and further information about travel medicine and infection.

The returned traveller and imported infections

The risk of acquiring any particular tropical infection depends on the area of the world visited, since many infections have a limited geographical range. Travellers who have been to lesser developed countries are more at risk than those who have visited more 'Westernized' nations. The risk also depends on the type of travel. Those who have stayed within major population areas in large hotels are less at risk than those who have travelled off the beaten track to rural areas. Not only will the latter have been more likely to have been exposed to insect vectors of disease and contaminated food and water supplies, but they may have been in closer contact with local people who might be harbouring unfamiliar infections. Finally, some women may have become pregnant while travelling and be concerned about the risks to the baby from drugs for prophylaxis or treatment, or from the effects of an infection in early pregnancy.

The risk of infection also depends on what precautions were adopted by the traveller both before travelling (e.g. immunizations), and while abroad (e.g. the use of chemoprophylaxis, insect repellents, food hygiene, sexual behaviour).

It is not necessary for a routine medical check-up to be arranged for all who have returned from a trip to the tropics.[17] In the absence of symptoms, the chances of finding any illness requiring therapy are small. It is a different matter, however, for those who have had any significant symptoms or change in general health while abroad or since their return. The symptoms of tropical diseases are not specific and individuals who have travelled are liable to all the infections seen in temperate climates (e.g. influenza, other viral infections, pneumococcal pneumonia, urinary tract infections), as well as to those endemic to the subtropics or tropics. The GP faced with symptoms in a returning traveller must not be blinkered and assume that the illness is something exotic: the usual range of 'temperate' infections must all be considered within a wider differential diagnosis.

In this section we will discuss the common symptom complexes presented by returning travellers to their GPs and the exotic infections that should be included within the differential diagnosis, in addition to the infections described within other parts of the book. Most patients with imported infections will have symptoms of fever, diarrhoea, jaundice, skin rashes, neurological or respiratory problems, either singly or in combination. In addition, there may be an eosinophilia found on a full blood count which may be further investigated in primary care. The general management of these presentations and of malaria is discussed below: details of some of the other important infections that cause them are to be found in the relevant chapters on body systems.

Fever

Fever is the most important symptom associated with recent travel abroad,[18] since it must always be carefully evaluated and, if the person has been to a malarial area (even if malarial prophylaxis has been correctly taken), malaria must be excluded with some urgency, since it can be rapidly fatal. *Fever in a traveller from an area where malaria is endemic is due to malaria until proved otherwise, whatever other clinical symptoms or signs may be present.*

Table 15.10 *The most important causes of fever in the returning traveller*

- Malaria
- Typhoid
- Dysentery (bacillary)
- Amoebic liver abscess
- Tuberculosis
- Hepatitis
- Dengue
- Visceral leishmaniasis
- African trypanosomiasis
- Brucellosis
- Leptospirosis
- Rickettsial infections (typhus, etc.)

Table 15.11 *Usual upper extremes of the incubation periods for the major tropical diseases*

Incubation period	Disease
Less than 14 days	Typhus and tick typhus
	Dengue
	Plague
	Enteric fever
14 days–2 months	*Plasmodium falciparum* (malignant tertian malaria)
	Scrub typhus
	Brucellosis
	Hepatitis A
	African trypanosomiasis
	Leptospirosis
More than 2 months	*Plasmodium vivax* (benign tertian malaria)
	Hepatitis B
	Tuberculosis
	Rabies
	Visceral leishmaniasis
	Filariasis
	Amoebic abscess of the liver

Most febrile illnesses, even in recent travellers to the tropics are never diagnosed and resolve spontaneously: they are probably principally caused by viruses. There are, of course, a number of other possible causes of fever. Some of these are extremely rare but the most frequent and important causes of fever in returning traveller are listed in Table 15.10. The diagnosis of other causes of fever can be aided by knowledge of the geographical area of exposure, the period since possible exposure (the incubation period of the various infections), and the immunization given and prophylaxis taken.

Although malaria, typhoid fever, tuberculosis, and infectious hepatitis are widespread throughout the tropics and must be considered in every febrile traveller, there are certain other infectious diseases with limited geographical distributions which only require consideration in specific instances. Some infections can be excluded if the period between leaving the endemic area and the onset of fever is longer than the extreme of the incubation period (Table 15.11). A history of being vaccinated against hepatitis B, hepatitis A, or yellow fever virtually rules these conditions out as the cause of fever. Typhoid vaccines are less effective, offering only about 70% protection.

Sometimes, the pattern of fever itself may be suggestive of a particular diagnosis: typhoid and typhus often cause a persistent pyrexia without any diurnal variation, an intermittent fever (where the temperature returns to, or below, normal between spikes) is seen in benign tertian malaria

Table 15.12 *Tropical infections associated with splenomegaly*

- Typhoid and paratyphoid
- Typhus
- Malaria
- Visceral leishmaniasis
- Leptospirosis
- Brucellosis
- Acute trypanosomiasis
- Relapsing fever

---

and sometimes in amoebic abscesses, and a relapsing fever, with several days of normal temperature between periods of pyrexia, is typical of certain *Borrelia* infections and dengue. The converse is not true; a specific pattern of fever is not always present in any one infection. Repeated rigors often accompany pyrexia due to malaria, typhoid, dengue,[19] and typhus but are also commonly caused by a number of non-tropical causes of fever such as bacteraemia (often associated with pyelonephritis, pneumococcal pneumonia, pyogenic abscesses, and cholangitis), and influenza.

The associated symptoms and signs are very helpful in determining the likely aetiology of fever in a recent traveller. Some of the more specific features (jaundice, diarrhoea, and neurological abnormalities) are dealt with in more detail below. Skin rashes of various types are not uncommon: maculopapular rashes are a feature of enteric fever, and petechiae may be seen in dengue and haemorrhagic fevers. Splenomegaly should always be sought: its presence is suggestive of a number of tropical infections (Table 15.12). Enlarged lymph nodes are palpable in such a wide range of infections that they are seldom of any diagnostic utility. An enlarged or tender liver, even in the absence of jaundice, may suggest a form of hepatitis (infective or alcoholic—individuals often over-indulge when on holiday) or an amoebic liver abscess.

The GP must always consider referral to a specialist centre for the returned traveller who is obviously ill. However, the common presentation of symptoms including fever to family doctors by this group of patients makes it impractical to refer them all. The clinical severity will be the major determinant but the GP should be very careful to exclude conditions such as malaria if investigations are to be undertaken in primary care. Discussion with the local microbiologist will prove invaluable in these circumstances. The laboratory tests that are requested should be tailored to the individual case but there are a number that ought to be considered minimal.

Examination of a blood film for malarial parasites is essential, and, if there is any possibility of exposure within the past two months (when life-threatening *Plasmodium falciparum* must be excluded), should be undertaken with extreme urgency. The blood film may also indicate the presence of trypanosomiasis or filariasis. A complete blood count with differential white blood cell count is usually helpful. An eosinophilia is a very useful pointer to the presence of systemic or gastrointestinal helminths, a neutrophil leucocytosis suggests pyogenic bacterial infection or an amoebic abscess, and leucopenia is a feature of many viral infections, visceral leishmaniasis, brucellosis, or enteric fever (typhoid). Other tests that should be performed, if there are particular historical, clinical, or laboratory clues to a particular condition are stool and urine microscopy (for parasites and/or their eggs) and culture, blood cultures, biochemical tests of liver function, a chest X-ray, and serological tests for specific organisms.

If the initial consultation fails to suggest a specific diagnosis, the patient is not believed to have a serious illness and, when necessary, a blood film has been declared negative by someone experienced in the diagnosis of malaria, then the GP may decide to observe the patient with an appointment for further review in 2–3 days. During the interval, the patient should be asked to keep a record of his/her temperature and to report any further deterioration in their health at once. Most of these patients will recover spontaneously. If there are any positive features on initial clinical examination, the laboratory investigations reveal significant abnormalities or the illness has persisted for more than a few days, then the patient should be referred urgently. Not everyone with an established diagnosis of a tropically acquired infection needs hospitalization: most patients with gastrointestinal infections, hepatitis, or vivax malaria can be managed as outpatients.

Malaria

Epidemiology

In ancient India malaria was known as the 'King of Disease'. It has plagued mankind since prehistoric times and despite intensive eradication programmes which have eliminated the disease in a number of countries in Europe and the Middle East, the disease remains endemic in some 100 countries or areas, placing almost half the world's population at risk. Malaria is distributed world-wide between the latitudes of 40 degrees north and 30 degrees south, generally at altitudes below 2000 metres. By 1965, India had reduced the number of cases from tens of millions to about 100 000, and in Sri Lanka only 17 cases were reported in 1963. However, this situation did not continue. In a population of some 12 million in Sri Lanka, in 1969, about half a million cases were reported. In India, approximately 6.5 million cases were reported in 1976. Tropical Africa is variously estimated to have 200 million infected people. The World Health Organization reported 270 million cases world-wide in 1989. Their programme to eradicate malaria has failed and been abandoned.[20]

Thirty million people visit malaria endemic countries from non-tropical countries each year. Cases of malaria in the UK are almost always imported: British people who originate from malaria endemic countries are at particular risk when visiting friends and relatives there.[21] If they were born abroad they will have decreased or lost any immunity and may be the group least likely to seek advice regarding prophylaxis. In the UK, between 1977 and 1990, the annual number of cases of imported malaria reported to the Malaria Reference Laboratory, London rose from 1529 to over 2000, with more than 50% due to *P. falciparum.* Between 1977 and 1993, 31 830 cases were reported of which 39% were due to *P. falciparum.*

Case history

One of the authors returned to work after a meeting where there had been a debate on how much to include about travel medicine. The administrator looked anxious and asked to discuss a private matter. Her husband had just returned from Nigeria where he had been visiting his mother. He saw his GP for flu-like symptoms after his return but one film for malaria parasites had been negative. He was reassured. However, he felt worse the next day and returned to the GP who admitted him to hospital for treatment of his falciparum malaria. His family were worried but they were also angry with him as he had resisted all advice to take prophylaxis on the basis that he was going home to a place where he had been happy and healthy. [The patient recovered and his wife has consented for the experience to be included here.]

There have also been occasional authenticated reports of patients who have contracted malaria although they have never left the UK. Such cases have all occurred in close proximity to airports and are presumably caused by infected *Anopheles* mosquitoes escaping from airliners and transmitting the disease to local inhabitants. In some cases, travellers arriving in the UK from another non-endemic country, have been infected in the aeroplane during a runway stop in an endemic country. Malaria is also very occasionally transmitted by blood transfusion, by needlestick injuries, or transplacentally, to produce congenital malaria.

Life cycle of malaria parasites

Four species of *Plasmodium* infect humans: *P. vivax* and *P. ovale* are the cause of benign tertian malaria, *P. falciparum* is the cause of malignant tertian malaria, and *P. malariae* the cause of quartan malaria. Infections due to *P. vivax* and *P. falciparum* are much more common than those due to the other two species. Malaria parasites replicate via an asexual cycle in humans and a sexual cycle in a female *Anopheles* mosquito. When an infected mosquito bites, parasitic forms called sporozoites are injected into the human. Within an hour or so these enter the parenchymal cells of the liver and there they multiply to form a tissue schizont containing numerous merozoites. One to two weeks later the schizonts rupture and the merozoites are released into the circulation. In *P. vivax* and *P. ovale* infections some of the sporozoites do not rupture, remaining in a latent form termed 'hypnozoites'. Within the circulation, merozoites attach to specific receptors on red cells (a different receptor for each species of *Plasmodium*) and enter the erythrocytes. The parasites then develop to form ring shaped trophozoites and multinucleated schizonts. In turn, these rupture to release more merozoites to infect further red blood cells. Within a few cycles the release of merozoites becomes

Table 15.13 *Clinical features of the four human malaria parasites*

Parasite	Disease	Incubation	Relapse	Chloroquine resistance
P. falciparum	Malignant tertian	12 days	No	Yes
P. vivax	Benign tertian	15 days	Yes 1–2 yrs	No
P. ovale	Ovale tertian	17 days	Yes 1–5 yrs	No
P. malariae	Quartan	8 days	Yes 1–50 yrs	No

synchronized (approximately every 48 hours for *P. falciparum, P. vivax,* and *P. ovale,* and 72 hours for *P. malariae*). After a while some of the merozoites do not enter red cells but develop into sexual forms or gametocytes which continue to circulate until ingested by a biting mosquito. The male and female gametocytes replicate in the sexual cycle to form sporozoites which enter the mosquito salivary glands ready to be transmitted to the next host.

Clinical features

Any patient returning from a malaria endemic area with a fever, regardless of history of chemoprophylaxis, should be considered to have malaria until proved otherwise.

The incubation period of malaria varies with the species of malarial parasites from 10 to more than 40 days, depending on the species of the parasite. For *P. falciparum* malaria it is usually 9–14 days, but may be longer, for *P. malariae* it is from 18 days to several weeks, and for *P. vivax* and *P. ovale* it is 12–18 days (but up to 12–15 months for some strains—especially if chemoprophylaxis has been taken). A study carried out at the London School of Tropical Medicine (R. Behrens, personal communication) determined that the time from arrival in the UK to presentation with malaria was on average 18 days, regardless of whether or not the traveller had taken malaria prophylaxis.

Infections with all four different malaria species have many features in common (Table 15.13). The most common presentation is with fever. This is the result of the release of each generation of merozoites into the circulation and hence starts irregularly but typically, within 2–3 days, settles into a pattern of paroxysms at intervals of 48 or 72 hours. The paroxysms begin abruptly with a feeling of intense cold and rigors followed by a rapid rise in temperature. After an hour or so there is a phase of delirium, burning skin, headache, myalgia, and other symptoms lasting for several hours and ended by intense peripheral vasodilation, sweating, exhaustion, and return of the temperature to normal. Diagnostic confusion with influenza is not uncommon. Splenomegaly and anaemia, largely due to haemolysis, are usually present and thrombocytopenia is common. The major clinical features of malaria are those of the complications: these are particularly associated with *P. falciparum* infections.

Plasmodium falciparum. This causes the most severe form of malaria and untreated is associated with an appreciable mortality. The fever is usually irregular, lacking the periodicity of benign malaria. Very high levels of parasitaemia can occur and the infected red cells adhere more easily to vascular endothelium, leading to vascular occlusion and tissue hypoxia. Almost any organ can be damaged or fail but a number of serious complications are common:

- *Cerebral malaria* (when the central nervous system is involved) is characterized by severe headache, increasing drowsiness and confusion, paralysis, and death. Seizures may occur and any coma lasting more than a few hours following a seizure is highly suggestive of cerebral malaria. It is associated with a mortality rate of up to 50%

- *Pulmonary involvement* with cough, haemoptysis, and acute pulmonary oedema

- *Splanchnic ischaemia* with abdominal pain, vomiting, and diarrhoea

- *Renal failure* due to acute tubular necrosis

- *Jaundice* due to haemolysis and/or hepatocellular dysfunction

- *Blackwater fever*, the trial of massive haemolysis, haemoglobinuria, and renal failure

- *Splenic rupture*, either spontaneous or following trauma

- *Fulminating disease*, resulting in renal impairment, pulmonary oedema, hypoglycaemia, spontaneous bleeding, hypotension, severe anaemia, and haemoglobinuria, is particularly common.

Individuals with heterozygous sickle-cell trait, thalassaemia, and glucose-6-phosphate dehydrogenase deficiency (G6PD) are partially protected from *P. falciparum* infection. Continual exposure to falciparum malaria in childhood produces partial immunity and hence many adult Africans have only mild illnesses when infected. This immunity is lost after a year or so of residence outside a malarious area. It is particularly important that UK residents who were born in endemic areas are aware of this fact so that before returning to visit their families they are urged to take malaria prophylaxis. It is the responsibility of GPs who care for such populations to ensure that the whole primary care team is informed about malaria prophylaxis and promotes it on all relevant occasions.

Plasmodium vivax and P. ovale. Individuals lacking the Duffy blood group antigen are naturally immune to *P. vivax* infection, since they also lack the specific receptor for merozoite attachment. These forms of malaria cause similar types of malaria with bouts of fever with a 48-hour periodicity. They are rarely severe since the parasites only attack immature red blood cells and parasitaemia is rarely above 1–2% of the red cell population. Merozoites may also be released from long-term hypnozoite forms of these parasites within the liver and benign tertian malaria can appear for the first time or relapse several months after leaving a malarial area. Irregular relapses may occur for up to five years. Mild jaundice may be present with frequent hepatosplenomegaly.

Plasmodium malariae. This uncommon form of malaria only infects ageing red blood cells. The fever has a 72-hour periodicity. There may be considerable anaemia and hepatosplenomegaly. The infection can run a chronic course with low grade fever and relapses occurring for up to 50 years from initial infection. The chronic immunological stimulation can lead to nephrotic syndrome.

Diagnosis

Malaria is very commonly missed and each year there are a number of avoidable deaths in the UK.[22] Eight people died from malaria in the UK between 1989 and 1990, all due to *P. falciparum*: 7 were acquired in Africa and the other in Oman. There were 1887 cases of imported malaria notified to the PHLS Malaria Reference Laboratory in 1994, of which 62% were due to *P. falciparum*: 9 people died. The key to diagnosis (the GP is often at the vital front-line) rests with a good history and a high index of suspicion. A study at London School of Hygiene and Tropical Medicine (R. Behrens personal communication) demonstrated that for non-fatal cases of malaria, the mean time from presentation to diagnosis was 4.8 days, whereas ultimately fatal cases were diagnosed less rapidly with a mean time from presentation to diagnosis of 6.8 days.

For practical purposes, confirmation of the diagnosis relies on detection and identification of the organisms in a properly stained blood film. High falciparum counts (more than 5% of erythrocytes parasitized) usually equate to clinical severity. Several smears should be examined and a negative report does not necessarily exclude the diagnosis, as prophylactic chemotherapy may suppress the parasitaemia. Occasionally, severely ill patients may have low levels of parasitaemia which are difficult to detect.

Treatment

Treatment of malaria requires killing of the erythrocytic stages of the parasite, in order to terminate the acute attack, together with eradication of any hepatic schizonts to prevent relapses. Several drugs can destroy asexual stages of the parasites.

Chloroquine is the most suitable drug for all forms other than falciparum malaria. Unfortunately, falciparum strains resistant to chloroquine are now widespread in Africa, South America, and Asia. For almost all patients with falciparum infection (the exception being those from Central America or the Arabian Gulf area) hospital admission for treatment with intravenous quinine sulphate, mefloquine, or a derivative of qinghaosu (e.g. artemether) is mandatory. Monitoring for complications and supportive measures are essential for the care of patients with severe (more than 5% parasitaemia) falciparum infections.

Additional supportive measures include blood transfusion (even exchange transfusion), the treatment and prophylaxis of hypoglycaemia particularly in pregnant women, care with intravenous fluids to prevent overload, and dialysis in the event of renal failure. Steroids for cerebral malaria and heparin in the prophylaxis of consumptive coagulopathy have not proved helpful.

Non-immune adults with benign forms of malaria should be treated with chloroquine. The dose used is chloroquine base, 600 mg (4 tablets of one of the standard preparations of chloroquine salts) immediately, followed by chloroquine base 300 mg (2 tablets) 6 hours later, and daily on days 2, 3 and 4. Partially immune patients need only receive 1 dose of 600 mg base. Children are given dosages in proportion to body weight.

Chloroquine will not eradicate hepatic schizonts and to prevent relapse of *P. vivax* or *P. ovale* infections, a course of primaquine needs to follow the chloroquine. Primaquine causes haemolysis in those with G6PD deficiency and so the patient's status must be checked before primaquine is given.

The returned traveller with diarrhoea

A large number of the 16 million annual travellers to the developing areas of the tropics and subtropics are exposed to food and water that are heavily contaminated with enteric pathogens. Most will lack any immunity to these pathogens and diarrhoeal illnesses are the most common infections acquired abroad: attack rates often approach 50%. The disease is particularly transmitted through fresh fruit or green vegetables, uncooked meat, and seafood. In most cases, the symptoms have subsided by return from business or holiday destination but all family doctors are presented at some time with patients whose symptoms have either continued on return or indeed have become much worse resulting in acute illness.

Most of the infections are also endemic in the UK (see Chapter 9) but the relative frequency of some is much higher in travellers. The predominant pathogen causing travellers' diarrhoea is enterotoxigenic Escherichia (ETEC) *coli*, with a minority of cases caused by *Shigella, Campylobacter, Salmonella,* viruses, or parasites (Table 15.14).

In the assessment of the returning traveller afflicted with diarrhoea a careful history and description of the diarrhoea is important and may help to indicate the most appropriate management. There are three main presentations of diarrhoea in travellers:

(1) acute watery diarrhoea,

(2) acute dysentery;

(3) chronic diarrhoea.

The most common presentation is that of acute watery diarrhoea. This

Table 15.14 *Causative organisms of travellers' diarrhoea*

Bacteria	Viruses	Protozoa
Escherichia coli	Rotavirus	*Giardia lamblia*
Yersinia enterocolitica	Calicivirus	*Entamoeba histolytica*
Shigellas	Enteric adenoviruses	*Cryptosporidium*
Vibrio cholerae	Norwalk agent	*Cyclospora cayetanensis*
Salmonellas	Astrovirus	
Clostridium perfringens		
Bacillus cereus		
Aeromonas		
Campylobacter		

is most frequently caused by enterotoxigenic *E. coli*, which accounts for approximately 50% of travellers' diarrhoea in Central and Latin America, Asia, and Africa. Symptoms often begin within the first week of the visit and, while usually short-lived, may persist for two or more weeks. Diarrhoea and abdominal cramps occur with malaise and nausea. Vomiting and pyrexia are uncommon. *Vibrio parahaemolyticus* and *Aeromonas hydrophilia* frequently cause illness in Bangkok and other parts of the Far East. Occasionally, cholera or cryptosporidiosis can be responsible for this form of illness in returning travellers.

Dysentery is less common. The most frequently identified causes are *Campylobacter jejuni*, *Salmonella* and *Shigella* species: occasionally *Aeromonas*, *Yersinia*, *Entamoeba histolytica*, and *Schistosoma mansoni* infections have been reported.

Chronic diarrhoea is uncommon following travel but when it does occur it can be very difficult to diagnose. Several organisms can be responsible; *Giardia lamblia* and tropical sprue are the most common problems but amoebiasis and schistosomiasis can also cause chronic or relapsing symptoms. It must also be remembered that an acute infection may precipitate an attack of inflammatory bowel disease or irritable bowel syndrome, or may lead to lactose intolerance, especially in infants.

Investigations are not required for cases of most cases of acute watery diarrhoea contracted overseas. Many cases will improve within a few days, either spontaneously or following suitable antibiotic therapy (see below). Furthermore, microbiological investigations are often unhelpful since the techniques needed for the detection of ETEC are not routinely available in most laboratories. In all cases of dysentery, however, microbiological investigation of the stool should be undertaken. Several specimens should be examined. Severely ill patients must be investigated and treated in hospital where close attention can be paid to electrolyte levels and to the state of hydration. Examination of warm stool taken in hospital during sigmoid- copy or colonoscopy may be necessary to identify the trophozoite stage of *Entamoebae histolytica*. A rectal biopsy may also enable schistosomiasis to be confirmed. It should be remembered, however, that the macroscopic and histological features of acute bacterial colitis cannot be distinguished with any confidence from those of idiopathic ulcerative colitis.

Patients with chronic diarrhoea also require investigation with repeated stool examinations. If malabsorption is suspected then referral to hospital for further tests is necessary.

In the home environment the patient should be carefully reviewed as dictated by the clinical condition. If there are any signs of dehydration (particularly in a young child) referral or admission to hospital should be considered.

Treatment

Although, as with other forms of enteric infection (see Chapter 9), the mainstay of treatment of patients with travellers' diarrhoea is rehydration, there are specific therapies that are of additional benefit. Loperamide (Imodium) has been shown to be of some benefit in reducing stool frequency and volume in those with non-inflammatory diarrhoea (the majority), and this allows travellers to continue with their planned itinerary. Hence, it should be advised for those with watery diarrhoea with no fever, and no blood or pus in the stool. However, any such preparations should be avoided in persons with features of dysentery, severe illness and in children.

If symptoms have lasted longer than two weeks and giardiasis is suspected it is reasonable to commence treatment with metronidazole pending the results of investigation. Either 400 mg, three times a day for 5 days or 2–2.5 g, once daily for 3 days. The latter dose may be repeated in one week. Patients must be told to avoid alcohol during treatment. Dosage should be reduced for children. Patients with moderately severe diarrhoea, particularly if there are dysenteric features are likely to benefit from empirical antimicrobial therapy and a 5-day course of a quinolone such as ciprofloxacin. All major pathogens that cause diarrhoea, whether by toxin production, mucosal ulceration, or penetration below the lamina propria are inhibited by quinolones at fairly low concentrations. These include *Shigella*, *E. coli*, *Salmonella*, and *Campylobacter*. Quinolones produce very high concentrations in the gut lumen, in the macrophages, and the mucosa. The additional benefit is that the normal bowel anaerobes such as *Bacteriodes* and *Clostridia* species are spared, limiting any overgrowth syndromes. The second choice in adults (it is less valuable because there is increasing resistance) is trimethoprim.

Trimethoprim is a better choice in children because of the concern of the effect of quinolones on growing cartilage. Where there is any doubt or concern overdiagnosis and management reference to an infectious diseases consultant should be made.

A number of drugs have been shown to be effective prophylactically against travellers' diarrhoea: trimethoprim, or a quinolone are the preferred options; but prophylaxis is best limited to those travelling for brief periods. Widespread

Table 15.15 *Principal parasitic causes of eosinophilia*

Bowel helminths	Tissue helminths
Roundworms (larval stage)	*Toxocara*
Hookworms	*Trichinella*
Strongyloides	Filaria
Whipworm	*Onchocerca*
Tapeworms	Loa loa
	Hydatid
	Schistosomiasis
	Liver flukes

use of prophylactic antibiotics in average holiday-makers is a sure recipe for the ultimate spread of resistance, not only in the enteric pathogens. Vaccines are also being developed against ETEC but are not yet available commercially. The newly developed oral cholera vaccine containing the B subunit of cholera toxin does protect against travellers' diarrhoea caused by ETEC that produce the very similar heat-labile toxin.

Eosinophilia

One of the more common problems encountered by a GP in the returning traveller or recent immigrant is an elevated absolute eosinophil count. Normally, there are up to about 400×10^9 eosinophils/l in the peripheral blood. The principal causes of an eosinophilia are various allergic conditions (both atopic and drug-induced) and parasitic infections (although certain uncommon neoplastic and rheumatological diseases are also associated with a raised eosinophil count). Parasitic causes are obviously of most importance in someone recently arrived from the tropics.

Eosinophilia is caused primarily by helminthic infections (and not by protozoans such as giardiasis, malaria, or amoebiasis), particularly those worms that spend some part of their life cycle in the tissues. The principal causes of eosinophilia are shown in Table 15.15. The risk of each of these in any particular individual obviously depends upon the exposure history (geography, time, activity).

The initial investigation of the individual with eosinophilia can be under-taken by the GP. After confirmation of an increase in the absolute peripheral eosinophil count above 450×10^9/L the initial investigations should include microscopical examination of stool specimens for ova, cysts and parasites (two or three specimens should be sent as excretion of ova may be intermittent), and urine specimens if there is potential exposure to schistosomiasis. It should also be recognized that the interval between infection (and often the appearance of eosinophilia as a result of migrating larvae) and detection of ova in stools or urine may be several weeks or months.

Further investigation of eosinophilia unexplained by the above simple, non-invasive investigations, should be undertaken after specialist advice has been sought. The tests employed will depend up the geographical and exposure history and may include serological tests for schistosomes, strongyloidiasis, and *Filaria*, and biopsies of small bowel, rectum, liver, skin, or muscle.

If, despite extensive investigations over several months, the cause for eosinophilia in an asymptomatic individual is not found, then it is unlikely that there is a significant health hazard present. Occasionally, a trial of therapy with thiabendazole is advised: this is to eliminate possible strongyloidiasis which can persist for decades and may become a threat if the person becomes immunocompromised at a later date.

Skin diseases

Skin diseases are very common in the tropics. The heat, dust, and high humidity predispose to infection of minor skin abrasions and wounds, including the bites of the numerous types of blood-sucking insects that may be encountered. Most of these superficial infections are caused by *Staphylococcus aureus* or *Streptococcus pyogenes* and are similar to those encountered in non-travellers. There are, however a number of specific tropical infectious diseases that involve the skin and that may be seen in returning travellers.

Jaundice

Jaundice after travel is most frequently due to hepatitis although it is important to remember that fever is unusual during the icteric phase of hepatitis and in any recent traveller with fever and jaundice, haemolysis due to malaria must be considered and appropriate investigations performed *immediately*.

The investigation of jaundice in the returned traveller or immigrant is otherwise similar to that of other patients. The type of jaundice, whether it is haemolytic, hepatocellular, or obstructive, needs to be established by means of biochemical tests of liver function and by ultrasonography. The type of jaundice will then determine the infections that need consideration and the further investigations indicated.

Neurological infections

Syndromes associated with infections of the central nervous system are described in Chapter 8. All the causes of meningitis, meningoencephalitis, and brain abscess described there are found in the tropics and subtropics. In addition, however, there are a number of other important causes of these symptoms that have a geographically limited distribution. A large number of viruses, transmitted by mosquitoes or ticks may cause encephalitis in travellers (Table 15.16).

Any acute febrile encephalitic illness with or without convulsions could

Table 15.16 *Important arthropod-borne infections of the central nervous system*

Vector	Disease	Geographical area
Mosquitoes		
	Japanese B encephalitis	India, South-east Asia, China, eastern former USSR
	Eastern equine encephalitis	Eastern and Southern USA
	Western equine encephalitis	Western USA
	St. Louis encephalitis	USA
	Venezuelan equine encephalitis	South and Central America; southern USA
	California encephalitis	Northern USA
	Murray Valley encephalitis	Australia, New Guinea
Ticks		
	Colorado tick fever	Western USA
	Tick-borne encephalitis	Central Europe, former USSR, Scandinavia

be a manifestation of cerebral malaria and this diagnosis should *always* be excluded as a matter of extreme urgency.

Referral of the returned traveller

It is perplexing for a GP to be confronted with a range of symptoms in a returned traveller which may be due to unfamiliar and potentially serious infections. Every doctor should make a mental note not to take short-cuts with these patients. Deaths from malaria with subsequent legal actions for negligence are reported every year. These events are devastating for patients and doctors alike. If there is any doubt about how to manage an infection in a returned traveller, discuss the case with an expert (see also Appendix 1).

APPENDIX 1

General information for travellers going abroad

How can current travel advice be obtained?

Health are professionals advising the public on health aspects of travel must ensure that the information provided is accurate and current.

The travel agent, while having a responsibility to the client can not be expected to provide other than broad guidelines. (For example, the author booked a holiday to Egypt and was given incorrect written advice by a nationally known travel agent that cholera vaccination is advised for that country.)

How then can the travelling public be provided with the correct advice? The onus mainly lies with the practice nurse or general practitioner.

Travellers may, of course, go direct to a specialized vaccination centre. However, most travellers will initially contact their GP's surgery. The level of sophistication of information will vary considerably depending on enthusiasm, training, and available information systems.

The various levels of information are:

Verbal
- From specialized centres
- Telephone: recorded tapes

Written
- Annual publications (e.g. the World Health Organization's 'Yellow Book')
- Monthly and weekly publications (e.g. *Pulse* and *General Practitioner* Journals)
- *Immunisation against infectious disease,* Department of Health 'Green Book' (HMSO 1996)

Electronic
- Discs. Computerized database. Care must be taken to use current information.
- Online via modem (e.g. Travax, British Airways Travel Clinics).
  These systems have the great advantage of rapid updating and improved accuracy.

Useful telephone numbers and addresses

British Airways Travel Clinics
Travellers may make an appointment for all, or part of a vaccination programme. Useful tested retail items and antimalarials are available. The very latest health advice for individual countries and regions is provided. Fees are charged for the service. For the location of the nearest clinic: Tel 01276 685040.

Hospital of Tropical Diseases Healthline
(Recorded advice, tailored to the destination, no longer free of charge: Tel 0839 337 733)

Travax
This a computerized database available from Communicable Diseases (Scotland) Unit, Ruchill Hospital, Glasgow (free of charge to NHS doctors). Provides regular updated information on immunizations and prevention of malaria: Tel 0141 946 7120.

Traveller database
This is a computerized database, updated monthly.

Pro Choice Applications Ltd
Trafalgar House
45 Halifax Road
Sheffield S6 1LA
Tel 0114 285 4443

Yellow fever registration
Addresses of yellow fever vaccination centres are listed in *Immunisation against infectious disease* (HMSO 1996); *Travel information for medical practitioners* (Department of Health). Doctors wishing to apply for registration at an official yellow fever vaccination centre may contact the following:

England
International Relations Division
Department of Health and Social Security
Room 554
Richmond House
79 Whitehall
London SW1A 2NS
Tel 0171 210 4850

Scotland
Scottish Office Public Health Unit
St. Andrew's House
Regent Road
Edinburgh EH1 3DE
Tel 0131 244 2178

Yellow fever vaccination certificates
These can be obtained from:

NHS Forms
Stationery Office Ltd Manchester
The Broadway
Chadderton
Oldham OL9 9QH
(Requests should quote 'Port 37' and the quantity required)
Tel 0161 683 2200; Fax 0161 683 2200

Vaccination and malaria prophylaxis advice
Hospital for Tropical Diseases (For malaria advice: Tel 0171 636 3924)
4 St. Pancras Way
London NW1 0PE
Tel 0171 387 4411

Scottish Centre for Environmental Health (SCIEH)
Ruchill Hospital
Bilsland Drive
Glasgow G20 9NB
Tel 0141 946 7120

Malaria Reference Laboratory
London School of Hygiene and Tropical Medicine
Keppel Street
London WC1E 7HT
(For malaria advice, recorded information, no longer free of charge: Tel 0891
600 350)

Medical Advisory Service for Travellers Abroad (MASTA)
London School of Hygiene and Tropical Medicine
Keppel Street
London WC1E 7HT
Tel 0171 631 4408; Fax 0171 323 4547
Tel answering for travel health line 0891 224 100

Regional Infectious Diseases Unit
City Hospital
51 Green Bank Drive
Edinburgh EH EH10 5SB
Tel 0131 536 6122

Department of Infection
Birmingham Heartlands Hospital
Bordesley Green East
Birmingham B9 5ST
Tel 0121 766 6611, Exts 4382, 4403, 4535

Liverpool School of Tropical Medicine
Pembroke Place
Liverpool L3 QA
Tel 0151 708 9393
Travel Health Advice Line 0891 172 111

Public Health Laboratory Service
Communicable Disease Surveillance Centre, Travel Unit
61 Colindale Avenue
London NW9 5EQ
Tel 0181 200 6868

Merieux Vaccination Information Service: Tel 01628 773 737
RADAR (Royal Association for Disability and Rehabilitation)
12 City Forum
250 City Road
London EC1V 8AF
Tel: 0171 250 3222
Fax: 0171 250 0212

Information for Diabetics
British Diabetic Association
10 Queen Anne Street
London WIN 0BD
Tel 0171 323 1531
(Travel guides are available for over 70 destinations for a nominal fee).

Medical information bracelets and necklaces available from:
- Medic-Alert Foundation: Tel 0171 833 3034; Fax 0171 713 5653

- SOS Talisman Co Ltd: Tel 0181 554 5579; Fax 0181 554 1090

The Blood Care Foundation
PO Box 7
Sevenoaks
Kent TN13 2SZ
Tel 01732 742427; Fax 010732 451199
(For a monthly or annual membership the foundation will supply properly
screened and tested blood world-wide in emergencies).

Emergency medical travel kits
Various kits are available and contain sealed sterile items of equipment such
as syringes, needles, suture materials, intravenous cannulae, sterile dressings
alcohol swabs, etc. These are advised for travellers in lesser developed
countries where medical hygiene is of a low standard. The kits carry suitable
identification to ensure their acceptance by customs officials. Some contain
letters (in several languages) addressed to customs officials, indicating that
the contents are for medical use only and are of no commercial value.

Suppliers
Philip Harris Medical Ltd
Hazelwell Lane
Stirchley
Birmingham B30 2PS
Tel 0121 433 3030
(Comprehensive kits suitable for a single person or a family, plus a larger
pack with transfusion fluid)

Medical Advisory Service for Travellers (MASTA)
London School of Hygiene and Tropical Medicine
Keppel Street
London WC1E 7HT
Tel 0171 631 4408
(Wide range of travel goods.)

Lifesystems
4 Mercury House
Calleva Park
Aldermaston
Berks RG7 4QW
Tel 01734 811 433
(Wide range of travel goods)

Safety and First Aid (SAFA)
59 Hill street
Liverpool L8 5SB
Tel 0151 708 0397

Industrial Pharmaceutical Services Ltd
Bridgewater Road
Broadheath
Altrincham
Cheshire WA14 1NA
Tel 0161 928 3672

Dixon Health Care
174–176 Hither Green Lane
Lewisham
London SE13 6QB
Tel 0181 852 0088

Williams Medical Supplies
Unit H6
Springhead Enterprise Park
Springhead Road
Northfleet
Kent DA11 8HD
Tel 01474 535 330/8

Homeway Ltd
West Amesbury
Salisbury
Wilts SP4 7BH
Tel 01980 626 361

APPENDIX 2

Travel clinic: patient record/questionnaire

Dr Smith
Dr Brown　　　　　Date　　　　　　　Newtown Medical Centre

Please complete a separate form for each traveller and hand it to the practice nurse who will inform you which vaccinations are required. If tablets for the prevention of malaria are required this form will be seen by your doctor who will then issue a prescription.

If possible, please allow 6 weeks before departure for completion of your holiday vaccination programme.

Name　　　　　　　　　Age　　　*Date of departure*　_____

　　　　　　　　　　　　　　　Date of return　　_____

Countries to be visited (in order)　　*Date*
1. _____　　　_____
2. _____　　　_____
3. _____　　　_____
4. _____　　　_____
5. _____　　　_____
6. _____　　　_____

Date of previous immunizations (if known):

Immunization	*Date*
Typhoid	_____
Hepatitis A	_____
Hepatitis B	_____
Yellow fever	_____
Tetanus	_____
Polio	_____
Meningococcus	_____
Japanese B encephalitis	_____
Rabies	_____
Tick borne encephalitis	_____

Allergies/reactions

Past medical history

Current medication

IT IS VERY IMPORTANT TO TELL THE NURSE IF YOU MIGHT BE PREGNANT

This section to be completed by the practice nurse or doctor
General holiday health advice given (to include):

- Accident prevention

- Food and drink

- Solar injury

- Safe sex

General advice about malaria prophylaxis given:

Yes/No

For the indicated journey, immunizations marked, are recommended:

Typhoid	_____
Hepatitis A	_____
Hepatitis B	_____
Yellow fever	_____
Tetanus	_____
Polio	_____
Meningococcus	_____
Japanese B	_____
Rabies	_____
Tick borne encephalitis	_____

Form to be retained in patient's notes. Advice to patient to be given in writing with copy in the notes.

References

1. Porter J, Stanwell-Smith R, Lea G. Travelling hopefully, returning ill. *BMJ* (1992) **304**: 1323–4

2. Darwood R. Preparation for travel. *Brit Med Bull* (1993) **49**: 269–84

3. Sloan D. Travel medicine and general practice: a suitable case for audit? *BMJ* (1993) **307**: 614–17

4. *Lancet* (editorial) (1992) **340**: 341–2

5. Mott A, Kinnersley P. Overprescription of cholera vaccine to travellers by general practitioners. *BMJ* (1990) **300**: 25–6

6. Moore P *et al.* Prophylaxis against hepatitis A for travel. *BMJ* (1990) **300**: 723–4

7. Bryan J, Nelson M. Testing for antibody to hepatitis A to decrease the cost of hepatitis A prophylaxis with immune globulin or hepatitis A *vaccines Arch Intern Med* (1994) **154**: 663–8

8. Tilzey A *et al*. Clinical trial with inactivated hepatitis A vaccine and recommendations for its use. *BMJ* (1992) **304**: 1272–6

9. Behrens R, Roberts J. Is travel prophylaxis worthwhile? Economic appraisal of prophylactic measures against malaria, hepatitis A, and typhoid in travellers. *BMJ* (1994) **309**: 918–22

10. Hawkes S, Hart G, Bletsoe E *et al*. Risk behaviour and STD acquisition in genitourinary clinic attenders who have travelled. *Genito Med* (1995) **71**: 351–4

11. Gillies P, Slack R, Stoddart N. HIV-related risk behaviour in UK holiday-makers (correspondence). *AIDS* (1992) **6**: 339–41

12. Dobson M. Vaccines, malaria and a host of resistance: 200 years after Jenner, the first malaria vaccine is now on trial. *BMJ* (1996) **313**: 67–8

13. Phillips-Howard *et al*. Risk of malaria in British residents returning from malarious areas. *BMJ* (1990) **300**: 499–503

14. Wiselka M J, Kent J, Nicholson K. Malaria in Leicester 1983–1988: a review of 114 cases. *J Infect* (1990) **20**: 103–10

15. Bradley D. Prophylaxis against malaria for travellers from the United Kingdom. *BMJ* (1993) **306**: 1247–52

16. Bradley D, Warhurst D. Malaria prophylaxis: guidelines for travellers from Britain. *BMJ* (1995) **310**: 709–24

17. Carroll B. Post-tropical screening: how useful is it? *BMJ* (1993) **307**: 541

18. Humar A, Keystone J. Evaluating fever in travellers returning from tropical countries. *BMJ* (1996) **312**: 953–6

19. Ramirez-Ronda C, Garcia C. Dengue in the Western hemisphere. *Infect Dis Clinics N Am* (1994) **8**: 107–28

20. WHO Malaria Unit: Global malaria control. *Bull WHO* (1993) **71**: 181–4

21. Bradley D, Warhurst D. Blaze M. Malaria imported into the United Kingdom in (1992 and (1993. *Commun Dis Rep Rev* (1994) **13**: R169–72

22. Svenson J, MacLean J, Gyorkos T. Imported malaria: clinical presentation and examination of symptomatic travellers. *Arch Intern Med* (1995) **155**: 861–8

CHAPTER SIXTEEN

Human immunodeficiency virus and AIDS

The acquired immunodeficiency syndrome (AIDS) was first described in previously healthy homosexual men in 1981 and is now recognized as being the most severe manifestation of illness resulting from infection with a retrovirus, now known as human immunodeficiency virus (HIV). The pandemic of infection due to HIV is the most dramatic epidemic of infectious disease in modern times and, despite major efforts, continues to progress world-wide and have an enormous impact upon health care provision. Although, in the UK, genitourinary medicine and infectious disease specialists have borne much of the responsibility for the clinical care of individuals infected with HIV, the infection and its ramifications impact on all involved in health care; general practitioners are increasingly involved in the management of such people. The complexities of the consequences of HIV infection are sufficient to warrant books of their own and hence this account cannot be very detailed and certainly not comprehensive: further details can be obtained from specialist texts.

We have, however, chosen to end this book about infection in general practice with a chapter on HIV infection because it serves as a paradigm for many of the principles we have discussed. It profoundly compromises the immune system itself, effective treatments and vaccines are still in the early stages of development, but it can be prevented by altering human behaviour. The mode of its spread leads to stigma and blame for some of those who are infected adding to the appalling toll of misery for patients and families who must watch previously fit young adults die. Ethical issues such as confidentiality are debated widely within the national press as well as the profession. Challenges for the primary health care team include learning to discuss safe sex without embarrassment with patients, learning how to discuss diagnostic testing and how to communicate the results, acquiring knowledge of previously rare infections and their treatment, and providing terminal care and family support. The important lesson learned from the study of this illness is that the treatment of infection is more than just selecting an antibiotic or ensuring immunization. It is also about health education and shared management of patients.[1]

AIDS

Definition

For surveillance and reporting purposes, the case definition of AIDS incorporates a variety of opportunistic diseases that may only need to be diagnosed presumptively in the presence of serological evidence of HIV infection.

Epidemiology

As of December 1995, the World Health Organization estimated that there had been a cumulative global total of nearly 6 million cases of AIDS. The number of reported cases was much less than this but many cases are known to go undiagnosed or unrecorded. Estimates of the prevalence of HIV infection are, of course, even more difficult to make, but the WHO figures suggest that at least 17 million HIV infections have occurred in adults since the start of the pandemic, to which can be added about 2 million children infected from perinatal transmission. Although the country reporting the highest total number of AIDS cases remains the USA (with an estimated 1.1 million HIV-infected individuals), it is believed that more than 50% of all HIV infections (11 million individuals) occurred in Africa. In some parts of Central Africa, 25% or more of the population have been found to be infected by HIV. Because of increased infant as well as adult mortality life-expectancy in Uganda had dropped to 37 years in 1994.[2]

As of February 1996, more than 12 000 cases of AIDS had been reported in the UK and more than half of these cases were known to have died. More than 25 000 cases of HIV infection are confirmed. Other industrialized countries from which large numbers of cases have been reported are France, Italy, Spain, and Germany (each of which had reported more cases of AIDS than the UK).[3] Although there are many uncertainties involved in the projection of the future of the pandemic, WHO has estimated that there will be a further 10–20 million new adult HIV infections during the 1990s, mainly in the developing countries, and 5–10 million children born with HIV, mostly in Africa. Of particular concern is the spread of infection in many Asian populations. By the year 2000, the sobering projections are of a cumulative global total of 30–40 million cases of HIV infection, 10 million adult cases of AIDS, and 10 million children orphaned as a result.

For the purposes of surveillance, cases of AIDS are classified into a number of risk groups or transmission categories. In 1995, the predominant risk groups for AIDS (and hence the groups with highest risks of HIV infection in the 1980s) in North America, Western Europe, and Australasia were men who had unprotected sexual intercourse with other men and injecting drug-users who shared injection equipment. In most of these countries, however, an increasing proportion of HIV infections are now resulting from heterosexual intercourse. This trend is reflected in an increase in the number of women with AIDS: 79 674 people were reported as having AIDS in the USA in 1994; 18% were women, a threefold increase on the proportion infected 10 years earlier. The greatest risk factor for heterosexual transmission remains unsafe sex and concomitant sexually transmitted disease. There is good evidence that consistent condom use confers a high degree of protection.[4]

Although men still account for more than 90% of all AIDS cases in the UK, reflecting the large number of cases in men who have sex with other men, there has been a small but significant increase over the past few years in the proportion of women with AIDS. Three-quarters of the HIV cases thought to have been acquired by heterosexual sexual transmission seemed to have been acquired following sexual intercourse abroad (largely in sub-Saharan Africa). In the USA, black and Hispanic people have higher relative risks of HIV infection and AIDS than do whites, particularly among the groups who report intravenous (IV) drug misuse, the use of crack cocaine or heterosexual contact with an IV drug-misuser.[5]

In sub-Saharan Africa, Latin America, India, and some Far-Eastern countries most individuals with AIDS probably acquired HIV infection via heterosexual sexual intercourse, often related to prostitution. The high prevalence of infection in many cities on these continents, together with poor sterilization of medical equipment and lack of screening of donated blood supplies, means that the potential for HIV spread by blood transfusion and needles is very real. With many women being infected, perinatal transmission is also any increasing problem. Children currently account for about 2% of the AIDS cases in the USA but between 5% and 25% of cases in some developing nations.

HIV

Virology and immunology

HIV is a RNA retrovirus of the lentivirus subfamily. Retroviruses contain an enzyme, reverse transcriptase, which transcribes the viral RNA into DNA. The DNA in then integrated into the genome of the host cell. Throughout the course of HIV infection there is an extremely high turnover of virus of up to 10 billion per day.

The virus itself is an icosahedral structure with external spikes made up of two viral envelope proteins gp (glycopeptide) 120 and gp41. The core of the virus contains several nucleocapsid proteins, the most important of which is p24, together with two copies of the viral RNA and the various viral enzymes, including reverse transcriptase.

One of the most important features of HIV infection is the persistence of infection despite the host immune response. The most important reason for this is that the target cells for HIV are immune cells possessing the CD4 surface glycoprotein molecule, to which the viral glycopeptide gp120 binds. Among the cells possessing the CD4 protein are helper T4 lymphocytes and macrophages. By integrating into the genome and establishing latency within these cells of the immune system, HIV is protected from the host defence mechanisms and can be transported around the body in an intracellular sanctuary.

Infection with HIV results in multiple effects on the immune system, but the most important is depletion of the helper/inducer T cells. This cell occupies a pivotal place in the immune response and loss of T4 cells has profound effects on the host's ability to combat infection. There is a wide variation in the rate of decline in T4 cell numbers among HIV-infected individuals and the mechanisms of T4 cell depletion and the viral or host factors which govern its rate are not clearly identified. What is clear, however, is that once the T4 cell count has fallen to less than 200/mm^3, then the individual is severely immunocompromised and development of opportunistic infection (and hence AIDS) probably becomes inevitable and imminent.

HIV also produces neurological disease: this is probably related to infected monocyte-macrophages within the central nervous system indirectly causing neuronal damage. The neurones and glial cells themselves do not appear to be primarily infected with HIV and the progressive neuronal loss is probably consequent on the release of toxic factors from macrophages.

Transmission

Sexual transmission is the predominant mode of HIV transmission, accounting for more than 70% of HIV infection worldwide. No sexual activity involving exposure to semen or blood is without risk. The risk of transmission from any single sexual contact, however, depends upon the specific sexual practice, the infectivity of the source individual, and possibly the strain of virus. Among homosexual men, receptive anal intercourse is more risky than insertive anal intercourse or fellatio. Among heterosexuals, bidirectional transmission of HIV can occur and the relative efficacy of male-to-female and female-to-male transmission is not certain, although data suggest that male-to-female transmission is about twice as effective as female-to-male transmission. In Africa, although the overall sex ratio of cases is 1:1, the ratio varies by age with high female:male ratios in the young and the opposite in those over the age of 40 years; these figures are similar to those of other sexually transmitted infections. The highest rates of transmission occur in those with other sexually transmitted diseases, particularly those causing genital ulceration. This probably reflects damage to genital epithelium (and hence easier transmission of HIV) and is not simply related to a larger number of sexual partners.

Epidemiological evidence also suggests that the infectivity of an individual may relate to their stage of HIV infection; the highest risks being once severe immunodeficiency has developed.

Transmission of HIV also occurs as a result of parenteral exposure to blood or donor organs. Intravenous drug abusers become infected from sharing HIV-contaminated needles or other equipment. Haemophiliacs given clotting factor concentrates and other individuals who receive HIV-infected whole blood, red cells, platelets, or plasma have an almost 100% chance of becoming infected. Gamma-globulin, albumin, plasma protein fraction, and hepatitis-B vaccine have not been implicated in the transmission of HIV. Screening of blood for HIV has almost eliminated the possibility of HIV transmission by transfusion. The rare exception is a donor who has recently been infected with HIV and has not yet seroconverted; the risk of this is probably less than 1 per million transfusions in the UK.

Virtually all the HIV infections that now occur in children are the result of vertical transmission from infected mothers. The current rate of maternal–fetal transmission is probably about 25%—rates vary in different studies from less than 15% in a European study to nearly 50% in a group of African infants. Transmission of HIV to the infant can occur transplacentally (true congenital infection), perinatally (probably the most important route, occurring via ingestion of maternal blood or maternal–fetal transfusion), or postnatally from breast-feeding. The likelihood of transmission probably depends on the stage of the mother's illness with highest rates during either primary infection or when disease is advanced (i.e. at times when the plasma virus titre is high).

HIV-infected individuals present no risk to others from their normal daily activities and contacts. There is no risk from the sharing of bathrooms, cooking utensils, cutlery, crockery, or other household, goods; and normal washing procedures with soap or detergent will suffice to decontaminate these items. The evidence for salivary transmission of HIV is nebulous at best and nobody ought to withhold mouth-to-mouth resuscitation from a person who has suffered a respiratory arrest. Those individuals who frequently have to perform such procedures, such as the members of rescue services, are given protective masks and resuscitation devices to reduce the remote risk to vanishingly small levels. Spillage of blood and other body fluids should be cleaned up with hypochlorite (1000 parts per million, ppm, for general cleaning and 10 000 ppm if organic material is present), which corrodes metal, or gluteraldehyde.

The risk of health care workers acquiring HIV from occupational exposure is very low; data from several studies suggest that the risk of seroconversion after needlestick exposure to blood from an HIV-infected individual is less than 1%. The risk of transmission can be minimized if health care workers adhere to the published recommendations and adopt standard precautions for all patients. Although many GPs have, as a result of HIV infection, now adopted procedures that prevent cross infection (e.g. use of latex gloves for the taking of blood and the stopping of resheathing of needles), such measures are still not universal and GPs need to develop rational and practical policies to protect themselves, their staff, and patients (see Chapter 2).

Prevention

The transmission of HIV by sexual intercourse can be reduced by a reduction in the number of sexual partners, particularly those whose previous sexual behaviour or history of drug-taking might have put them into a group with increased risk, and the use of condoms. Certain sexual practices are less risky than others: so-called 'safer sex'. Within this category are oral sex (although HIV transmission has been reported in individuals who have only engaged in oral sex with their partner), mutual masturbation, and other forms of non-penetrative sex.

Individuals who are misusing drugs by injection whether intravenous or subcutaneous ('skin popping') are often much more difficult to counsel since complete withdrawal from the habit is often an unrealistic objective. Needle exchange schemes have been introduced to many areas with the aim of exchanging dirty needles, syringes, and other equipment (the 'works') for clean items. These individuals also need counselling about safer sex practices and the dangers of using prostitution as the means of financing their drug habit.

Diagnosis

The diagnosis of HIV infection is most easily accomplished by detecting antibodies to various viral antigens, particularly p24 and gp41 (one of the envelope proteins), by means of an enzyme-linked immunosorbent assay (ELISA). Such tests are highly sensitive and specific: the specificity is enhanced further by performing a number of different tests or by using a very highly sensitive technique such as Western blotting. Viral antigen detection and quantification of HIV load by measurement of HIV RNA concentrations is also possible but are not yet widely available tests.

Following HIV infection, a period of viraemia and p24 antigenaemia can be detected within 1–4 weeks and lasts for several weeks. This is followed by the development of antibodies to HIV envelope and core proteins within 3–12 weeks of the infection. The serological response to HIV (and presumably infection with HIV) is lifelong. As the disease progresses to AIDS, however, the viral antigenaemia reappears and, as it does, the antibodies to p24 decline and disappear; antibodies to the envelope proteins remain detectable.

Investigations

The testing for HIV infection may occur as part of a screening process or in an individual. Screening is routine among donors of blood, organ, or sperm and may be offered (after informed consent) in some instances, such as certain antenatal clinics in areas or populations with a high incidence of infection. At present, however, screening of the general UK population is not advocated since the prevalence of infection is very low and hence screening would not be cost-effective. In addition, a positive test might well lead to social discrimination and severe psychological disadvantages for the individual. Anonymous screening of populations, whereby blood samples obtained for other purposes are tested, enables the prevalence of HIV infection to be monitored and the pattern of the epidemic to be followed. The disadvantage is that no information about risk factors can be recorded and positive individuals cannot be traced and offered therapy.

The testing of individuals for HIV infection is a contentious point. It may be undertaken in an individual who has symptoms suggestive of HIV infection, or who is concerned to know their serological status, or as part of an insurance medical or entrance visa requirement for certain countries. For whatever reason it is important to ensure that appropriate counselling is offered, that the patient's consent for the test is obtained, that privacy is available and that absolute confidentiality is maintained. Pretest counselling involves a discussion of sensitive and personal matters relating to sexual practices and providing the individual with information about the meaning and potential consequences of the test. One of these is the possible future need to apply for life insurance, because although attitudes are changing, many British insurance companies still ask an applicant whether they have ever had an HIV test rather than whether they have ever tested positive. The apparent need for insurers to know that an applicant previously tested negative for HIV deters many from being tested in general practice unless a discussion of how records of the consultation and result of the test will be recorded. Such difficulties do not arise if the HIV test is undertaken at an anonymous testing site such as a genitourinary medicine clinic. Until recently, the cons of being HIV tested often outweighed the pros but improvements in the management of early HIV infection are beginning to tip the balance in favour of increased testing.

HIV testing should always be preceded by pretest discussion in order to prepare people for the social, psychological, and legal consequences of a positive test. A very careful social and sexual history should be taken, slowly and sensitively. Time spent building up trust at this stage will be of inestimable value in the future should the test result be positive.[6]

Agreement to testing for HIV should be based on informed consent and the areas covered in this process should include an understanding of how the virus is acquired and transmitted and the fact that confidentiality will be the highest priority. An interval of 12 weeks should elapse between the episode relating to possible HIV infection and testing thus allowing for measurable level of HIV antibodies to develop.

During counselling, relationships should be considered including the decision of who needs to know and why. Preparation for a positive result is part of the counselling process and an explanation of how follow-up care would be arranged should this be required.

The patient should be given the earliest possible appointment to return for results and these should ideally be given by the same person who did the counselling. It is better not to give a positive result at the end of the week when there may be no support available; rather wait until Monday, and then offer an appointment for the following day to continue discussion and to offer support.

Later counselling may include issues surrounding:

- Old or new sexual relationships
- Telling family and friends
- Decisions regarding pregnancy
- Anxiety over minor infections and drug treatments
- Legal matters (e.g. drawing up a will; arrangements for orphaned children)
- Coping with extreme ill health and possible disfigurement
- Death and dying at a young age

Counselling people who are worried about HIV infection is a skilled task and should not be undertaken without training and a real understanding of the many factors involved, including the accuracy of the test and methods for confirming a positive result (see p.000 on testing).

HIV and infection

Several systems are used to classify the various manifestations of HIV infection and disease. The one still used most widely is that published in 1987 by the Centers for Disease Control in the USA which is based on clinical criteria and divides individuals with HIV infections into four groups. There are drawbacks to this system in that the categories do not necessarily reflect disease progression and neither is it predictive. A simpler system is now often used that classifies HIV-infected patients according to a mixture of clinical and laboratory parameters.

Primary infection

Between 1 and 8 weeks after initial infection with HIV, one-half to two-thirds of individuals develop an illness that resembles infectious mononucleosis with fever, sweating, rash, sore throat, and lymphadenopathy. Acute neurological manifestations including aseptic meningitis, encephalitis and myelopathy have also been described. These symptoms coincide with seroconversion to HIV-antibody.[7]

Early HIV disease

Once the seroconversion illness is over, an infected individual enters a so-called 'asymptomatic' phase, during which symptoms related to immunodeficiency are absent. A number of minor illnesses can occur, however. About 50% of HIV-infected individuals develop a syndrome of lymphadenopathy at two or more extrainguinal sites which lasts for at least 3–6 months and for which no cause can be found. This is defined as persistent generalized lymphadenopathy (PGL) and is a very sensitive marker for HIV infection.

The glands are rubbery, discrete, non-tender, up to 2 cm in diameter, and found particularly in the cervical, axillary, and occipital areas. Asymmetrical and rapidly enlarging lymph nodes should prompt a search for other processes. PGL is not a marker of disease progression and most patients can be managed expectantly.

Thrombocytopenia (TCP) occurs much more commonly in HIV-infected individuals than in the general population. It can occur at any stage of HIV infection and in all 'risk groups', but usually first occurs in the absence of other symptoms. It has a relatively benign prognosis with bleeding of any consequence rare. In a minority of individuals HIV-related TCP (HIV-TCP) spontaneously remits. The pathophysiology of HIV-TCP is controversial and may indeed differ between infected individuals. The management of HIV-TCP is usually supervised by hospital specialists and if therapy is given (and for many patients it is unnecessary), then prednisolone and/or zidovudine (see below) are the most effective options. Splenectomy may be indicated for those failing on chemotherapy: this operation does not appear to accelerate the progression of HIV disease.

Intermediate HIV disease

Oral disease of various sorts is often seen as HIV infection progresses. Candidiasis is the most common oral lesion and is similar in appearance to that seen in other individuals with thrush, although it is often more severe. *Candida* oesophagitis, manifested by dysphagia and substernal pain may complicate oral thrush, particularly in late HIV disease. Oral candidiasis may respond to therapy with topical nystatin or amphotericin but most patients require therapy with ketoconazole or other systemic treatment. Sometimes long-term prophylaxis with ketoconazole or fluconazole (which is much more expensive) is needed. Fluconazole is usually required for oesophageal infection. About half of HIV-infected individuals with oral candidiasis will progress to AIDs within 12 months.

Hairy leucoplakia consists of white, furry, linear lesions, usually situated on the lateral margins of the tongue. It is believed to be caused by Epstein–Barr virus and can be treated with oral acyclovir. It is asymptomatic but is a useful prognostic indicator in HIV infection, almost 50% of affected individuals progressing to AIDS within a 16-month period.

A distal peripheral neuropathy is a common feature of the later stages of HIV infection, affecting up to 30% of individuals. It causes painful dysesthesia and sensory impairment without much motor weakness. It is due to axonal degeneration and the outcome is poor.

The constitutional symptoms of intermediate HIV infection are fever, malaise, night sweats, diarrhoea, and weight loss. The cause of these symptoms is often obscure and they may be related not only to HIV infection but to psychological factors or intercurrent illnesses. Their presence should prompt a careful search for evidence of opportunistic infection or malignancy.

Dermatological manifestations are common during this stage of HIV infection. Troublesome herpes simplex virus infections, particularly perianal lesions in homosexual men, can cause significant tissue destruction. One or more episodes of herpes zoster and multiple lesions of *Molluscum contagiosum* are the result of decreasing immunological responses to viruses. Similar deterioration in immune function also leads to tinea infections of the skin and nails, cutaneous candidiasis, folliculitis, and seborrhoeic dermatitis, which is very common and presents as a scaly red rash on the scalp and face. Severe psoriasis can also occur, either as a flare-up of previous disease or *de novo*.

The period of time between initial infection with HIV and the development of AIDS in adults has a mean of about 10 years; in contrast, in infants the mean incubation period is as short as 2 years. The risk of disease progression increases with the duration of infection, with a rate of about 4–10% per annum (although a low rate of progression is seen for the first few years after infection). The factors influencing the activation of latent HIV infection (and hence the progression of illness) are the subject of intense research but are still poorly understood.

Late HIV disease (AIDS)

Late HIV disease is associated with severe immunosuppression and the appearance of opportunistic infections. As many HIV-associated infections result from the reactivation of latent pathogens, the frequency of the various opportunistic infections differs according to the geographical locality and the previous places of residence or travel of the patient. The likelihood of individual infections also depends to a certain extent on the severity of the immune deficiency, some, such as cytomegalovirus retinitis and *Mycobacterium avium* complex (MAC) infections occurring predominantly when the CD4 cell count has fallen to very low levels (below 100 cells/mm^3).

Brief details of many of the various opportunistic infections found in AIDS are given in other chapters and will not be repeated here.

Disseminated infection with organisms of the MAC occurs at some time, in up to a third of patients with AIDS. It usually causes fever, weight loss, night sweats, refractory anaemia, and persistent diarrhoea. Culture of blood or stool may be positive and the organisms are usually easily visible in enormous numbers in the bone marrow, lymph nodes, or liver biopsies. The prognosis is poor. Rifabutin and the new macrolides, azithromycin and clarithromycin, show some promise in the treatment of MAC infection but the optimum therapeutic regimen is still unclear.

Tuberculosis is also becoming quite common in individuals with HIV infection, both early and late. In the early group the infection is usually pulmonary and relatively easy to treat. In late HIV disease, the tuberculosis is often disseminated and the prognosis is poor: although the tuberculosis responds to conventional therapy, the average survival is less than one year.

Patients with HIV infection are also at increased risk of certain malignant neoplasms, particularly Kaposi's sarcoma and high grade lymphomas of B-cell origin. Kaposi's sarcoma (KS) is a multifocal malignant tumour of the vascular endothelium, possibly arising from lymphatic endothelium. It is almost exclusively seen in homosexual men and its incidence seems to be decreasing. There has always been considerable evidence that KS in AIDS is caused by a sexually transmissible agent other than HIV (probably transmitted by oro-anal contact in gay men), but the nature of this agent was only determined in 1996, with the discovery of a hitherto unknown human herpesvirus, now termed 'Kaposi's sarcoma-related virus (KSRV)' or 'human herpesvirus type 8 (HHV-8)'. The lesions of KS in AIDS are usually multiple and involve any area of the skin, commonly with involvement of the gastrointestinal tract and/or lungs. The skin lesions start as small flat reddish-purple areas, progressing to raised painless plaques and nodules. The individual lesions often follow the lines of skin cleavage. Palatal and gingival lesions are commonly present and tissue oedema occurs when the legs or face are heavily involved. KS is rarely fatal and treatment is usually only recommended for localized lesions that are causing particular problems (ulceration, bleeding, difficulty eating, etc.). Low voltage irradiation is generally used for such lesions. Cytotoxic drugs (vincristine and liposomal daunorubicin) and interferon therapy are not widely used in the UK, since any remission is often short-lived and accompanied by unpleasant side-effects from the drugs.

Primary lymphoma of the central nervous system is not uncommon in patients with AIDS; nearly half of those with symptomatic HIV infection who survive for three years on zidovudine will develop non-Hodgkin's lymphoma. It is usually a multicentric B-cell tumour that grows rapidly and is associated with a poor prognosis. Epstein–Barr virus nucleic acid sequences can be found in some tumour cells. In some patients, radiotherapy can help.

Mortality

Patients with HIV infection and AIDS only require admission to hospital if there is an acute clinical illness. For much of the time they can be kept out of hospital with their care provided equally well by the GP as by the out-patient clinic of a hospital. Patients who are asymptomatic but known to be HIV antibody-positive need to be reviewed regularly every 3–6 months and can be asked to return earlier if there any medical, psychological, or social problems. At regular reviews arrangements can be made with local laboratories for blood specimens to be sent for the monitoring of immunological decline (either by sophisticated techniques or by simple screening tests such as the full blood count and ESR). As patients become more unwell with persistent generalized lymphadenopathy (PGL) and the AIDS-related complex (ARC), then although short periods of hospital care may be required for specific investigations, most therapy and care can continue to be administered by the GP.

The diagnosis and initial treatment of most opportunistic infections and tumours that define the progression to AIDS needs to be undertaken in hospital, and preferably in a unit with some experience of the condition. Chemotherapy for opportunistic infections will normally need to be continued indefinitely and much of the prescribing and monitoring of this can be undertaken by the GP. Even intravenous treatment with, for instance, ganciclovir or foscarnet for cytomegalovirus retinitis can be given at home by means of a Hickman line and liaison with the hospital pharmacist.

Therapy and vaccine[8]

The drug used most extensively in the treatment of HIV infection is zidovudine, an inhibitor of the reverse transcriptase enzyme of the virus. Studies have demonstrated that zidovudine therapy in patients with late HIV disease (after the development of opportunistic infections or other symptomatic complications) delays the progression of HIV infection, decreases further opportunistic infections, and results in prolonged survival. There is significant improvement in the cognitive function of those with HIV-related dementia and in thrombocytopenic patients the platelet count is often increased. Studies suggested that symptomatic patients with a CD4-lymphocyte count of less than 500/mm³ or asymptomatic patients with a CD4-cell count of less than 200/mm³ benefited from zidovudine therapy, with a slowing of the fall in CD4 cells and significantly fewer patients progressing to AIDS. A dose of 500 mg daily seems to be just as effective as higher dosage and is associated with fewer side-effects. Bone marrow suppression is the most serious adverse effect. The resultant anaemia may necessitate transfusions, a reduction in dosage, or therapy with recombinant erythropoetin. Neutropenia is the most frequent dose-limiting toxicity. Nausea, headache, myalgia, and insomnia are common during the first few weeks of therapy but are usually temporary and seldom limit therapy.

The extent and duration of the response to zidovudine are, however, limited. HIV strains resistant to the drug appear within 6 months or more of therapy and, after a number of trials, the recommendation was to change anti-HIV therapy to other antiretroviral drugs such as the reverse transcriptase inhibitors didanosine (ddI), zalcitabine (ddC), lamivudine (3Tc), or stavudine (d4T) after 8–26 weeks of zidovudine. Didanosine is not myelosuppressive but causes pancreatitis and peripheral neuropathies; the latter is also the dose-limiting toxicity of zalcitabine and stavudine. Lamivudine seems free of major toxicity.

Studies in 1995 and 1996 have changed the fundamental concept of antiretroviral therapy. One group of studies have clarified the dynamics of HIV infection; it is estimated that the mean rate of HIV replication is 10 billion new viruses each day with a rate of CD4-cell destruction of about 1 billion cells daily.[9, 10] This enormous viral turnover, coupled with a high rate of spontaneous mutation of HIV, rapidly creates a population of at least 10 million genetic mutants, many of which are resistant to one or more of the drugs listed above.

Two large clinical trials of zidovudine monotherapy versus combinations of zidovudine and either ddI or ddC have shown that for patients who have never received nucleoside therapy, combination therapy was significantly more effective than monotherapy, possibly as a result of delaying emergence of drug resistance. These data have led to a far more aggressive approach to therapy, with the use of drug combinations for patients starting therapy and a shift in opinion towards starting therapy at an earlier stage of the illness. None of these developments is without considerable increase in costs which will have to be publically debated as priorities are decided within the finite resources of the health service.

Other compounds such as non-nucleoside reverse transcriptase inhibitors and protease inhibitors are steadily being introduced. Such is the pace of change that recommendations regarding therapy for HIV infection can become outdated within a matter of months. Currently, there are a number of different HIV vaccines undergoing development. The majority of these are prophylactic vaccines designed to prevent an individual being infected by HIV, but others are designed to have therapeutic benefits for those already infected. The obstacles to the development of any of these vaccines are immense, one of the most important being the enormous variation of HIV strains and the inability, at present, to identify a highly conserved area of the virus surface protein that will induce neutralizing antibodies. It is not necessary to discuss in detail the vaccines under study; suffice it to say that several different approaches have reached the stage of animal studies and phase I and II trials in humans. It will not be until large phase III field trials, with their considerable logistical difficulties and great expense, have been performed in countries where there is a high incidence of HIV infection, that the potential efficacy of any candidate vaccine can realistically be determined. Such answers are still at least several years away and it is unlikely, even with favourable results, that an effective preventative HIV vaccine will be readily available within the present decade.

Case history

A 25-year-old single woman returned to UK following the break up two years previously, of a long-standing relationship with a European. She had recently received a letter from her former male partner indicating that he was HIV positive. Her first reaction was to ignore this as there had been an acrimonious split-up in the relationship but after further thought she remembered, that prior to their relationship, he had been an intravenous drug user. She telephoned the local AIDS helpline and was advised to consult the clinical nurse specialist in HIV, AIDS, and sexually transmitted diseases at the local genitourinary clinic. Detailed discussion took place and, following comprehensive pretest counselling, HIV testing was carried out. While the result was available the next day, Friday, the specialist nurse counsellor postponed the consultation until after the weekend. The patient attended to hear that the test result was positive. Her immediate reaction was to hasten to the local nursery school to collect her 2-year-old son in order that he should also be tested. The test proved negative. The patient initially declined to tell her GP that she was HIV positive. However, after some weeks she agreed that this action would be appropriate, providing the information remained confidential to her doctor and her HIV status was not known to any other members of the practice staff. The patient told her doctor about her HIV-positive result. He was more than a little surprised and with some degree of anxiety noted from her record, that over the past few months he had carried out cervical cytology, examined a bleeding haemorrhoid, and excised a mole from her back.

Points for discussion

The following are suggestions for discussion: the GP and his/her attitude to HIV-positive patients; confidentiality arrangements in general practice; and HIV test results should not be given on a Friday (suicide risk, HIV is a lonely diagnosis).

References

1. Smith S, Robinson J, Hollyer J *et al.* Combining specialist and primary health care teams for HIV positive patients: retrospective and prospective studies. *BMJ* (1996) **312**: 416–20

2. US Bureau of the Census. Center for International Research. Population trends, Uganda. Washington (1994)

3. European Centre for the Epidemiological Monitoring of AIDS: *AIDS surveillance, EC & COST countries* (no. 29, March (1995)). Paris (1995)

4. Vincenzi I. for the European Study group on heterosexual transmission of HIV: A longitudinal study of human immunodeficiency virus transmission by heterosexual partners. *N Engl J Med* (1994) **331**: 341–6

5. Edlin B, Irwin K, Faruque S *et al.* Intersecting epidemics: crack cocaine use and HIV infection among inner-city young adults. *N Engl J Med* (1994) **331**: 1422–7

6. Department of Health. *Guidelines for pre-test discussion on HIV testing.* PL/CMO/(96)1 London: Department of Health (1996)

7. Jolles S, Kinloch de Loes S, Janossy G. Primary HIV-1 infection: a new medical emergency? *BMJ* (1996) **312**: 1243–4

8. Weller I, Williams I. Ups and downs—and ups in the antiviral therapy of HIV infection. *Genito Med* (1996) **72**: 2–5

9. Wei X, Ghosh S, Taylor M *et al.* Viral dynamics in human immunodeficiency virus type 1 infection. *Nature* (1995) **373**: 117–22

10. Ho D, Neuman A, Perelson A *et al.* Rapid turnover of plasma virions and CD4 lymphocytes in HIV-1 infection. *Nature* (1995) **373**: 123–6

EPILOGUE

We have come full circle in this account of infection and its impact on the human world. HIV/AIDS can been used as a paradigm to reflect the myriad of issues raised by patients who acquire an infection. This is because its acute and chronic aspects, its multisystem involvement, and the ethical and social issues surrounding it echo many aspects of other infections.

At one level this book can be taken as a catalogue of disasters, as an 'historical' account of organisms which have gained distinction from among the thousands of species in the microbiological world for their capability and impact in causing disease in humans. On another level, it is, of course, an account of human response to such events. This response has been offered in a number of different ways. Scientifically, expressed as efforts to identify and give account of aetiological agents, their epidemiology, and the natural history of infections; medically, by attempting to elucidate strategies relating to prevention, control, and treatment of infections; and compassionately, by emphasizing that at all times the scientific and medical response must be tempered by a perspective of the whole person and not just the system affected by the disease process. We believe that it is this triad of responses to patients with infection which results in their most effective management. It will ensure that the patient—and not the process—will determine the direction that management and its ultimate outcome will take.

INDEX

Note: Page references in **bold**
indicate chapter headings.